A STRANGER IN THE FAMILY

A
STRANGER
IN THE
FAMILY

Culture, Families, and Therapy

Vincenzo DiNicola

W. W. NORTON & COMPANY

New York   London

I am grateful to the original publishers for permission to reprint material in the following chapters. Much of this material has been extensively reworked and modified.

Chapter 1 is based on two chapters published in other works: Brunner/Mazel (DiNicola, 1994), American Psychiatric Press, Inc. (DiNicola, in press). Parts of chapter 3 were adapted from several other works: *Systèmes Humains* (DiNicola, 1985d), *International Journal of Family Psychiatry* (DiNicola, 1986), American Psychiatric Press, Inc. (DiNicola, in press). Chapter 4 is based on several previous publications: *International Journal of Family Psychiatry* (DiNicola 1986), *Transcultural Psychiatric Research Review* (DiNicola, 1988a), Brunner/Mazel (DiNicola, 1994), American Psychiatric Press, Inc. (DiNicola, in press). Parts of chapter 5 appeared in different forms in other works: Éditions Douglas (DiNicola, 1992), American Psychiatric Press, Inc. (DiNicola, in press), APA Press (DiNicola, 1996). Parts of chapter 6 appeared in different forms in other works: *Journal of Strategic & Systemic Therapies* (DiNicola, 1985a), *Transcultural Psychiatric Research Review* (DiNicola, 1990b), Éditions Douglas (DiNicola, 1992), American Psychiatric Press, Inc. (DiNicola, in press). My memoir (chapter 11) was published in Italian in an earlier version: *Terapia Familiare* (DiNicola, 1995a).

First Edition

For information about permission to reproduce selections from this book, write to Permissions, W. W. Norton & Company, Inc., 500 Fifth Avenue, New York, NY 10110.

The text of this book is composed in Palatino
Composition by Bytheway Typesetting Services, Inc.
Manufacturing by Haddon Craftsmen
Book design by Susan Hood

Library of Congress Cataloging-in-Publication Data
    DiNicola, Vincenzo F.
        A stranger in the family : culture, families, and therapy /
    Vincenzo DiNicola.
            p.   cm.
        Includes bibliographical references and index.
        ISBN 0-393-70228-6
        1. Family psychotherapy.   2. Psychiatry, Transcultural.
    I. Title.
    RC488.5.D55   1997
    616.89'156 — dc21   96-40310   CIP

W. W. Norton & Company, Inc., 500 Fifth Avenue, New York, N.Y. 10110
                    http://www.wwnorton.com
W. W. Norton & Company Ltd., 10 Coptic Street, London WC1A 1PU

1 2 3 4 5 6 7 8 9 0

We are born, so to speak, provisionally, it doesn't matter where. It is only gradually that we compose within ourselves our true place of origin so that we may be born there retrospectively and each day more definitely.

—*Rainer Maria Rilke*

Alla mia madre e alla nostra famiglia in Canada
(To my mother and to our family in Canada)
Ao meu pai e a toda minha familia no Brasil
(To my father and all my family in Brazil)
and to Italy, our birthplace

Lebeiti haruchani be'eretz Israel
(To my spiritual home in the land of Israel)

And to my wife, Vittoria Lopez
and our children, Carlo Dante and Nina Mara,
who connect me to all the parts of my family
and together compose my true place of origin in this
world

FOREWORD

"Between Two Chairs"

"When I left Italy at the age of 20, I was the first to leave my home town to emigrate to South America. I didn't want to spend my whole life working the land, like my brothers. I wanted to study; my teacher had spoken with my father and encouraged him to let me continue with my studies. But at home, they needed another pair of hands for the family fields, although I didn't want to bow my head and break my back, wasting my life on a land that offered nothing. I wanted to see the world and so I left. First I emigrated to Venezuela, later to Argentina, and then to Brazil where I settled down to have my second family.

"Professor, at 20, when you're young, you can make mistakes and I didn't have anyone who could advise me to do this or that. Life taught me what to do. But do you think that has Vincenzo forgiven me? The thought of my son was in head for many years. Later, I searched for him in Canada and in England . . . Professor, believe me that when I left Italy, I didn't know that my wife was expecting a baby! I learned about Vincenzo much later, from my family in Italy. I loved my wife very much, but our families pitted us against each other. But tell me, do you think that Vincenzo has really forgiven me?"

This is a fragment of an intimate and heartfelt conversation I had with Giuseppe, Vincenzo DiNicola's father, in August of 1996 while he was driving me and my son Diego from the airport in São Paulo, Brazil, to his house outside the city. Vincenzo and his half-sister Silvana, who had left from the airport in another car, were anxiously waiting at home. Due to Giuseppe's torrent of confidences, we missed our exit off the highway more than once, and we arrived quite late in the evening. In spite of my fatigue after a long flight, I was very touched to hear the voice of a father who finds his son after 40 years. And even more so because over the last 10 years, I had the occasion to follow Vincenzo's movements, first within him and later more openly, in his search for his father.

Simply and without rhetoric, Giuseppe's words allow us to feel the weight of a grief that lasted half a lifetime, words that powerfully evoke the essence of his story. It's the humanity of his account—stirred by unforeseeable events and the years slipping by—that gives meaning to these events, even when they appear to be incomprehensible or contradictory. As Silone (who is cited in the book) affirms, each of us has the right to tell our own story in our own way. The key is not to let the story stay buried inside us and to find the right moment with the right person whom we can trust to let it out.

The moment was right for me too: it was very gratifying that my 16-year-old son was there with me, sitting in the back seat of the car but totally caught up in this story of Giuseppe's youth—a hard youth, far from classrooms and the security of a happy childhood among the affections of family and friends. A story similar, in fact, to that of many emigrants dislocated from their origins to reconstruct the present day after day in another place, seated uneasily ''between two chairs.''

For several years, I worked as a social psychiatrist with Italian-American families in a community mental health center in the South Bronx and as a consultant to a junior high school with many Black and Puerto Rican students. These adolescents and their families frequently expressed the feeling of being torn ''between two cultures.'' This had a very negative meaning for them, mixed with feelings of humiliation and anger, as if each person's identity was suspended between two forces perennially at odds with each other. At the same time, I was able to experience the vital energy that springs up when space and value are restored to their roots, especially when they appear to be lost or cut off. In short, it is possible to reconcile ourselves with the present, even a very difficult one, to the extent that we feel—or can recapture—the security of the cultural and family values that nurture us.

In theory, this ''in between'' position of emigrants—in between their society of origin and their host society—or of those who belong to a cultural minority, can be considered an added resource that offers more than one choice. This fosters a greater mobility between two alternatives, allowing movement from one space to the other and from one language to another—very useful skills for establishing social relationships in a new world. In reality, this advantageous position exists only when we can move easily from one chair to another, without worrying about losing our original position. Curiosity is the vital spring that encourages us to come into contact with diversity, as DiNicola insists, while tolerance is merely the way to remain closed up in our own worlds.

On one side, we see in psychiatry that social prejudice tends to marginalize everything that presents itself as different, creating through discrimination and poverty the conditions of chronic patienthood for individuals with mental disorders and relational distress. On the other side are what DiNicola calls "invisible" but very real forms of social pathology: the fear of losing one's roots; the hidden loyalties that nestle within every story of uprooting and emotional cutting off; the illusion of suspending time; diversity perceived as a threat to one's own existence; the sometimes exasperated defense of our own traditions; and love confused with the need to control others. These emotional situations render being caught between two cultural communities among the most serious existential predicaments.

These are the human predicaments discussed in this volume, which is as valuable as it is unique. DiNicola offers culture as the hinge of human relations. The family's "presenting culture," as he maps it out at the beginning of this long voyage, "is the royal road for understanding 'mind,' 'self,' and 'identity,'" where we encounter the strange and the familiar, interweaving a dance that allows us to embrace differences and to live with diversity. DiNicola's learned and multifaceted argument, based on the concept of "multiple descriptions," stimulates our need for an open professionalism that unites our knowledge without confining it in "technocratic" or sectional interests. The author succeeds in creating an imaginary dialogue among family therapists, transcultural psychiatrists, and child psychiatrists, so that the families, cultures, and children we encounter in this book come together in the therapeutic space, joining hands.

But at the same time, DiNicola invites us to search for therapeutic resources in our own growth experiences, in the recognition of our personal gaps as points of departure to "make sense" of family stories. The last chapter, "Strangers No More," achieves the high point of the book, synthesizing both personal and professional concerns in the construction of the family therapist's competence.

A Stranger in the Family is a fundamental volume that proposes the basis for a new way of thinking and practicing for family therapy, reintroducing affect and meaning into the systemic paradigm. In many ways, this is a book that breaks the mold, provocatively confronting the conformity and technocracy of many books and schools of family therapy which ignore or underplay culture, ethnicity, race, class, religion, or other social variables. DiNicola has the courage to highlight these fundamental but relatively unexplored themes and to assert that we cannot treat mental disorder—an individual's psychological disturbance and relational distress—without framing it in the "presenting culture" of the family and, therefore, within its social and institutional contexts. Out of these concerns, he has constructed cultural family therapy for the North American context.

In the early 1980s, the first work on the themes of ethnicity and the family life cycle appeared. According to Celia Falicov (1995), this "ethnic-focused" position highlighted the "regularity" of certain features—thoughts, behavior, feelings, customs, and rituals—of the particular ethnic group being observed, producing what DiNicola calls "static snap-shots" of families and cultures. In this view, family diversity is generated by ethnicity.

Falicov (1995) describes two other possible approaches to family diversity. In the "universalist" perspective, families are considered more similar than different (and contextual variables such as race, gender, and ethnicity are considered irrelevant compared to basic processes presumed to be common to all systems). This contrasts with the "particularist" perspective, wherein the specific features of families make them unique and different rather than alike (the specific internal world of the family is responsible for the family's destiny, downplaying the impact of social inequities and social change on the development of the family itself). As DiNicola teaches us, this binary contrast between universal and particular features of social life has been a core debate in transcultural psychiatry.

Cultural perspectives in family therapy are now clearly advancing. DiNicola's thinking goes well beyond the limitations of an ethnic focus or binary contrasts, to present a multidimensional and comparative approach to families and culture. Using the postmodern notion of "multiple descriptions," DiNicola brings several levels of "strangeness" into focus: the alienating symptoms of mental illness, the family members as cultural outsiders in society, and the family therapist as an outsider to the family. We need, the author states, to imagine a new vocabulary for cultural predicaments that have been invisible to us. Words like "strategy," "ethnicity," and "paradox," for example, should be replaced with others, such as "cultural translation," in order to help people find words for their own pain in their own language, "metaphor," which allows us to enter into the "web of meaning" of other lives, "family myths," which help us to understand the cultural transmission of stories from generation to generation, and "curiosity," which may lead to understanding and perhaps to acceptance.

Cultural family therapy is not presented, then, as an effective new "technique" to use in our encounters with other family cultures. Rather, understanding the experiences of migration and "cultural change," developing sensitivity to the pain and humiliation of "liminal people," and conducting "threshold therapy" as described by DiNicola represent an opportunity for the therapist's growth and a cultural challenge to rediscover the human and spiritual values immanent in the encounter between the strange and the familiar. But how can therapists stay in touch with their own personal, gender, and cultural integrity and, at the same time, listen to the language of other cultures? An attentive and curious reader may find her own personal answer to this question between the lines of this text.

—*Maurizio Andolfi*, M.D.
Director, Academy of Family Psychotherapy,
Professor of Psychology, University of Rome

CONTENTS

A STRANGER IN THE FAMILY

"I am a stranger and a resident among you . . . "
—Genesis 23:4

INTRODUCTION

"Every Exit Is an Entrance Somewhere Else"

My aim in this book is to open space for people who have been treated like minor characters in the drama of family therapy. In doing so, I will put onto center stage all sorts of strangers in society, families of diversity, and their human predicaments—cultural issues that have been ignored, neglected, and discounted in family therapy. In the tragicomedy, *Rosencrantz and Guildenstern Are Dead*, Tom Stoppard takes two bewildered minor characters from *Hamlet* and thrusts them onto center stage. But their destiny is not to be found there, so we meet them "off-stage" trying to find meaning in their absurd existence:

> We keep to our usual stuff, more or less, only inside out.
> We do onstage the things that are supposed to happen off.
> Which is a kind of integrity, if you look on every exit being
> an entrance somewhere else. (Stoppard, 1967, p. 28)

By narrating family stories and elaborating conceptual tools for cultural family therapy, I hope to demonstrate that when we meet people in cultural transition who face doors closing on them, we can help them open other doors in their new worlds. And, as new experiences call for new descriptions, we need to imagine a new vocabulary for cultural predicaments that have been invisible to us. New clinical problems arising from the ever-changing diversity of human experience demand fresh analogies and metaphors. The language of family therapy has become encrusted with outdated concepts or notions that carry too much baggage and so must be refreshed. Some of the words that no longer describe my thinking

1

or my practice are: "strategy" (a term from war studies and game theory which creates opponents rather than *collaboration* and *negotiation*; see Chapter 1); "ethnicity" (which creates outsiders rather than acknowledging that all *cultures* have a history and a geography and a figure/ground relationship to one another; see Chapter 2); "enmeshment" (this is the *familism* of traditional societies seen out of cultural context; see Chapter 7); and "paradox" (why give people absurd puzzles to solve when we can help them construct more meaningful *metaphors* to transform their experiences?—see Chapter 10). This kind of word-weeding helps us build what I call the postmodern language of therapy (DiNicola, 1993).

———

> Family therapy is the starting point for the study of ever wider social units.
>
> —Mara Selvini Palazzoli
> (1974/1963, p. 241)

Selvini Palazzoli's quote has been an inspiration to me from the early days of my training in family therapy and transcultural psychiatry. Like her, I was attracted to family therapy "to bridge the gap between sociology and psychiatry" (Selvini Palazzoli, 1974/1963, p. 251). When she wrote this more than thirty years ago, Selvini Palazzoli lamented the practice of treating families in relative isolation. This book offers ways to end that isolation by (re)placing families and the practice of family therapy in cultural context.

Selvini Palazzoli, who lives and works in Milan, also represents a connection to Italy (my country of origin), to child psychiatry (my chosen profession), and to the foundations of family therapy and the women who nurtured me (she was my first mentor in family therapy). Her quote serves as a continual invitation to expand my thinking and my work beyond these starting points. Doing so is the product of a lifelong engagement with the predicament of strangers. This predicament has been articulated as "the needs of strangers" by Canadian humanist Michael Ignatieff (1986) and cast as a dialogue between "aliens and alienists" (an archaic term for psychiatrists) by British transcultural psychiatrists, Roland Littlewood and Maurice Lipsedge (1989). The people whom American philosopher Richard Rorty (1989) describes as "strange people, strange families, strange communities" are, in my formulation, "strangers in the family."

This phrase, which I have chosen as the title of my book, is polysemous—which means, I hope, that it will be pregnant with numerous associated and constructed meanings for the reader. It is modeled on other books that I admire. Natalia Ginzburg's (1989/ 1963) reminiscence of her Italian Jewish family, *Lessico Familiare*, plays with layers of meaning in each word ("family sayings, familiar words"). Another title, *Thinking through Cultures*, richly conveys Richard Shweder's (1991) profound argument that psychology and culture are intimately interwoven. Upon reflection, it seems that authors choose polysemous titles when they straddle diverse fields or when they want to go outside the established mold to break the frame. This makes them liminal texts—at the threshold of different worlds, or at least different descriptions of the world—just as many of the stories in this book describe liminal people.

In referring to "a stranger in the family" (also the title of Antonella Trevisan's story in Chapter 8), I mean that when a family therapist meets a family across cultures to deal with a psychiatric problem, several levels of strangeness may be discerned: (a) the alienating symptoms of mental illness (re)presented by one or more members of the family; (b) the family members as cultural outsiders in society; and (c) the family therapist as an outsider to the family and perhaps to the family culture, entering this alienated family. My hope in such therapeutic encounters is to make these experiences less strange and more familiar, as the family adapts to its predicament. In other words, by enhancing strangeness, by opening up the many experiences of strangeness in family life, I offer a road to adaptation (within the self and the family) and acculturation (in society), which ultimately means making the strange more familiar.

DEFINING FAMILY THERAPY

Why practice family therapy? I am surprised at how rarely this question is asked nowadays. *Family therapy is the space that we open to explore the possibilities of the family.* My definition of *the task of*

family therapy is to give structure and meaning to a family's predicament.
It is not our task alone—it is explored in narrative genres such as
autobiography, journalism, film, and fiction. This exploration occurs in therapy (that is, we need therapy) when it does not happen
anywhere else. It provides guidelines for investigation and tools for
change. Family therapy offers (re)descriptions of human predicaments and tools for inventing new metaphors for family experiences. This, above all, states the argument for the *relevance of family
therapy*: not because families have problems, or because the family
is an especially salient context for children and other dependent
members, or even because outcome studies support the claims of
family therapy, but because it is *a compellingly meaningful way to
ground the work of therapy*. Family life, to echo Carl Whitaker's seminal idea, is the crucible of our personal experiences. Family therapy
implicitly acknowledges what psychologists Jerome Bruner (1990)
and Richard Shweder (1991) and philosophers Charles Taylor
(1989) and Richard Rorty (1989) have made explicit: that psychology
must be based on social life, giving primacy to systems of meaning.
Our experience of mind—human consciousness—emerges *through*
social interactions. Consciousness is culture, one of the integral
sources of the self. "Identity" is formed within and through the
informing contexts of family and culture. The "self" we seek is
culturally constructed and socially distributed. As family therapists,
we seek "mind" through context and relationship. As cultural family therapists, we find the royal road for understanding "mind,"
"self," and "identity" in the "presenting culture" of the family.
Constructed this way, cultural family therapy is my contribution to
a cultural psychology and to a psychiatry of meaning.

"AN ART OF LENSES": CONCEPTUAL TOOLS
FOR CULTURAL FAMILY THERAPY

In Antonioni's film *The Passenger*,[1] there is a tense encounter between an African leader and a jaded British journalist who con-
fronts him:

Interviewee: Mr. Locke, there are perfectly satisfactory answers to
all your questions. But I don't think you understand how little

you can learn from them. Your questions are much more revealing about yourself than my answers would be about me.

Journalist: I meant them quite sincerely.

Interviewee: Mr. Locke, we can have a conversation—but only if it's not just what you think is sincere, but also what I believe to be honest.

Journalist: Yes, of course, but . . .

The interviewee stands up and turns the camera around onto the interviewer.

Interviewee: Now, we can have an interview. You can ask the same questions as before.

Cultural family therapy turns the camera around: same questions, different perspective—what Lynn Hoffman (1990) calls "an art of lenses." All the innovations of family therapy are an attempt to change lenses and perspectives: inviting the client's family members into the therapeutic space, working with co-therapists, teams, and the one-way mirror, sending messages from the other side of the mirror, reversing the mirror with reflecting teams, employing narratives such as letters and family stories, and a more radical change—the collaborative use of the therapist's personal and cultural resources with families.

Cultural family therapy is an interweaving of stories (family predicaments expressed in the narratives of family life) *and tools* (clinical methods for working with and making sense of these stories in cultural context). By interweaving stories and tools, cultural family therapy is aimed at understanding *and* change. Neither one alone suffices, as each of them produces only part of the solution. Examples of emphasizing understanding include such hermeneutic approaches as psychoanalysis and interpretive anthropology. Examples of emphasizing change include strategic family therapy, behavior therapy, and psychopharmacology. Salvador Minuchin has likened the family therapist to the anthropologist who must "join the culture" he comes to study (Malcolm, 1978). Minuchin's insight points to the parallels in "meeting strangers," whether in a cultural encounter as an anthropologist or across family cultures as a family therapist. Nonetheless, there are differences. As Mara Selvini Palazzoli (1986) wrote, unlike the anthropologist studying a tribe or the work of sociology, family therapists are asked to effect changes. Because we are asked to intervene, our task as clinicians is much different: for us being inside or outside the family culture is a tool and not a goal. The goal is therapeutic change, the transformation of experience.

Cultural family therapy is a synthesis of family therapy and transcultural psychiatry, a synthesis that can be very fruitful for both the families who come for help with their cultural—that is, *human*—predicaments and for the growth of both fields. As a result, I am addressing two somewhat different kinds of readers: clinicians such as social workers, psychologists, psychiatrists and others who work with families, and students of culture, including medical anthropologists and sociologists, cross-cultural psychologists, and transcultural psychiatrists. My goal, then, is to orient cultural scholars to some key ideas in family therapy and therapists to selected concepts about culture. As a result, different readers will have varying needs and different ways of reading this book.

Throughout the book, I have woven over two dozen family "stories," varying from brief clinical vignettes and cameo portraits to longer and more detailed multigenerational narratives. I also introduce and elaborate my conceptual "tools" for cultural family therapy. Most chapters introduce and illustrate one or two new tools, which are labeled and described in detail. By "tools" I mean the actions and thoughts of the therapist—what philosopher Michel Foucault (1980) calls a "tool-kit." Some of my conceptual tools are actions, such as "spirals"—my way of conducting collaborative interviews. Others are more like lenses that change the focal length of our gaze or color what we see, such as "masks"—which help us to see the cultures that we all carry, either as costume or camouflage. These tools are informing perspectives that are conceptual and metaphoric, in that they invite us to think differently about families and cultures as systems (see Falicov, 1988; Rosenblatt, 1994).

MAPS FOR THE READER

Some of the different ways to read this book, therefore, are to choose family stories from the Index of Family Stories, or to choose conceptual tools, briefly described below. The book is divided into three parts, each with a theme. Each chapter has a brief overview of its key ideas at the beginning; the scholarly context—references and brief explanations of issues in the text—are collected in notes at the end. Key words and ideas from each chapter are also collected in a glossary at the end of the book. Here is a brief overview:

PART I: MEETING STRANGERS

Chapter 1: The Strange and the Familiar
Stories: "The Frozen Sea Within Us," "Two Old Men,"
"The Berlin Wall"
Tool: Spirals

I imagined Chapter 1 as an overture, sounding the main themes of the whole book: I introduce the concept of intercultural consulting, stories of families moving across cultures, the problems and promises of translation, and the personal nature of therapy for all of us. The first of my conceptual tools is called "spirals" in my clinical shorthand, by which I identify a way of meeting strangers through negotiation and collaboration.

Chapter 2: Cultural Family Therapy: A New Synthesis
Story: "The Many Faces of Self-Starvation"

In this chapter, I outline my synthesis of family therapy and transcultural psychiatry and review problems with family therapy's use of cultural concepts. To prepare the way for culture-responsive family therapy, I discuss the need for multiple descriptions of predicaments, two basic therapeutic temperaments (technocratic and phenomenological), and problems with family therapy across cultures. In closing, I contrast "paradigm" with "syntagm," a fresh approach that is sensitive and responsive to each family as a unique culture.

Chapter 3: The Presenting Culture
Stories: "Meeting Strangers/A Familiar Stranger," "Racism in the Family," "A Latin Temperament," "Elephant Boy"
Tools: Masks, Roles

In this chapter, I update my synthesis of family therapy and transcultural psychiatry by outlining some major issues in cultural studies and cultural aspects of family therapy. It is written for therapists who are less familiar with this territory than cultural scholars. It reframes what the presenting issue is in therapy—neither persons nor predicaments narrowly understood but the "presenting culture." This leads to a discussion of my second conceptual tool, which I call "masks"—cultural costume and camouflage. How the therapist positions himself in relation to the family is captured by my third tool, "roles"—those of insiders and outsiders. For cultural scholars, I have tried in this chapter to harness their complex and sometimes contradictory work to a clinical task.

PART II: ON THE THRESHOLD: LANGUAGE, IDENTITY, AND CULTURAL CHANGE

Chapter 4: Beyond Babel
Stories: "Unlovable," "Drifting Apart," "The Japanese Earthquake," "Mother's Space," "A Private Language"
Tool: Codes

This chapter looks at the work of both therapists and cultural scholars from the point of view of language and translation. I have made translation the key metaphor and tool for cultural family therapy. I review translation across cultures and exciting developments in translation theory. I give working definitions of translation; its applications to therapy is my fourth conceptual tool, "codes." Cultural and therapeutic translation are illustrated with several clinical vignettes.

Chapter 5: Changelings
Stories: "The Story of an African Harlequin," "A Caribbean Cordelia," "A Train of Traumas," "Culture Is Not a Dirty Window," "A White Boy Who Thought He Was Cree"
Tool: Cultural Strategies

This chapter brings together the themes of this book so far in an examination of identity and cultural change. The royal road for understanding "mind," "self," and "identity" is in the "presenting culture" of children and their families. In this chapter, *changelings*—children and their families undergoing cultural change—are explored in five stories of migrant children and the issues for identity and adaptation that emerge while working with them in therapy. The fifth conceptual tool of CFT is the negotiation of "cultural strategies" that children and families use for adaptation and acculturation.

Chapter 6: Threshold Therapy
Stories: "An Acoustic Mask," "Mum's the Word"
In this chapter I call for a study of *liminal people* and *transitional states*. Following a review of the relationship between culture and mental illness, *culture-change syndromes* are defined and illustrated through two stories of children with selective mutism. Cultural family therapy with changelings or liminal people may be described as *threshold therapy*. Conclusions are drawn from the relational and cultural study of development and of mind.

Chapter 7: Stones and Bridges
Story: "Conspiracy of Silence"
This chapter examines "The Myth of Independence" as a connecting theme in Western psychological theories and therapies. Aspects of the myth of independence are outlined to show the pervasive implications of this concept. Two aspects are explored in depth: (1) how independence has become enshrined as an ideal goal in Western family therapy, and (2) how this differs from two other societies—India and Japan.

Chapter 8: Stones Without Bridges
Stories: "A Stranger in the Family," "The Past Is a Foreign Country," "From the Cradle," "A Pain with No Name"
Tool: Bridges
In this chapter, I present four "orphan cases." In each case, the impediments to working more fully with the clients' families limited the elucidation of their predicaments. Cut off from a more complete relationship to her family and society, each of these individuals suffered in a unique way. They illustrate the psychological, social, and cultural implications of the myth of independence, which identifies my sixth conceptual tool, "bridges"—understanding cultural aspects of the family life cycle.

PART III: FAMILIES AS STORYING CULTURES

Chapter 9: The Garden of Forking Paths
Story: "Above My Heart, Above My God"
Tool: Stories

This chapter illustrates the use of the conceptual tools of CFT in family narratives. "Stories," my seventh conceptual tool, examines the evolving narrative of family life and therapy as a garden of forking paths. Here, I complete the story of the Shami family, introduced in Chapter 1. Their story demonstrates all the tools presented so far—spirals of negotiation, cultural translation, and playing with roles, masks, cultural strategies, and bridges.

Chapter 10: The Web of Meaning
Story: "I Am Myself What I Have Lost"
Tool: Multiple Codes (Metaphor, Somatics)

Metaphor and its power to transform experience is the subject of this chapter. Metaphor allows us entry into the "web of meaning" of other lives, an alternative to narrower views of family therapy. A Portuguese immigrant family's story illustrates the possibilities of narrative transformation through my eighth conceptual tool, "multiple codes." These are the complex messages encoded in metaphor (figurative language) and somatics (embodied meaning), illustrated by the Figueroa family's experience of loss, pain and overcoming. The chapter closes with an overview of the key metaphors for culture, families, and therapy constructed throughout this book.

Chapter 11: Strangers No More
Stories: "Strangers No More," "Cinema Paradiso"
Tool: Suturing

The final chapter tells one more family story: my own. It comprises several narratives: a memoir of the journey to meet my father in Brazil, how I stitched the fragments and "outtakes" of my father's life into a portrait of my parents' marriage to create a coherent narrative of my family, concluding with reflections for therapists about how we heal ourselves. It is interwoven with the story of the Sicilian boy, Totò from the film *Cinema Paradiso*—an illustration of intertextuality. If family predicaments are "stories gone awry," then "suturing," the ninth and final conceptual tool I offer, is cultural family therapy as story repair. Although it may seem that this is family therapy without a therapist, a closer reading will show that much therapeutic work preceded—and followed—this momentous journey.

———

Even though this book opens with themes of strangeness and alienation, deepened with stories of "changelings" and "orphans," the stories of the Shami family and my own family sustain my belief in the transformative possibilities of cultural family therapy. I am an Italian who lives in Canada writing for a North American audience. As a sojourner in several other countries—England, Israel, the United States, and Brazil—I know enough about them to have my own perspective on their problems and enough respect to understand that each society needs to find its own solutions. After a study of the books that these societies have produced about family problems, I have concluded that there can be no comprehensive text on this subject. Furthermore, since each society has its own model of intercultural relations, each society needs to write its own books, for each generation. I hope this book will find some use in parts of my society, but I fully expect that the solidarity required by intercultural communication will mean that other books will be needed by people in other societies. To paraphrase Canadian media maven Marshall McLuhan, this book is a probe, not an answer.

My purpose is not to alleviate our anxieties about strangers by searching for universal human qualities but to find ways to embrace differences and to live with diversity. In North America, those of us who have a complex personal identity are continually faced with questions about where we fit. I hope to challenge the North American stereotype of assimilation, which sets out implicit rules for dealing with such situations. This stereotype assumes that migrants and minorities are refugees of some sort, for political or economic reasons, who gratefully give up their attachments to other places and other ways of being. It has become a common refrain to bemoan "hyphenated" Canadians or Americans. This is an absurd imposition of cultural categories. To the question, "Are you Italian or Canadian?" my response is "I'm Jewish." To the question, "Are you a family therapist or a child psychiatrist?" my response is "I'm a psychologist." I feel like Groucho Marx—as soon as you create a category I want to bust out of it. Provisionally, I describe myself as having an Italian heart, an Anglo-Saxon brain, and a Jewish soul; I'm working on integrating something Afro-Brazilian into the mix.

Just as I do not make assimilation my personal goal, I do not ask for tolerance, which I believe is a false sentiment. To ask for tolerance presupposes a discomfort with difference. My own attitude is not one of discomfort: I accept difference, sometimes I enjoy it; at times it arouses a critical reaction in me, but almost never indifference. I try to bring to my differences with other people a sense of curiosity.

Curiosity is more useful and edifying than tolerance. Curiosity may lead to understanding and perhaps to acceptance. Tolerance is indifference: why should it matter to you that I am this way in the world? In North America, tolerance is a middle-class value nurtured by liberal ideals. Fortunately, I was not raised with this kind of constraining sentiment, which discourages asking important questions. And I am troubled by the notion that some questions should not be asked because we may not like the answers—this is the heart of theocracy and fundamentalism, fascism and totalitarianism of all forms, which are anathema to an open society (Popper, 1945). An open society demands that questions be posed openly and honestly. To be sure, timing and context, the form and syntax of a question cannot be separated from its substance, but neither should such considerations smother curiosity.

Under some circumstances, I respect the choice not to answer a question. For instance, my curiosity shuts down if I am so affronted by a question that I cannot maintain my integrity. This is an acknowledgment that even curiosity has limits, that opening some doors inevitably closes others. It may be hard to maintain curiosity about views that undermine what Richard Rorty calls the "final vocabularies" forming the bedrock of our values. Despite the fact that I have migrated across countries and cultures all my life, rarely have I felt my "final vocabulary" so threatened. Seldom has it been necessary to resort to the extreme recourse of shutting down a dialogue. One way I keep from shutting down is to adopt an ironic, postmodern stance. This allows me to maintain personal commitments while being open to how other people define themselves. It keeps my curiosity alive by reminding me that identities shift, collide and overlap, submerge or dominate, coalesce and create new syntheses.

When Italian writer Ignazio Silone (1949) was defending the way his beloved *cafoni*—"know-nothings"—speak in his novels, he responded in the simple prose that was his strength. He chided his critics that as we (he was speaking for the poor people of our region) do not come to Rome to tell you how to speak, you should not tell us how to talk in Fontamara. Silone (1949, p. 31, my translation) concluded: "Each of us has the right to tell our own story in our own way."

In letting people tell their own stories, we become an audience for those stories. This is a gift we give each other. To be an audience is not a passive process, but a very active one of constructing the meaning of what the other person wishes to convey. My "audience" (understood as an active listening process) extends beyond (re)constructing what families are saying to actually editing their stories. While journalists and anthropologists take as their trade the accurate (re)presentation of others' experiences (if such a thing is possible—and many thoughtful practitioners of these professions think it is not), therapists are authorized to help families negotiate change points in their lives. But being an editor of family stories gives me large scope to make my own meanings. As a person, I am a storyteller with my own tale to tell. I consider this both inevitable and necessary. In fact, I can think of no better reason to work with other people: the effort to understand each other gives meaning to our lives, a process from which we all grow and gain.

———

"For God's sake, open the universe a little more!"

This book "pushes the envelope" on the therapeutic frame. If family therapy expanded the frame of individual psychotherapy, cultural family therapy stretches it even further into the social surround. There is a beautiful, haunting image in Saul Bellow's (1982) novel, *The Dean's December*, where the central character hears a dog barking wildly. In an imaginative reconstruction, the man understands the barking as a protest against the limits of dog experience: "For God's sake, open the universe a little more!" In bringing this image to our attention, Salman Rushdie (1991a) reminds us that Bellow is not just talking about dogs and that "the dog's rage, and its desire, is also mine, ours, everyone's" (p. 21).

I believe that the effort to expand one's narrative voice is what makes us human, building the solidarity that connects each of us to a community, making us larger than ourselves, working across differences for the sum of our alliances. This is why I close the book with my own encounter with an alien part of my self, a self that lived apart from me in Brazil, who speaks and dreams in Portuguese, and "only dances samba," as Brazil's Antonio Carlos Jobim sang. Being human is an endless effort to collect our distributed selves from all the locations where they are scattered, forging them into a more coherent account of who we are.

So my choosing to include this part of my story is an "act of meaning," to use Jerome Bruner's (1990) wonderful expression for it, opening up my universe a little more. And I hope to convince you that it is not an "act of courage," as many commentators have generously suggested, but a necessary part of my argument for cultural family therapy. Therapy is not, for me, only a collection of tools and techniques, which appeals to our technocratic society. I also wish to explore the phenomenology of each family's experience. When I am with a family, I do not wish to act as if I am hidden and mute behind the mirror, but personally visible and professionally active in front of the family. To do otherwise is to gloss over the therapist's own personal, family, and cultural being.

Why does this book give so much attention to narrative genres, such as ethnography, autobiography, fiction and film? Narrative teaches us how to understand ourselves and others by (re)description. It increases solidarity by decreasing the cultural and social distances between us and them. When the vagaries of the real world overwhelm me, I take to the imaginary worlds of literature, music, and cinema to learn and to practice other possibilities. Some favorite writers, cited here and there in this book, have charted amazing places for the mind to travel—Natalia Ginzburg (an Italian Jew), Jorge Luis Borges (an Argentinian), Alice Walker (an African-American), Milan Kundera (a Czech who lives in Paris), Margaret Laurence (a Canadian who lived in Somalia), Richard Rodriguez (an American of Mexican parentage), Evelyn Lau (a Chinese-Canadian), Salman Rushdie (an Indian/Pakistani who lives in England), Gwendolyn MacEwen (an Anglo-Canadian poet and short-story writer), and Derek Walcott (a Nobel Prize-winning Caribbean poet and playwright from St. Lucia who lives in the United States).

An alternative is to actually travel to other places where we can learn new things or practice newer parts of ourselves. One of Hungarian-Jewish physicist Leo Szilard's (1963) personal commandments was to "Go into solitude or among strangers, so that the memory of your friends does not hinder you from being what you have become." The consultations and other therapeutic encounters recounted in this book were conducted in various cities where I have lived and during visits to other family therapy centers where I was making a stranger of myself.

Come join me on the journey!

—Vincenzo DiNicola
Kingston, Ontario

A NOTE ON LANGUAGE

You have taught me language; and my profit on't
Is, I know how to curse . . .

> —Shakespeare,
> *The Tempest*, Act I, Scene i

This book was written in English, which has the equivalence of a mother tongue for me. That is to say, I understand all the nuances of how strangers are cursed, a valuable education for a cultural family therapist. Some of the material is translated from other languages. Wherever published English translations are available, those versions are used; otherwise, I have rendered some of the French, Italian, and Portuguese quotations into English myself. In fact, I am tempted to describe myself not as the author but the translator of this book, which is congruent with my whole argument and with the postmodern notion that you, as reader, are your own author, free to make your own constructions. Given the subject matter of this book, there are numerous foreign names and phrases, locations, and references. I have resisted the temptation to make them so accessible that we lose the sense of encountering something foreign and new.

I did the editing of this book largely under the influence of Brazil's Antonio ("Tom") Carlos Jobim (1924–1994), who composed lyrical, languid *sambas*, a kind of tropical blues. Jobim provided me with key metaphors for my work, such as *desafinado*, "out of tune." The family stories and vignettes in this book may strike the reader as incomplete. I have resisted the urge to close on paper what remains open in their lives. As I suggest in the postscript to my memoir in Chapter 11, the difference between fiction and reality is that fiction has to make sense; at any given time, real life is often fragmentary and incomplete, waiting for the meaning to be made. I was inspired by Jobim's celebrated duet with Elís Regina on *Águas de Março*, "The Waters of March," a stream-of-consciousness exchange of voices in a palette of impressionistic hues, at times just trading one-word images:

> *E pau, e pedra, e o fim do caminho . . .*
> It's a stick, it's a stone, it's the end of the road . . .

When I refer to professional work, I have adopted the following conventions: "clinician" refers to any practitioner of an established mental health profession (e.g., psychiatry, psychology, social work) doing general work such as assessment; "therapist" refers generically to psychotherapeutic activities; "family therapist" refers specifically to therapeutic work with families; "social scientist" refers to academic scholars and researchers in fields such as anthropology, cognitive science, history, linguistics, psychology, sociology, and translation theory.

I have resisted changing these conventions at the behest of any newly-minted "traditions." I am writing about family therapy, a term that, as American journalist Janet Malcolm (1978) noted, sounds like a job description for a funeral home director. Whether you call yourself a "systems consultant" (as Luigi Boscolo and Gianfranco Cecchin do, see Boscolo et al., 1987, p. 24) or you refer to your professional activities as therapeutic conversations or story-editing, I take it that we still have a lot in common.

When I refer to families in treatment, I have chosen to call them "clients," as this term seems to have achieved the greatest degree of acceptance among a variety of therapists in North America. I use the term "patient" to identify the situation of a person with identified medical or psychiatric problems. Since one of the themes of this book is plural identities and multiple descriptions, I am suggesting that someone is a "patient" when being treated for schizophrenia and a "client" when engaged in family therapy.

On the subject of identities, I have tried to give to each individual or family story a meaningful context—where individuals or families are from, their expressed customs and beliefs, where and when they were treated, and of course, a name. While wishing to respect the confidentiality of my clients, I believe it is important to give people a name. So, although I have changed the names and other identifying features of these families, I have found equivalents that stay close in spirit to their cultures of origin. I have also adopted Italian family therapist Maurizio Andolfi's custom of giving each session or story a title, often expressed in what I call "concrete metaphors" (see Chapter 6).

Each society offers different constructs for giving persons their identities. In general, the people in this book are not constructed racially in the American sense of the term, which is to say, whether they are Black, Latino, White, Asian, and so on. Canadians look at identity in terms of national origin, often reduced to spoken language; our major categories are English, French, and Native. Here, the contrast of the "two solitudes" of the European founding peoples, English and French, overwhelms all other constructs. Thus, an Italian family in Montreal is "English," while a Haitian family is "French." This dichotomy eventually inspired an attitude of "a pox on both your houses" from the rest of us, opening space for other pluricultural, multicentric experiences in Canada. The identities of the families in this book are an encounter between what they have imported from other places and what their host society offers them.

In the literature of anthropology and transcultural psychiatry, there is, as yet, no consensus on key terms. Again, I have adopted conventions that work best for the present purposes: "culture" is central to the work of anthropology (and defined in Chapter 2); "cultural" is an adjective used to describe specific cultures, whereas "intercultural" seems most appropriate when describing meetings between two different cultures, as in "intercultural encounters." The German psychiatric pioneer Emil Kraepelin coined the term "comparative psychiatry," a tradition honored by my teacher, the late British/Canadian psychiatrist H. B. M. Murphy (1982) in his textbook, but the field I trained in was called "transcultural psychiatry" at McGill University, emphasizing the comparative study of mental illness in different cultures and their healing practices. Working in the American Midwest, psychiatrist Armando Favazza (1986) calls it "cultural psychiatry," emphasizing the cultural context of all psychiatric work, while American anthropologist-psychiatrist Arthur Kleinman (1977), whose early research focused on Chinese presentations of depression, wrote about "the new cross-cultural psychiatry," emphasizing uniqueness and differences between cultures rather than universality and similarities. Throwing his net even wider, British psychiatrist Suman Fernando (1988) calls for a "socio-cultural psychiatry," arguing that what is needed "is not the cultural psychiatry of anthropologists or family therapists" (p. 104). To a great extent, these (re)definitions are polemical exercises, an example of what I call the "bootstrap complex," the wish to create a new tradition.

And now for the dreaded English pronouns (I didn't invent the language, I just live here). I have adopted a variety of approaches to this problem. First, I have tried to write in a way that addresses people with curiosity and respect about who they are. Second, I have tried to be accurate and specific when referring to known individuals. Third, whenever I refer to general cases—therapists, say—I use male pronouns. Why? This is part of my hermeneutic or interpretive stance, which holds that there are no privileged positions, only particular contexts embedded in history, culture and language. By writing as a male therapist, I am acknowledging that I am a man and cannot speak for women. What I can and do offer is my interpretation of the experiences of a number of women in this book, but that is quite different from trying to be either all-embracing or gender-free. As a man, I am neither.

When I have written articles and chapters with female pronouns, editors and readers could not follow the flow, given my masculine name. I quite enjoy reading work by women who write with female pronouns, but it is not a voice that I can adopt authentically. I am attracted to the postmodern construction "s/he" but it seems to underscore the ambiguity of sexual roles and to challenge gender stereotypes somewhat more than conveying the simple message of "he and/or she," which is inelegant. I have tried numerous experiments—not only with gender but with age (writing from a child's perspective) and culture (writing from the perspective of someone from a culture other than the ones I know intimately).

These remain experimental dialogics, at least in my present narrative voice.

To quote, yet again, my dear *paisano* or countryman, Ignazio Silone (1949, p. 31)—

> *Si lasce . . . a ognuno il diritto di raccontare i fatti suoi a modo suo*

> Each of us has the right to tell our own story in our own way

—this is mine.

ACKNOWLEDGMENTS

This book has its origins in my postgraduate training in psychiatry at McGill University, where I devoted myself to the dual foci of family therapy and transcultural psychiatry. My mentor and friend throughout my training was Raymond Prince, M.D., then Director of the Division of Social and Transcultural Psychiatry. Dr. Prince was continuously open to my explorations as I began to integrate cultural aspects of psychiatry with family therapy, culminating in my thesis for the Diploma in Psychiatry at McGill, "Family therapy and transcultural psychiatry: An emerging synthesis" (DiNicola, 1985b, 1985c), published as a two-part overview in the journal of which he was editor, *Transcultural Psychiatric Research Review*. Many of my key ideas were sketched out in that publication. I thank another teacher and friend at McGill, Dr. Laurence Kirmayer, the current editor, for permission to use material from it and other essays of mine in that journal.

At the time, my main influences in family therapy came from two Italian training centers—Milan and Rome. I immersed myself in the work of the Milan Group and began a long friendship with Mara Selvini Palazzoli, M.D., of the University of Milan. Her response to my proposed synthesis of transcultural psychiatry and family therapy was very encouraging (Selvini Palazzoli, 1986). My contacts with the Nuovo Centro per lo Studio della Famiglia (New Center for the Study of the Family) in Milan over the years have been professionally instructive and personally nourishing. At the same time, I began to be interested in the work of Maurizio Andolfi, M.D., of the University of Rome, who taught me that "Rome is not a suburb of Milan." I trained with him through workshops and visits to his training center in Rome. With both of these Italian family therapists who have an international focus, I worked on developing a culturally-responsive approach to family therapy. Their influences are echoed throughout this book in numerous ways, including consultations with them and interpretations of their published work.

Part of the message of this book is that no one and nothing can grow and change in a vacuum. I want to acknowledge the invitations, support and instructive feedback from colleagues to whom I presented much of the material in this book. The presentations I made to the following groups were particularly important in the evolution of my work (some of them were published):

- American Orthopsychiatric Association Annual Meeting, Toronto, Ontario, 1984 (DiNicola, 1985d)
- Canadian Psychiatric Association Annual Meeting, Quebec City, Quebec, 1985
- Douglas Hospital, McGill University Dept. of Psychiatry, Montreal, Quebec, 1988. Ellen Corin, Ph.D., an anthropologist at McGill University, invited me to present my family work in an anthropological perspective (DiNicola, 1988b) on which Chapter 1 is partly based.
- Society for the Study of Psychiatry and Culture (SSPC) Annual Meeting, Farnham Castle, Surrey, England, 1989 (DiNicola, 1990a)
- World Congress of Psychiatry, Athens, 1989
- Institute of Family Therapy, London, England, 1990
- Sixth Annual Conference, International Counseling Center, Washington, D.C., 1991
- Ethnicity and Family Therapy Conference with Monica McGoldrick, Allan Memorial Institute, McGill University Department of Psychiatry, Montreal, Quebec, 1991 (DiNicola, 1993)
- Quebec Association of Marriage and Family Therapy, Montreal, 1992
- Ethnocultural Aspects of PTSD and Related Stress Disorders, WHO/NIMH/VA Institute, Honolulu, Hawaii, 1993. I am grate-

ful to Tony Marsella, Ph.D., a leading cross-cultural psychologist, for inviting me to this key meeting (DiNicola, 1996).

- Family Therapy Program, University of Calgary, 1995 (DiNicola, 1995b)
- World Congress of Social Psychiatry, Rome, 1995
- Loss and Family Resources Residential Practicum with Maurizio Andolfi, M.D., Sardinia, 1995
- Second Brazilian Congress of Family Therapy, Gramado, RS, Brazil, August 1996

All of the families in this book were seen with family therapy teams. I want to thank my supervisors, colleagues and trainees in numerous institutions for their support and feedback over the years. Ronald Feldman, M.D., and Gerald Wiviott, M.D., of McGill University, supervised my therapy with several of the families in this book. Among many colleagues, it is a pleasure to name a few: John Theis, Ph.D., Chair of Psychology at the University of St. Jerome's College, Waterloo University, enriched me with sage advice and inspired me with his consultations and co-therapy with the Shami family (discussed in Chapters 1 and 9) during his sabbatical in family therapy with me at the University of Ottawa. Two other colleagues have actively worked with me as review readers and cultural consultants throughout my writing: Tazuko Shibusawa, L.C.S.W., a Japanese family therapist and doctoral student at UCLA, and Nasreen Khan Roberts, M.B., B.S., a Pakistani child psychiatrist at the University of Calgary.

For two chapters, I owe special thanks. I would like to thank Mara Selvini Palazzoli and Raymond Prince for their dialogue and comments on earlier versions of Chapter 7 on "The Myth of Independence." My memoir in Chapter 11 has a history of many encouragements. Maurizio Andolfi, who first encouraged me to embark on the journey to meet my father, invited me to write my memoir for a special issue of *Terapia Familiare* on the identity of the therapist (DiNicola, 1995a). My memoir also appeared as a prepublication excerpt from this book in *The Family Therapy Networker* and I am very grateful to Rich Simon, Ph.D., and his staff for their tremendous care in shaping the final version for publication. I also wish to thank Karl Tomm, M.D., for the opportunity to present my memoir to a reflecting team at the University of Calgary, and Carol

Liske, Ph.D., editor of *The Calgary Participator*, for permission to rework a version that first appeared in English in her newsletter (DiNicola, 1995b). Special thanks are due to two fine teachers: Barry Thorne, Ph.D., of the English Department at Queen's University was enormously helpful in giving shape and structure to my narrative, and Raymond Reed, M.A., my high school English teacher, who has nurtured my love of language and literature for the past twenty-five years.

Susan Munro, my editor at Norton, has been the most patient of souls as she waited for my manuscript. Her gentle advice guided me toward a more coherent whole. She is a kind of Zen master of editing—patient, nonattached, open to the author's world. Wendy Gollogly, my resourceful administrative assistant, juggles my competing duties admirably to create the time and space necessary for reflective writing.

Throughout the evolution of this book, my own family provided the intimate context for my growth and change. I have been continually supported and enriched by my mother and my wife and children, who often join me on my cultural pilgrimmages around the world—from my spiritual engagement with Israel to my personal and cultural explorations of Brazil. Together, we live in our own pluricultural, multicentric world, created not out of material artefacts, but out of our own lives. My wife, Vicky Lopez, who was born in Montreal, is a descendent of Spanish Jews who migrated to southern Italy during the Inquisition. Like literary theorist George Steiner (1975), Vicky is a language student (and teacher) with no mother tongue, as she glosses fluently among Italian, English, and French. Our children, Carlo and Nina Mara, attend bilingual Roman Catholic schools, the faith of their grandparents, while a *mezuzah* (parchment scroll) made of Murano glass from Rome's main synagogue adorns the lintel of the door to my study, where I keep my collection of books on Italian Jewish life and my *talith* (prayershawl) and *tefillin* (phylacteries) from Mea Shearim in Jerusalem.

Finally, my thanks to all the families who, in their pain, took pains to teach me about their cultures around the world.

Part I

MEETING STRANGERS

In my utopia, human solidarity would not be seen as a fact to be recognized by clearing away "prejudice" . . . but, rather, as a goal to be achieved. It is to be achieved not by inquiry but by imagination, the imaginative ability to see strange people as fellow sufferers. Solidarity is not discovered by reflection but created. It is created by increasing our sensitivity to the particular details of the pain and humiliation of other, unfamiliar sorts of people.

—Richard Rorty,
Contingency, Irony, and Solidarity
(1989, p. xvi)

Chapter 1

THE STRANGE AND
THE FAMILIAR

*Intercultural Encounters among Families,
Therapists, and Consultants*

And in your excitement at the trip, the last thing in the
world that would occur to you is that the strangest glimpses
you may have of any creature in the distant lands will be
those you have of yourself.

—Margaret Laurence,
The Prophet's Camel Bell
(1963, p. 1)

*T*his opening chapter is an "overture" to the book, sounding the major
themes that follow. I introduce the experience of intercultural consulting by exploring translation—not just as a practical problem or technical
task in family therapy—but as a key metaphor of human communication. I
do this by offering both literary and therapeutic encounters as examples
of narratives. Family therapy has recently added to the older notion of
"punctuation" (see Simon et al., 1985, pp. 284–285) the metaphor of
family life as a "narrative" (Parry & Doan, 1994). The family narrative
or tale, originally written and edited by the family, may be rewritten and
co-edited with therapists and consultants. Doing so requires a way of
negotiating cultural encounters through spirals, the first conceptual tool I
introduce for CFT. In other areas of social science and the humanities, the
narrative metaphor has been made concrete (what Gregory Bateson called
"a metaphor that is meant") by referring to lived experience as a "text."

27

Applied across cultures, translation is another dimension of this textual reading of family life. Cultural and therapeutic translation are necessary decoding tools for the text of the family narrative to be understood. Without this dimension of cultural translation, the intercultural consultation experience remains alien, fragmentary, and incomplete.

FROM FAMILY SAYINGS TO FAMILY MYTHS

There are five of us children. We live in different cities now, some of us abroad, and we do not write to one another much. When we meet we can be indifferent and aloof. But one word, one phrase is enough, one of those ancient phrases, heard and repeated an infinite number of times in our childhood . . . would make us recognize each other in the darkness of a cave or among a million people. These phrases are our Latin, the vocabulary of our days gone by, our Egyptian hieroglyphics or Babylonian symbols. They are the evidence of a vital nucleus which has ceased to exist, but which survives in its texts salvaged from the fury of the waters and the corrosion of time. These phrases are the foundation of our family unity which will persist as long as we are in this world and which is recreated in the most diverse places on earth . . .

—Natalia Ginzburg
(1989/1963, pp. 23–24)

We all begin with the private language of the family, what Natalia Ginzburg calls the *lessico familiare*. The translation of this phrase as "family sayings" misses her *double entendre* or pun on *familiare*. Her meaning might be better translated by the pairing, "family/familiar"—emphasizing both the biological and social connectedness of family members. This shared early experience is the basis of the family myth (Ferreira, 1967).

We move from family sayings to family myths—an organization of our experiences and our worlds. Like young children moving out from a secure home base to progressively wider and unknown places, we move from the familiar to the strange, seeking to familiarize even the most foreign experience. As our world expands, we develop another layer of sayings and myths: we move to community and to culture. And we develop a cultural identity and the cultural costume that accompanies it. Cultural costume is made up of the sayings and the mythology from the larger community in which the family lives that defines its experience (DiNicola, 1986; Friedman, 1982).

This growth can also make familiar parts of ourselves and our worlds foreign. Every door we open is both an entrance and an exit. To move beyond the familiar and the established self is to enter a dance of polarities: the dance between self and other is a pivot between the strange and the familiar, between personal and social being, and a fluid switch of perspectives between insiders and outsiders.

For people who live in cultural communities with a continuous history, all these elements of identity may appear to form a seamless whole. From the familiar to the strange, each individual and each family constructs a composite identity of personal and social being (Harré, 1979, 1984). But in a world of immigrants, shifting boundaries, refugees, and rapid cultural change, these different elements can create a veritable Babel of confusion (Berry, 1992; DiNicola, 1985b, 1985c, 1986, 1992, 1993). Let me give an example from therapy.

"The Frozen Sea Within Us": A Russian/Jewish Family Comes Out of Hibernation

Montreal in the early 1980s. A mixed Russian/Jewish family, the Mandels, are in therapy. The client is a 12-year-old boy, Nikolai, who is brilliant, quirky, and troubled. He carries disturbing, violent imagery in his head. The father, a Russian Jew, is an electronics engineer from Moscow. The mother, ethnically Russian (not Jewish), is a costume and set designer who has worked in theater and cinema. They are very cultured, literate people whose rich understanding of the world outside their apartment contrasts starkly with their relative lack of insight into their own lives.

For this reason, I tried to give meaning to Nikolai's violent ideation by referring to Franz Kafka, a writer whose life was marked by ambivalence and lack of individuation from his parents. The situation of Kafka's life led to ambivalence: he was a Czech Jew living in Prague, writing in German. Critics have said that his disturbing writing prefigures Nazism and the Holocaust (Pawel, 1984).

In a letter to his friend Oskar Pollak in 1904, Kafka wrote that what were needed were "books that grieve us deeply, like the death of someone we loved more than ourselves, like being banished into forests far from everyone, like a suicide. *A book must be the axe for the frozen sea within us*" (italics added). Using a literary reference that this family could appreciate, I presented Nikolai's troubling mental imagery as a response to the frozen sea of his family.

Perhaps the family sea had been frozen over by ambivalence and neglect. The parents had never resolved their ethnic and religious differences, so they are torn as to which community and which religion to join. In the official atheism, classlessness, and denial of ethnicity of the former Soviet Union, these had not been pressing issues for them. When they stepped out of that orbit, however, all these issues came out of hibernation. They had considered emigration to Israel, but the mother was not Jewish and she and Nikolai would have to convert. After they settle in Montreal, Nikolai experiences painful alienation at the French public school that all immigrants must attend in Quebec. After some family deliberations that restage their dilemmas, the boy is enrolled in a Jewish private school where the other children are from observant Jewish families. Instruction is in English, French, and Hebrew. Again, the boy encounters problems: he is not considered Jewish (which is a matrilineal religion); nevertheless, he comes home from school with enthusiasm for religious observances that are neither understood nor followed at home. This sets off the ancient conflicts between the two sides of his family.

How can this child absorb a religion that is not truly his own within a family that has not resolved its core religious and ethnic identities? The city they live in plays out the parents' private divisions in a battle over the language of instruction for immigrant children. It must be French, but some families opt out by sending their children to private schools where both English and French are taught. (For historical and cultural background on this situation in Quebec, see Richler, 1992.) The family members' confusion is potentially amplified by their encounter with a therapist who is also an immigrant to this city and has one foot in Christianity by upbringing and another in Judaism by adoption. Lastly, I am committed to working with the family, while my supervisor/consultant is a psychoanalyst who works within an individual perspective.

These shared experiences encoded in language and in family and cultural myths shape both personal and social being. When new experiences are encountered in the form of new words, people, and places, there is an experience of strangeness. Nikolai came from a family that had not resolved important differences in their families of origin. I suspected that they left the Soviet Union partly to escape these unresolved differences. If so, their new encounters only enhanced Nikolai's confusion and mistrust. My supervisor/consultant formulated Nikolai as a child developing the characteristics of a "borderline personality," with a profoundly disoriented core identity. I agreed that he was much like Kafka, torn between alliances and lacking an age-appropriate identity that was stable and distinct from his parents. In Kafka's case, this literally followed him to his grave: he is entombed at the Strasnice Cemetery in Prague with both his parents where the tombstone bears all three names (see Pawel, 1984). If my supervisor's developmental hypothesis is correct, did Nikolai's identity confusion generate his other, interpersonal conflicts? Or did his confusion have its origin in confounding experiences within his family? If the latter is correct, then those confounding experiences may continue to be generated and played out within the family, amplifying Nikolai's confusion and alienation.

The impact of migration is another and more significant consideration for this family. A Canadian study of Soviet Jewish immigrants and their children (Barankin et al., 1989) shows that children are doubly exposed to the direct impact of migration on themselves and to the adaptational difficulties of their parents. The study also highlighted the adaptive capacities of these families and outlined protective factors that can help immigrant children to be resilient and can be used therapeutically.

In this family's odyssey, each society offers different definitions of key aspects of their lives. At one time in their former Soviet home, the Mandel family's ethnic and religious differences were in "hibernation" (later, being Jewish in Russia became much more problematic). Even considering a life in other societies (such as Israel) roused them like a bear from a long sleep—urgent and ominous. The family's encounter with a new multicultural society had brought the family's identity issues out of hibernation after several generations, but their adaptive responses are still frozen over. Focusing only on individuals or family interactions here is too narrow. We need the larger contexts of culture and society to meaningfully restage the Mandels' personal, family, religious and cultural dramas.

THE FAMILY THERAPIST: A STRANGER IN THE FAMILY

When strangeness comes in the form of an encounter with a family therapist, several levels of strangeness may be discerned. One or more family members are behaving strangely; they may have become estranged from themselves or from other family members; the family turns to outsiders or strangers with an experience of strangeness within the familiar. In Nikolai's family, for example, his parents recognized that within their familiar experiences with each other, something different and strange was occurring. Nikolai was increasingly "estranged" from them. The family turned with this puzzle to a real stranger outside the family—a family therapist. There came, in turn, other strange aspects of their encounter with a therapist: negotiating new and difficult tasks through a newly acquired language in a cultural context that was alien and sometimes hostile to them.

A family therapist joins these strangers in search of the familiar and the reassuring. My definition of the task of family therapy is to give structure and meaning to a family's predicament. In Luigi Pirandello's play *Six Characters in Search of an Author* (1952), the characters are members of a family who come in search of the playwright (who they fear has abandoned them) to complete their story so they can find the meaning of their existence. Nikolai's story is a troubling one for me. When it was time for me to move on to another rotation in my psychiatric training, my supervisor would not agree to transfer the case to another institution. So this story (like many others) has no ending for me. At times, this family visits me in the middle of my work with other families to ask me about my commitment to what I am doing and to finish the task I started with them.

The therapist may or may not be successful in alleviating their suffering or in giving meaning to their story, but families inevitably suture the story of therapy and of the therapist into the narrative of their lives. Even the most reluctant families have stories to tell about previous encounters with therapists: the personality, the quirks, the beliefs, the perceived successes or failures of their encounter with the therapist all become part of the history and mythology of the family.

When therapy falters or fails, we should consider expanding the therapeutic system with other meaningful connections for the family (e.g., a grandparent) or with a consultant. When I am brought in as a consultant, I listen to stories about other therapists with great interest, looking for clues about how my own encounter with the family may be understood. It is also worth noting because families are sometimes successful in casting a previously negative therapeutic experience in different, more positive terms. I find this exhilarating because this often demands a whole new vocabulary—"New experiences call for new descriptions" (DiNicola, 1993, p. 49). I wonder what story Nikolai's family would tell about our unfinished therapy?

THE CONSULTANT: ANOTHER STRANGER

Given the complexities of working with families across cultures and languages, family therapists frequently need consultants as cultural brokers or as resources on specific aspects of a family's predicament such as posttraumatic stress. (In many cases in this book, I was sought out primarily as a cultural consultant, notably in the case of the Shami family, told further on in this chapter.) Into this complex story, the consultant is brought as one more stranger, creating yet another level of strangeness. What the consultant can do is open the system up for the introduction of novelty. If the family members are open to new experiences, this will be incorporated into their history and their repertoire of skills in a helpful and positive way. If not, this new stranger will be dealt with in the family's usual way: treated as an outsider to maintain rigid boundaries, as a witness to confirm survivorhood, to legitimize and validate their pain, and their reasons for prizing it and retaining it.

Of course, the therapist may have his own reasons for not changing and for experiencing the consultant as an unwelcome stranger.

In fact, the consultant can be approached by the therapist for all the same reasons that families come into therapy, including ambivalence about change. A common reason for a consultation is for validation for the therapy to continue on the same tack, rather than change direction. ''Am I doing the right thing?'' the therapist asks the consultant.

In order to understand what a cultural consultant can offer a therapist working across cultures, we need an overview of what interventions family therapists have available to them. In my reading of the field (DiNicola, 1990e), family therapy interventions are ways of feeding back, transmitting, or transforming the information obtained from the family and the therapeutic systems. With all their interventions, family therapists do three simple things: (1) enhance uncertainty, (2) introduce novelty, and (3) encourage diversity. The family in therapy may use these therapeutic messages to structure their experience and to make meaning of their predicament.

If we understand the consultant as a stranger visiting the therapeutic system (family plus therapist), an obvious role for the consultant is to *introduce novelty*. The consultant imports information from the outside. This is an active, sometimes directive role of the consultant who uses herself as a source of information for this family. In the encounter with families across cultures, the consultant may be culturally different from the family, the therapist, or both. When the consultant is culturally different from the family, this gives her great freedom to make radical redefinitions, to bring in almost anything from outside the system.

When the consultant is culturally similar to the family, the therapist, or both, but the family is situated in a new society, this gives her the opportunity to *enhance uncertainty*. Information already in the family or therapeutic system can be released, as it is reflected back to the family, who hear it as ''news.'' The news allows family members to experience the problem differently, making them uncertain of their solutions.

Any combination of differences or similarities among the family, therapist, and consultant can be used to *encourage diversity*. Old information is perceived as new (i.e., transformed) or new information is received into the system by its members. This is beyond introducing novelty from the outside: the family members try out new definitions, roles, and behaviors for themselves. This is especially helpful for families who see new situations as threats rather than opportunities.

THE ARRIVAL OF THE CONSULTANT AT
THE CASTLE OF CROSSED DESTINIES

One of the guests drew the scattered cards to himself, leaving a larger part of the table clear; but he did not gather them into a pack nor did he shuffle them; he took one card and placed it in front of himself. We all noticed the resemblance between his face and the face on the card, and we thought we understood that, with the card, he wanted to say "I" and that he was preparing to tell his story. (Calvino, 1977, p. 6)

A consultant arrives at a family meeting much as the knight in Italo Calvino's tale arrives at a castle. She finds people whom she does not know (the family) assembled by a host (the therapist). The castle (the treatment context) is to some greater or lesser extent unknown to her, as are the circumstances which have brought these people together (the histories of the family and the therapeutic systems). The knight (the consultant) does not know why she is really there or what may emerge.

The knight must rely on language and other shared symbols to communicate and understand the stories of the host and the other guests. The possibilities would appear to be endless, but the opportunities, the time, and the tools may be limited. Furthermore, the knight finds that she cannot speak (the consultant may not speak the same language as the family members or the therapist).

Using the analogy of the arrival of the knight at the castle with the consultant's work in a therapeutic system, three questions come to mind: (1) Where do you start? (2) How do you stay on track? and (3) How can you tell where you are going (if you have not been there before)?

1. *Where do you start?* Can the seemingly endless variety of human stories be told with a limited number of symbols or cards? If the consultant is a stranger to the world of the family, the therapist, or even the society in which the therapeutic system has been constructed, is there some set of family stories for the consultant to fall

back on for guidance? Although the consultant meeting a new family across cultures may feel as though she is in a labyrinth of endless blind alleys or a territory without a map, she has her own personal resources to fall back on. No one starts with nothing. The consultant cannot be a blank screen, without a personal, family and cultural history. Furthermore, there is no value-free social science, psychiatry, or therapy. The goal is not to be neutral or unbiased, but to make one's practices culturally informed.

Three strategies can help to make the consultant more culturally responsive. First, by acknowledging certain starting points, the consultant can proceed by the method of differences: is this the same or different from what I have encountered before? Second, the consultant can take the attitude of asking the family and therapeutic systems to instruct her on these differences and enter a cultural encounter. Third, and above all, the consultant needs to have a sense of irony about her own starting points and about the systems she is about to enter. Without irony, the consultant risks the arrogance of imperialism (my culture is dominant and superior), the naiveté of common sense, which assumes universalism (everybody does supposedly basic things in more or less the same way), or the circular and impotence-inducing stance of extreme cultural relativism (every cultural group is distinct and must be understood on its terms, as explained by its own people).

2. *How do you stay on track?* If the consultant is to enter a cultural encounter, can it be only a one-way street? If one is foreign to the environment one visits, can one truly understand others without revealing something of oneself? It is actually very difficult in the face of cultural differences not to tell something of one's own story. Even at scientific meetings dealing with empirical research on ethnocultural factors in psychiatry and therapy, presenters openly discuss their own involvement in their work or reveal it indirectly by their choices of terms, methods, and how they evaluate their results.

My assumption is that one cannot conduct therapy as a one-way street, with the flow of information from family to therapist or consultant. Yet the individual psychotherapy tradition has led many therapists to feel uncomfortable with understanding their social roles in therapy and to reject self-disclosure as therapists. One strategy for managing these concerns is to employ the perspectives of insiders and outsiders (DiNicola, 1985c, 1986). These perspectives offer a useful way to map the relationship between the therapist and the family. In turn, one can map the relationship of the family and the therapeutic system to the society at large and to the consultant. For example, immigrant or refugee families may see themselves as outsiders to the society. However, their goal may be to integrate into their new society or to hold themselves apart. This may have implications for how they see therapists and consultants. Immigrants and refugees with an integrationist view are inclined to be accepting of authority figures and health care providers in their new society (Berry, 1992).

The therapist and the consultant can learn to use different personal qualities and identifications to adopt a role that will meet the family's needs. In different situations, we all occupy both insider and outsider roles; neither is superior, both can be useful. As an insider, the therapist or consultant takes a position of shared common experiences with the family. The advantage is that one can acknowledge what is shared and act accordingly. There is an atmosphere of working together, especially when the family and the therapist or consultant are different from the host society. This occurs for me when I am treating an Italian family or any family when we define ourselves as immigrants in Canada and discuss our reactions to Canada and other Canadians.

As outsiders, the therapist and consultant can be explicit about their differences or inequalities in relation to the family. The advantage with this perspective is that one can take either the posture of an expert or a one-down position by acting as cultural outsider. For example, while acknowledging individual experiences, one can discuss common reactions that immigrants or refugees have in coming to a new country. Alternatively, one can emphasize the uniqueness of their experience and invite family members to be experts on their own culture and their own journey of change.

Of course, taking these different perspectives enhances the experience of irony in both the individuals and the systems. By experimenting with multiple identifications, the consultant can help the therapist to expand his/her repertoire of therapeutic resources. Observing this process, family members can model the growth of the therapist by expanding their views of themselves as individuals and as a family. Over the course of therapy, by seeing many possible insider and outsider perspectives, a family may also start to play with such definitions, seeing them as more fluid and open to change.

This parallels the model of the therapist's role in the family articulated by Andolfi and his colleagues (1989). First, the identified client is detriangulated by taking him or her out of the center of all interactions. This allows the therapist to occupy that role for a time. Later, as the family has new experiences through therapy, the family can give up their need to have anyone (including outsiders) play such a role.

The most intriguing example of this is Andolfi's use of the child as a co-therapist (Andolfi, 1994). Sometimes, Andolfi works through the identified client on a telephone or intercom while he observes the family behind a one-way mirror. This more directly challenges the distinction between being inside (healthy, part of, same as) and outside (unhealthy, separate from, different than) the family.

3. *How can you tell where you are going (if you have not been there before)?* Does each of us hold enough of the cards to tell our own story or to see it played out in the hand of another player? If you do not have a great deal of experience, how can you recognize the patterns and connect them to each other and to yourself?

> I open my mouth, I try to articulate words, I grunt, this would be the moment for me to tell my tale, it is obvious that the cards of these other two are also the cards of my story, the story that has brought me here, a series of nasty encounters that is perhaps only a series of missed encounters. (Calvino, 1977, p. 99)

One answer to this question is to use cultural consultants when working with families across cultures. Therapists not only hear the tales of other people, but also do their work because they have forgotten their tales, confused them in the telling, or wish to be freed of them like the knight in Calvino's tale. Therapists cannot simply put aside their lives while working; for example, they may seek a consultation during a time of personal crisis and change. This may be used creatively and therapeutically for the family and the therapist. As another stranger, the consultant occupies a liminal position. From this place at the border or on the boundary of therapeutic experiences, the cultural consultant can help the therapist to redefine himself (or opt for congruence), to enter a new experience (or define himself by renouncing it). Therapists who are more interested in the phenomenology of family experiences are more likely to enter this space. This is the so-called madness of psychiatrists and the craziness of doing therapy: to explore one's own madness by immersing oneself in the madness of others, to redefine oneself by repetition and re-exposure, to learn new words by attending to the lost meanings of old ones, and to find one's place by leaving it for the experience of new places.

A MODEL FOR CULTURAL FAMILY THERAPY (CFT)

CFT is an interweaving of family stories (predicaments expressed in the narratives of family life) and conceptual tools (lenses, metaphors, and clinical methods for working with and making sense of these stories in cultural context). Over two dozen family stories are told in this book and nine conceptual tools for conducting CFT are outlined. Although each new conceptual tool is introduced separately and illustrated in family narratives, in practice they are all intimately interwoven. "Spirals," the first conceptual tool for CFT, is a description of how to negotiate cultural encounters. Cultural and therapeutic translation, part of a clinical tool I call "codes," are briefly introduced and illustrated through two family consultations.

SPIRALS: FAMILY THERAPY AS A CULTURAL ENCOUNTER

At the heart of CFT is a cultural encounter between the family and the therapist. This encounter is a special instance of the family's cultural experience in a new and potentially alienating society. It can also be a provocative and demanding experience for the clinician. In my construction of this relationship (DiNicola, 1985c, 1986,

1993, 1994, 1996, in press), everything can be negotiated between the family and the therapist. The therapist must be attentive to the family's definitions of self and family as well as to what constitutes problems and solutions in the family's world-view. What demands even greater flexibility and therapeutic resources is that the therapist must be prepared to examine, adapt, or even discard the usual assumptions, methods and goals of therapy.

Spiraling is a way of conducting the interview in which you gently skirt around the issues and let the family members lead you to what they are looking for: how they define themselves, how they define the problem, and what sorts of solutions are acceptable to them. This illustrates what I mean by seeing therapy as a social construction rather than assuming you share the family's definitions or know things about them because of some cultural ''snap-shot'' you have of them. I call this a *spiral* because you circle, gradually getting closer and closer until you end up at something that is understood by both therapist and family. By then you have together defined all the terms and you know the implications of each term and each intervention.

This tool was shaped by my adoption of the Milan group's interviewing style (''hypothesizing-neutrality-circularity''; see Selvini Palazzoli et al., 1980) and the notion of ''openings'' described by Luigi Boscolo and his associates (1987). It is also informed by anthropological literature on how families meet indigenous healers.[1] There is a kindred approach in the narrative therapy of Michael White. White (1995) refers to his way of interviewing as ''re-authoring'' or ''re-storying,'' guided by two concepts—*landscapes of action* and *landscapes of consciousness* or meaning (which he adapted from Jerome Bruner). In describing how he uses these two concepts in sessions, White refers to a ''zig-zagging process.'' He moves back and forth from one landscape to the other, emphasizing that he does not follow any formal sequence or paradigm. What I am calling ''spiraling'' incorporates White's notions of landscapes and more. I am not just zig-zagging across conceptual landscapes, but also moving among roles, masks, codes, and other tools that I will describe.

Spiraling is a process that moves across time as well. What Salvador Minuchin calls ''joining'' in family therapy, I call ''meeting strangers'' in cultural family therapy. This spiraling process is not just done once and then you move on—you keep doing it, negotiating, collaborating. Solidarity is built moment by moment, session by session; it can never be assumed. You never step into the same river twice. Other waters and still other waters flow on. Spiraling does not so much lead to other work, as it is the product of the other work. So through all the cultural and therapeutic translation that the cultural family therapist does, he is spiraling, building solidarity.

CULTURAL TRANSLATION

The fundamental attitude and the most basic tool in CFT is cultural translation. *Intercultural communication and translation*, as practiced in transcultural psychiatry and in CFT, is the elucidation of an individual's or a family's idioms of distress, explanatory models of illness, and perceived predicaments using family members, culture brokers, and other informants when useful, and language translators when necessary, in a collaborative effort. Stripped down, it is the effort to help people find words for their own pain in their own language.

Cultural translation is a much more workable attitude than cultural relativism or tolerance. Relativism and tolerance do not invite an encounter but mutual indifference. Conducting therapy requires a more active involvement motivated by curiosity about differences or the desire to build bridges across differences. The effort to translate and work across differences (rather than tolerating them), encourages both parties—families and therapists—to relinquish clichés, myths, and stereotypes to explore together new perceptions, explanations, and ways of being.

THERAPEUTIC TRANSLATION

Once the therapist acknowledges that meeting families across cultures is always a cultural encounter and facilitates cultural translation for expressing their predicaments, the task is to move on to a translation of their distress into the language of therapy. *Therapeutic communication and translation* is the process of rendering an individual's or a family's idioms of distress, explanatory models of illness, and perceived predicaments into therapeutic idioms.

Together, cultural and therapeutic translation are part of the conceptual tool I call "codes" (discussed in greater detail in Chapter

4). Decoding—the use of cultural and therapeutic translation—leads to a double description of their predicament for each family: their own private language for their pain and a more public, possibly more accessible therapeutic language. This process of double description in family and therapeutic languages also underscores that CFT is a collaborative effort among family members and therapists.

"LOST ACROSS CULTURES, FOUND IN TRANSLATION": CONDUCTING CULTURAL FAMILY THERAPY (CFT)

To illustrate the use of these tools in conducting CFT, two encounters with families in therapy across cultures and across languages are presented below. The first encounter is a single consultation session that took place in 1987 during a practicum in family therapy for an international group of family therapists at the Institute of Family Therapy in Rome with Dr. Maurizio Andolfi.[2] In this case, the meaning was conveyed not entirely *with* words, but perhaps *through* the words, even *in spite of* them. We could say that the meaning of this encounter was lost across cultures but found in translation. When, during the practicum, the visiting trainees became concerned that they could not understand all the interactions of the Italian families, Andolfi would say: "Forget the words, pay attention to the process."

The second encounter was a year-long course of therapy conducted at the Family Therapy Program of the University of Ottawa in the early 1990s. We will be introduced to the Shamis, an Arabic immigrant family, whom we will revisit in Chapter 9. Their family story serves as the "frame story" for this book, like the story of Scheherezade in the *Thousand and One Nights*, who kept the emperor Shahryar awake night after night by telling tales to avoid being executed. In a very real way, the sessions with this family forestalled unpleasant social consequences for them while we were searching for better solutions.

"The Berlin Wall": A Consultation in Rome

Summer 1987. I consult to an Italian family therapist working with a family from Rome, the Savellis. Claudia, the identified client, is a

25-year-old woman accompanied in this session by both parents and two older sisters. I am presented as a Canadian of Italian origin with some knowledge of Italian but more comfort with English. For this reason (and for the other practicum trainees behind the mirror), we use a professional translator. The therapist explains the reason for this consultation to the family.

Therapist (in Italian): The Professor is visiting from Canada . . . Dr. Andolfi and I find ourselves in a situation we don't understand very well. We're at a moment of great confusion; we feel bankrupt. Therefore, we've asked the Professor to give us a consultation.

Imagine my experience: everything that is said has to be translated. Although I can follow both languages, I have to wait for each message to be translated before I can respond in English. The session is effectively linguistically duplicated or *double-coded* (in sociolinguistics, a language is a "code").

At first I find the process of translation frustrating because it slows down the pace of the session. However, double-coding gives me the opportunity to process the session through two languages and two cultures. Sometimes, I do not agree with the translator's choice of words or images to convey the meaning. I find myself looking for my own versions of what I am hearing.

After a while, I take advantage of my own experience to connect with what the family is presenting to me. In his brilliant theory of translation, Douglas Robinson (1991) calls this intensely personal, mediating experience of the translator the "somatics of translation." Although it is not immediately evident in any bizarre behavior or words from Claudia, the identified client, there are many tortuous, verbally indirect interactions. I feel a split between words and feeling in this family. I understand the words but not the feelings. The overall impact is confounding, as though we are in a fog. Since this is a family with a schizophrenic member, it is probably not accidental that misunderstandings between words and emotions arise among them. I begin to experience a connection with Claudia. The double-coding that is going on for me in the session in Italian and English, my need to wait for and react to the translation, and at the same time my doubts about the accuracy of the translation are clues to the client's verbal confusion and the family atmosphere of fog.

I begin to feel that Claudia is also experiencing confusion and fog. I begin to hear her words as attempts to capture two different, perhaps incompatible, worlds. Then it hits me: she is also double-coding. Her slowness, her tortuous delivery, her odd way of phrasing and rephrasing expressions are her attempts to articulate divergent experiences (inside herself or within the family). This also explains my own language discomfort. At first, I doubted my fluency in Italian because of her unusual expressions; then I questioned the translator's accuracy. However, the translator's real mistake is in trying to convey something "sensible" in English rather than allowing the client's idiosyncracies to come through from the Italian. All of this is amplified by the fact that the other family members have also adopted a somewhat indirect and evasive manner of communicating (which was also glossed over by the translation).

As to the content of the session, at the beginning there is discussion of the missing male members of the family and what this means. Since the Italian therapist is a woman, I decide to use my presence as a man to side with the baffled and ineffectual father. I want to know why he is alone with all these women and why the other men in the family (his sons) are not there with him. I consciously choose to work with splits in this family. So far, I have noticed two: the split between words and feeling (the original definition of schizophrenia, which in Greek means "split mind") and the split between women and men in this family. And of course, all the people present have been going through a third: the split between Italian and English. As the session proceeds, another split becomes clear between the children who have done well, married and moved out, and the two remaining at home, Claudia and Marco. The parents, especially the mother, express great interest, to the point of intrusiveness, about what Claudia and Marco think.

At this point, I decide to reflect with the therapist about what I have heard so far. In what follows, keep in mind that my part of the dialogue is in English, the others speak in Italian, and each statement has to be translated.

Dr. DiNicola: I'm impressed by two ways in which people can be together in this family. . . . One way is to look successful, to be married and to have children, and to live nearby. The fact that they feel successful seems to give them permission to share what they've done with the family. But the two who are at home have a much more subtle way of being with their parents. They live at home and keep their thoughts to themselves.

So my thought is to ask the parents: what do they prefer—to know their children at arm's length or to have their children at hand and not know them?

Therapist: I think it's true about the affection that circulates between parents and children. What makes us go on in therapy, Dr. Andolfi and I, is this energy that's circulating in the family. But at the same, there's something that I call "a mystery." This mystery's like a forbidden area, as though somebody, something *(the translator misses the therapist's metaphor of a wall)* would prevent anyone who gets even a little bit close to the family from getting closer so that they can touch the family.

Dr. DiNicola: Do you mean that for everybody or do you have certain people in mind?

Therapist: I feel that especially for Marco. I feel that Marco is like somebody who's being locked up . . . walls have been built up around him. *(Her Italian expression,* murato vivo—*"walled in alive"— is much more graphic, like "buried alive.")*

Dr. DiNicola: I feel a kind of concern and tenderness from you toward Marco.

Therapist: Yes, it's terrible to see such a young life, with such strong and fresh feelings, dying day by day.

Dr. DiNicola: You know him so well from one meeting?!

Therapist: No, I know him from what they told me about him. I feel now that the bricks that they put up around Marco are not real bricks.

Dr. DiNicola: Did the family put these "bricks" up around him?

Therapist: A little bit. This was done by each one of them a little bit. One day one brick was put by a member of the family, another day another brick was put by another member of the family, and one day they discovered they had put up a wall.

Dr. DiNicola: That's what happened in Berlin. That's how they built the Berlin Wall. It's been in the news while I've been here in Italy. They're trying to tear it down.

To capture all these splits, I chose a concrete metaphor for this family and my experience with them—"the Berlin Wall" (this was before the fall of the Berlin Wall in 1989), building on an image used by the therapist. Notice that the translator did not use the word "wall." If I had been not following the dialogue in Italian, I would have missed this rich metaphor. The wall is an image of divisions in the family between women and men, sickness and health. As often happens in families with a schizophrenic member, there is a pseudo-protective attitude toward a schizophrenic member. Cloé Madanes (1980) calls such attitudes "protection rackets." While there is protection going on, it is aimed at the rest of the family, especially the siblings, not at the identified client. This may be a clue as to why the other siblings are absent. Parents of schizophrenic offspring sometimes are afraid of the unaffected siblings becoming "contaminated" by the "sick" one. Later, trying to connect Marco's absence and the wall built around him, I ask the family, "Is the wall there to keep somebody in or to keep people out?"

Mother: It was built to keep people inside, but I can't imagine that a family would build a wall to keep a son inside . . . Marco only came once, but he's exactly the one who's in the family, who still lives with us.

Dr. DiNicola: To whom is he being loyal by not coming today?

Mother (quickly and assuredly): To his own ideas.

Dr. DiNicola: Do his ideas also belong in the family?

Mother: No, they are his own personal ideas.

Dr. DiNicola: He is a very interesting person, Marco, because he is the one who is most "inside" the family and his ideas don't belong to the family!

Mother: The therapist knows that Marco has his own ideas and doesn't share ours about doing family therapy, and so on. She knows that Marco came only once just because he had promised to come, but they never succeeded in having him come again.

Dr. DiNicola (to Claudia): Do you and Marco live at home . . . all the time?

Claudia (attentive but silent, long delay, then responds almost painfully): Yes.

Dr. DiNicola: Why do you delay? Do you have other things on your mind?

Claudia: I was thinking about things that didn't pertain to this, but I don't know . . . I was thinking about things of my own . . .

Dr. DiNicola: Ah! . . . Do you, like Marco, also have ideas that you don't necessarily share with the family? Have the parents noticed that?

CLAUDIA (SITS SILENTLY, REFLECTING, GIVES NO RESPONSE)

Mother: Yes, especially now, she keeps a lot of things to herself. Of course, all children have areas that they keep secret from parents. But we have noticed just recently that she has more secrets from us.

These exchanges reflect the family's preoccupation with what Claudia and Marco are thinking, what is going on inside them. They want therapy to get their thoughts out into the open. The therapist has also become caught up in this "mystery." So I elaborate the metaphor of the wall to help the family describe the different behavior of Claudia and Marco, rather than challenge it.

Dr. DiNicola (to the therapist): I said there may be two ways of being in this family . . .

(To the whole family): Walls can be symbolic, not real. You can even walk through them.

(Facing the parents): And I think that whoever built the wall did it out of tremendous caring.

(PAUSE FOR TRANSLATION)

Maybe the wall serves to mark off where the fears belong and to protect some of the children who have done well.

(PAUSE FOR TRANSLATION)

(Turning to the older sisters): So you're in West Berlin and that requires one way to live.

(PAUSE FOR TRANSLATION)

(Turning to face Claudia): And I think that Claudia and Marco are in East Berlin, where to survive you have to keep your thoughts to yourself.

(Pause for translation)

(*To everyone*): And that's just what Claudia and Marco have done.

(Pause for translation)

Building a metaphor. Reflecting on this session after almost a decade, I am struck by how alive it still is inside me. I am struck by how attentive we need to be to conduct therapy. And not only across cultures. Do we listen closely enough to nuances in therapy when we share the same language? When the translator missed a single word—"wall"—its *absence* in her English translation alerted me to its importance. I was waiting for it and when I did not hear it, it offered me a tiny opening, a keyhole, into the therapeutic process. Word by word, a metaphor was carefully built up, refined, and elaborated with the therapist and the family members. We became co-architects of the metaphor (and thereby of the session). From the Berlin Wall (which is a space divider), we traveled East and West, and discussed how the parents could visit both sides using visas (exploring mutually estranged territory). They all participated in giving life to this inanimate wall. It became a systemic metaphor not because of the qualities of the word "wall" but because the "wall" was passed around like a marker on a board game, with everyone using it in a different way to talk about their relationships, including the therapist.

Notice that with the wall we created space for Marco. By talking about the wall, we built windows and doors into it. At least in this session, Marco was no longer *murato vivo*—"walled in" or "buried alive." We listened to each person's experience as if it made sense: Claudia and Marco have their reasons for keeping their thoughts to themselves, the parents have their visas for crossing boundaries, the siblings need the wall to protect them from their fears, and the therapist may now use the wall to explain why she feels there is a "mystery," why the therapy is "confused" and "bankrupt." Talking about the wall gave all present a common experience. This is the beginning of a therapeutic translation of their experience as a family, building toward the metaphoric transformation of their experiences towards health (see Chapter 10).

IMPLICATIONS OF TRANSLATION IN THERAPY

The translator's experience instructs us that in the attempt to translate across cultures, many insights may be garnered. The attempt to chart a one-to-one mapping of experience between cultures reveals some features common to both worlds but, more importantly, the distinct features that make a particular family's world unique. This is just as true for ethnography, where a comparative encounter between cultures teaches us something about each culture, as it is for cultural family therapy, where we meet each family as the bearer of a unique set of personal, family, and cultural myths.

Translation across languages is notoriously difficult, hence the adage from Italian—*traduttore, traditore*: translator, traitor. There is always the danger of mistranslating or reducing the other's person words into something closer, less alien to your own language and experience. But this is a counterfeit; cultural encounters are about the alien and the strange, not glosses on the familiar. Anthropologist Mary Douglas (1975b) suggests that if we do not examine what we find obvious or "self-evident," then "our only recourse . . . is to translate from other cultures into our own" (p. 277). The more familiar the translation is made to seem, the more we impose our provincial point of view on other cultures. "So the consequence of good translation," Douglas concludes, "is to prevent any confrontation between alien thought systems" (1975b, p. 277).

Translation is a metaphor for communication and for relationships. When astute observers from the social sciences and the humanities pay attention to culture, they not only deal with translation but conclude that it is fundamental to all human communication. In his seminal work on language and translation, George Steiner (1975) states:

> a human being performs an act of translation, in the full sense of the word, when receiving a speech-message from any other human being. In short: *inside or between languages, human communication equals translation.* (p. 47, italics in original)

Translation is so fundamental that it has become the key metaphor for all my clinical work. In subsequent chapters, I will deal with translation at greater length, discussing translation theory and my approach to cultural translation and therapeutic translation. Meeting strangers, whether across cultures or other differences, always involves a process of double-coding, of making comparisons, of translating. For these reasons, I concluded from my first experiences with cultural family therapy that ''All therapy is a form of translation—of language, of culture, and of family process'' (DiNicola, 1986, p. 189).

''Two Old Men'': Co-Editing A Family Story

A consultant from Beirut. Ottawa, early 1990s. The Shamis, an Arabic immigrant family from the Middle East, were referred to me by both the court and the child welfare system. Samya, a 13-year-old girl, had made inconsistent allegations about physical and sexual abuse at home and in her community. No one had been able to get at the ''truth,'' although some of the officials eventually acknowledged cultural differences in the construction of appropriate personal and family boundaries and in the perceptions of abuse.

My contract with the referring agencies and with the family was not to discover the ''historical truth'' but to help the family heal whatever trauma had occurred and their suffering by helping them relate their ''narrative truth.''[3] The family was extremely angry with the Canadian authorities over the allegations, the removal of their daughter, and her alleged promiscuity and rape while she was kept in a group home. By the time I met them, they had great difficulties accepting the good will of anyone involved in their case.

The nodal point in my work with this family occurred at the very beginning. The problem was how to begin family therapy with people who were both hurt and angry. How does one enter a family system characterized by ''familism'' (a family-centered way of being), enhanced by its encounter with an individualistic culture and made rigid by accusations of child abuse?

My approach was to ''go with their culture.'' I asked the parents what their view of the problem was and what solutions would be acceptable to them. The key question was: if a family problem occurred in Lebanon, to whom would you turn for help? Their answer was clear: to the elders of the family. Following their own preferred solution, I invited them to bring the child's grandparents to a session. After some discussion, we learned that Samya's maternal grandfather was visiting the family in Ottawa from Beirut. Using their own metaphors, I referred to this person as "the head of the family" and their "moral leader." They felt obliged to comply with my request because this view of the grandfather as a moral leader was culturally sanctioned. I then reframed their predicament not as a psychiatric problem or a protection issue but as a "cultural question," which the father qualified as a "human question." This is an instructive reframing; for the father, his culture is universal and therefore "human" rather than Arabic or Islamic. This is a characteristic of many traditional societies. Even after living in Canada's pluricultural society for decades, my grandmother, who is from a small mountain town in central Italy, refers to people as *cristiani*; for her being Christian and being human are synonymous.

When the grandfather arrived at the next session, I received him with great ceremony as the head of the family. As he spoke only Arabic, we communicated through a family member, although we faced each other directly the whole time. My message was simple: he was the old man (leader) of the family and I was assigned by the courts as the old man (specialist) for therapy. As one old man to another, I wanted to consult with him about how to help his children, Samya's parents. He nodded with understanding. He had a clear-headed view of the problem: "The girl's father," he said, "is trying to raise his family in Canada the way we do in Beirut." Although he was visiting Canada for the first time and had never been outside of Lebanon before, he stated with authority that "Canada is a different place with different rules."

This created a therapeutic opening for me. Surely few "Canadian" therapists would have had the knowledge or authority to make such a statement or have it accepted by the family. The old man of the family gave me the authority to help his children and grandchildren live in Canada by a new set of rules. This also offered a bridge for the intergenerational tensions felt by Samya and her siblings in trying to be dutiful traditional Arabic children at home while living in the pluralistic Canadian society.

What followed was an intense year of family therapy. Many difficult issues were encountered, but the family was able to develop trust in the treatment team. (We will meet Samya and her family

again in Chapter 9. Their changing predicaments and their therapeutic transformations serve as connecting threads for my discussion of cultural family therapy.)

THE TRANSLATOR'S TURN: "I ALSO TRY TO TELL MY TALE"

In Calvino's (1977) novel, there is a chapter called, "I Also Try to
Tell My Tale." Calvino the story-teller also needs to tell his story.
And I believe that the tale of the therapist or the consultant is in all
the stories of their families in treatment and in their selection of
stories they choose to tell. The professional handicap of the therapist or the consultant is the story of their therapeutic impasses, the
stories that they repeat and revisit in their efforts to master them.

As for my own tale, the key metaphor for my life and my work
as a psychiatrist and therapist is translation. For many years, my
professional experience has been to translate others' experiences.
Sometimes, this is quite literal, as my encounter in Rome demonstrates. But even when working in one language understood by all
present, I will turn to a co-therapist or a family member and ask
that person to "translate" what someone has just said. Or, if I feel
that something I have said is obscure or misunderstood, I will ask
if someone is willing to translate my thoughts into different words.
When a co-therapist is present, this is a useful way to expand the
possibilities in a given message (enhancing uncertainty or encouraging diversity) by having my co-therapist interpret and add his or
her own thoughts. Often, a family member will come to my rescue
when I request an interpreter. I am especially intrigued by how well
young children and other unexpected translators (such as "mute"
siblings and other "uncooperative" family members) can perform
this task.

This is a form of reflection within the session I used long before I
read about Tom Andersen's (1991) interesting work with reflecting
teams. I have called these reflections "translations" (in the American film Being There, a simple gardener is turned into a political
phenomenon when the Washington power brokers translate his
simple phrases into spin-doctored political prescriptions) or used
terms from theater and cinema such as "asides" (when one charac-

ter speaks but other characters do not hear, common in Shakespeare's plays) and "breaking roles" (when an actor turns to speak to the audience, memorably in the British movie *Alfie*). Through these translations, asides and role changes in the course of a session (which can be understood as the introduction of novelty, the enhancement of uncertainty, and the encouragement of diversity), one can also discern peering between the art and the artifice of language and therapy, the "translator's turn" (Robinson, 1991).

My own diverse experiences constantly bring me back to a common thread, to my point of origin, even as I draw farther away from it in time, in distance, and in the nature of my activities. After many attempts at redefinition, many detailed investigations and attempted solutions, I recognize my own story more clearly in the stories of my families in therapy. The experiences brought to me resemble more and more a series of tarot cards, or perhaps my favorite books and films, with their familiar faces and well-known tales. "I have seen this face before, I have heard this story," I say to myself, only to recognize, some time later, that the family was a mirror held up to my own face.

And so Nikolai's story, "The Frozen Sea Within Us," is part of my story, about living in different, sometimes incompatible worlds. His presence in my life is a reminder of all the tasks I have left unattended and incomplete and, more painfully, of the cherished people I leave behind each time I move. It is also a personal reminder of the limits of the therapist's power and influence, a lesson reinforced by Joel Elizur and Salvador Minuchin (1989) in their self-critical review of the real social context of family therapy.

"The Berlin Wall," my consultation with the Savelli family in Rome, is also part of my story, representing the rigid boundaries between incompatible systems (that may collapse for a time). This encounter illustrates my notion of family therapy as cultural translation. "Two Old Men," an early session with the Shami family, is my most successful attempt to integrate two cultures in therapy and to harness the authority that a traditional society invests in the elderly to solve complex family problems in a pluralistic society. Furthermore, I was able to move beyond translation to actually become a co-editor of the family story. It represents my construction of therapy in postmodern society (see DiNicola, 1993). This means constructing a framework that allows people to live more comfortably with social contradictions and cultural diversity while respecting the private values that give meaning to their lives.

I have spent a good deal of time translating words and emotional worlds, working carefully to convey experiences from one culture in the language of another. Like Calvino's silent knight communicating with tarot cards, I have been forced to expand my therapeutic resources through consultations with others. And the only available vehicle for all of this is language, which confounds and divides us like the Tower of Babel (which toppled because people could no longer understand each other's tongues) and reaches across differences like the Rosetta Stone (that was the key to the translation of hieroglyphics and the whole civilization of ancient Egypt). The Tower of Babel and the Rosetta Stone are two contrasting images of human communication. One is the image of the problem; the other the image of the solution. Through language, in the translation and editing of family stories, I feel that I can arrive at some provisional peace with my intercultural and other liminal experiences at the borders of human interactions:

> Thus I have set everything to rights. On the page, at least. Inside me, all remains as before. (Calvino, 1977, p. 111)

Chapter 2

CULTURAL FAMILY THERAPY

A New Synthesis

Family therapy provides one of the most fruitful areas of cooperation between psychology, psychiatry and medical anthropology.

—Cecil Helman,
Culture, Health and Illness
(1994, p. 291)

In this chapter, I outline my synthesis of family therapy and transcultural psychiatry, sketch out the main themes of transcultural psychiatry, and review problems with family therapy's use of cultural concepts. To prepare ourselves for culture-responsive family therapy, I address the need for multiple descriptions of predicaments, discuss two basic therapeutic temperaments (technocratic and phenomenological), and review problems with the portability of family therapy across cultures. I close by asking if we can give up our cherished "paradigms" for a more phenomenological approach that is sensitive and responsive to each family as a unique culture. In this approach, we would meet each family with a fresh approach each time—a "syntagm."

A NEW SYNTHESIS

Concepts are required which can aid the understanding of the relationship between the family and the wider culture and which can account for the "movement" that occurs between the two. Geertz's (1973b) concept of culture as a "web of meaning" is important here because it leaves room for variations within the same culture.

—Rosine Josez Perelberg,
"Familiar and Unfamiliar Types
of Family Structure" (1992, p. 115)

When *Ethnicity and Family Therapy (EFT)*, edited by Monica McGoldrick, John Pearce, and Joe Giordano, was published in 1982, a wave of recognition went through the family therapy community: here was something that was undeniably part of what family therapists saw and dealt with, but no one had before presented a paradigm for working with ethnicity in family therapy. Monica McGoldrick especially has a talent for identifying critical issues at the edge of the family field and bringing them to the center. She has done this with genograms, the family life cycle, ethnicity, and feminist issues.

Family therapists were generally receptive to and positive about *EFT*. As I was beginning my training in both transcultural psychiatry and family therapy at McGill University in Montreal, *EFT* brought together all my interests. My review (DiNicola, 1984a) was a rave. Students of culture, however, expressed reservations and were generally far less positive. On balance, its strength was in bringing culture into the discussion about families; its weakness was in its "static snapshots" of cultural communities. Ironically, the best chapters in the book are the ones that illuminate the book's weaknesses by criticizing the cross-cultural perceptions of other people through cultural myths: Carlos Sluzki on "the Latin lover revisited" (1982) and Edwin Friedman on "the myth of the shiksa" (1982).[1]

On the heels of the emergence of this landmark text and other thoughtful publications, such as Celia Falicov's *Cultural Perspectives in Family Therapy* (1983), I proposed a synthesis of family therapy and transcultural psychiatry based on their mutually enriching perspectives. In a detailed two-part overview (DiNicola, 1985b, 1985c), I suggested that conceptually both fields produce diversified information of breadth, like the wide-ranging fox, rather than the depth produced by the burrowing of the single-minded hedgehog in mainstream psychiatry research or individual psychotherapy.[2]

My proposal can be summarized briefly:

A synthesis of cultural and family studies has the potential to enrich both fields. Transcultural psychiatry was lacking a clinical model while family therapy was enlarging its scope. Although no therapeutic or clinical approach had been able to incorporate the cultural observations of transcultural psychiatry and anthropology, I proposed that as a treatment model, family therapy is broad enough to encompass cultural observations. For transcultural psychiatry, family therapy can be a clinical tool for cultural research, using the family as a window on cultural processes. Family therapy, on the other hand, was ready to expand its field of observation to the larger contexts of ethnicity and culture. Transcultural psychiatry offers family therapy a comparative tool to pose questions about family functioning in different cultures, testing the limits of its models and suggesting necessary adaptations of its techniques across cultures.

This proposal got notice from both sides of the synthesis. Despite the positive reception of my thesis (and subsequent papers and presentations) from both family therapists and cultural scholars, there has not been a broad acceptance in the family field of the salience of culture beyond the recognition of cultural groups who have distinct problems or who demand a voice. In the United States, family therapists were interested in what cultural methods I could suggest or devise (see Falicov, 1986), while cultural psychiatrists were encouraged by a tie-in with therapy and sought greater clinical relevance in my synthesis ''for all individual patients and not merely for those that are 'different''' (Favazza, 1986, p. 87). In Britain, influential social and cultural psychiatrists expressed support for my proposed synthesis, while articulating critiques about family therapy's use of culture (Fernando, 1988; Helman, 1994).

TRANSCULTURAL PSYCHIATRY

This book is an extension of my synthesis of family therapy and transcultural psychiatry to illustrate my model of cultural family therapy. In this chapter, I will examine the problems with family therapy's use of culture and the foundations of family therapy in light of new social realities, arguing for a new story for family therapy based on the metaphor of the "family-as-culture." As my analysis of these problems is from the perspective of transcultural psychiatry, a brief sketch of transcultural psychiatry is in order.

Transcultural psychiatry has strong Canadian roots, with many international branches. The term "transcultural psychiatry" was coined in the 1950s by a group of psychiatrists led by Eric Wittkower at McGill University in Montreal who formed a team of researchers and established a newsletter (later *Transcultural Psychiatric Research Review*) to share their findings. H. B. M. Murphy (1986) noted in his history of the the development of the field that:

> The choice of the term "transcultural" caused some debate, since "cultural," "ethno-cultural," "cross-cultural," and "comparative" could also have been used, each carrying a somewhat different connotation. The "trans" part of the term even caused some unease, since it appeared to imply that the field would be concerned only with features that transcended cultural boundaries, not those that remained within them; but on the other hand it could be taken as implying intercultural comparison. (p. 13)

At the outset, according to Murphy (1986, p. 13), the field catered to three main target groups: (1) researchers interested in the influence of culture on mental health, (2) clinicians who found Western psychiatric teaching unsuited to practice in societies with very different cultural contexts, and (3) social psychiatrists seeking to add an international dimension to their concerns. The McGill group led by Wittkower and later the Transcultural Section of the World Psychiatric Association chaired by Murphy chose to bring together the first two concerns.

Raymond Prince, director of social and transcultural psychiatry at McGill in the 1980s, offered a broad and practical definition: transcultural psychiatry is concerned with the comparison of mental disorder among different ethnic groups and/or cultures.[3] In Prince's view, transcultural psychiatry deals with three areas:

1. Cultural variation in psychiatric symptomatology and diagnosis (comparative psychiatry),

2. The study of culture-bound syndromes (discussed in Chapter 6),
3. How culture affects healing practices (such as indigenous healing practices).

Prince's third point has the most salience for family therapy. One implication is that all explanations of mental illness arise from what anthropologist Clifford Geertz (1983) calls "local knowledge" and that all therapies are what I call "cultural products," not just indigenous healing practices. Another implication is that all therapy needs to be culturally informed.

Emphasizing epidemiology (the study of the distribution of illness), Murphy (1982) called his landmark text, *Comparative Psychiatry* (the international and intercultural distribution of mental illness), which he defined as "the study of the relations between mental disorder and the psychological characteristics which differentiate nations, peoples, or cultures," whose "main goals are to identify, verify, and explain the links between mental disorder and these broad psychosocial characteristics" (p. 2). This important aspect of the field emphasizes objective population research using a comparative approach with little direct focus on or applicability to the problems of individuals or families who come for our help. With this objective stance, comparative psychiatry leans to the *etic* viewpoint, which calls for the researcher to develop an analytic structure from the outside with concepts and criteria assumed to be "universal."

From the beginning, though, transcultural psychiatry was also interested in *emic* perspectives—generated within the specific culture in question. Questions from the "emic" viewpoint in transcultural psychiatry include: What is the experience of mental illness in a particular culture? How is it expressed by the members of that culture? How is it explained by them? And what sorts of healing practices do they turn to for help?

"THE NEW CROSS-CULTURAL PSYCHIATRY"

Weighing in with impressive credentials in both psychiatry and medical anthropology, Arthur Kleinman (1977) of Harvard University, who founded the journal *Culture, Medicine and Psychiatry*, criticized the "old transcultural psychiatry" as being preoccupied with "universals" across cultures, notably externally-imposed Western psychiatric categories (the "etic" approach). In its place, Kleinman proposed a "new cross-cultural psychiatry," an interdisciplinary framework drawing on the rapidly expanding discipline of medical anthropology along with newer methods in psychiatric epidemiology. Kleinman emphasized a more "emic" approach, arguing that concepts of mental health and illness are culturally based and that concepts and therapies should be drawn from local cultures to be effective.

By the mid-1970s, transcultural psychiatry had evolved from being a minor research subspecialty of psychiatry into a vigorous, multidisciplinary, and at times contradictory field of cultural studies with numerous journals and transcultural psychiatry societies in several countries.[4] This growth threatened to split the field into "emic" (culture-specific) and "etic" (comparative and universalist) wings.

Fortunately, the split has not occurred for several reasons. First, these controversies invigorated academic debates and stimulated even more research in the field of cultural studies, often capturing mainstream attention in academic journals and among clinicians. Kleinman (1988) addressed core issues in general psychiatry from a cultural perspective in his book, *Rethinking Psychiatry*. Second, the "etic/emic" distinction and Kleinman's contrast of the "old transcultural psychiatry" versus "the new cross-cultural psychiatry" are forced dichotomies that have led to a more comprehensive synthesis of approaches by both researchers and clinicians. Third, more psychiatrists in developing countries are speaking for themselves, as are advocates for minorities and immigrants in developed countries, resulting in more practical applications of cultural studies to real-world concerns. Furthermore, transcultural psychiatry has matured greatly in the last ten years, with greater clinical applications than ever. Last, these academic debates have largely obscured a more significant shared problem, that of facing up to the effects of cultural traditions on both mental illness and therapies in all societies. While in the past, Western transcultural psychiatrists preoccupied themselves with exotic mental disorders in other cultures (in the study of culture-bound syndromes), we are now recognizing the cultural shaping of illness in our own backyard with illnesses such as anorexia nervosa (explored later in this chapter and in

Chapter 6). Equally compelling are the problems associated with rapid cultural change (culture-change syndromes) experienced by immigrants and refugees, such as selective mutism (the subject of Chapters 5 and 6). To put it simply, cultural psychiatry should begin at home (Murphy, 1977).

The view that emerges from cultural psychiatry in the 1990s is of a processual understanding of culture *situated in* and *created by* the social world of families and other interpretive communities. With this growing emphasis on meaning-making and the social construction of reality, culture is a process "located not in the minds of individuals, but *between* people, in the medium of intersubjective engagements" (Lewis-Fernandez & Kleinman, 1995, p. 434). This leads to the view of illness as embodied experiences based in biology *and* shaped by cultural processes. And cultural psychiatry emerges as the discipline that can examine the connections between social worlds and embodied illness.

PROBLEMS WITH FAMILY THERAPY'S USE OF CULTURE

We are increasingly becoming a world of migrants, made up of bits and fragments, from here, there. We are here. And we have never really left anywhere we have been.

—Salman Rushdie
(quoted in Marzorati, 1989, p. 100)

While continuing to be enthusiastic about the synthesis of family therapy and transcultural psychiatry, I also took stock of the mounting criticisms. Critiques focused primarily on one book—*Ethnicity and Family Therapy* by McGoldrick and her associates (1982). The most detailed cultural critique came from anthropologist Tullio Maranhão (1984), writing in *Culture, Medicine and Psychiatry*. Maranhão's critique of *EFT* is often cited and amplified by other cultural scholars (see Helman, 1994; Kareem & Littlewood, 1992). When I presented my model of cultural family therapy at the annual meeting of the Society for the Study of Psychiatry and Culture (SSPC) in Surrey, England (DiNicola, 1990a), I concluded with a critique of family therapy's cultural analysis, which I have expanded below. It speaks to the problems that were crystallized by *EFT*, but also goes beyond that volume to both theoretical and clinical practice issues.

These concerns sometimes arise because cultural issues are often ignored altogether. Many books on family therapy still do not mention culture, ethnicity, race, class, religion, or other social variables. Only since the 1980s have sex-role differences been addressed, and the social realities of economics, sexuality, and new family forms have been oddly left out of the family portrait. Sometimes, culture is misconstrued. When culture is invoked at all, the scholarly apparatus (ideas, language, methods, research findings) of anthropology or transcultural psychiatry is rarely used. One critic concluded, ironically and provocatively, that family therapy doesn't need anthropology (Maranhão, 1984). At other times, family therapy simply discounts culture, reframing social and cultural issues as family problems.

Numerous problems have been identified in the approach to cultural diversity represented by *EFT*. They are broken down into five problem areas.

"ETHNICITY"—HOMOGENEOUS, STATIC, TROUBLESOME

"Ethnicity" is a limited construct to imagine cultural diversity. As Edward Said (1994) concludes in his study of culture and imperialism, "No one today is purely *one* thing. Labels like Indian, or woman, or Muslim, or American are not more than starting-points, which if followed into actual experience for only a moment are quickly left behind" (p. 336).

1. *Homogeneity assumption.* Families of a given cultural community are all assumed to share certain features, regardless of social class, religion, educational, employment, and urban-rural differences. This homogenization is represented in many critical accounts by the use of the term "ethnicity," which is felt to create or reinforce stereotypes.

2. *Static snapshots.* In *EFT*, mini-ethnographies are offered as "static snapshots" of ethnic groups in larger societies, assuming they are valid generalizations, missing individual and family subculture differences. This picture is not only static in place, but in time as

well; family therapy has often lacked a historical context for its understanding of the family. Furthermore, such snapshots are used as guidelines for the conduct of therapy.

3. *Diversity as a disease*. Family therapy seems to treat cultural diversity as something to "cure" (Maranhão, 1984).

"ASSIMILATION"—PRESCRIBING
A MAINSTREAM MODEL

"Assimilation" is the presumed goal and model for how immigrants or minority members enter their host or dominant culture.

4. *Assimilation assumption*. In *EFT*, the dominant assumption is that immigrant and minority families can and want to become part of the United States through the only model that emerges: assimilation into the "melting pot." As Maranhão reads the text, "the function of family therapy is to facilitate this process of cultural adaptation in the Babel of ethnicities that is America" (1984, p. 272). This is the trap of many accounts of ethnicity, multiculturalism, and race relations in the United States and Canada: they polarize the discussion in terms of assimilation versus estrangment, as with bilingual education.

5. *Model of acculturation*. Mainstream family therapy assumes that assimilation is the goal of therapy, rather than the more complex realities lived by many outsiders to the cultural mainstream. There are many ways to enter another culture, from total immersion and assimilation (giving up one's former language, culture, and identity) to a kind of cultural apartheid (socially or internally imposed). There are also many confused, estranged, and lonely people who lose (or never attain) the cultural resources of their original culture and never really achieve a grasp of the language, culture, and habits of their new society.

6. *Acculturation rates*. The transcultural psychiatry literature demonstrates that the individual members of immigrant families have differential rates of acculturation and different personal goals (e.g., El-Islam, 1983; El-Islam et al., 1986), which can be understood as the collision or overlap of two or more different cultural maps of the family life cycle.

CULTURAL DISTINCTIONS—WHO WE ARE,
WHY WE ARE HERE, HOW WE TALK

"Objectification" of others, outside the dominant culture, means ignoring diversity among cultural communities and their distinctive identities as expressed in their values and their shared symbols and languages.

7. *Immigrants vs. refugees.* Mainstream family therapy has taken almost no notice of refugees, torture victims, and PTSD, lumping them all together with immigrants or "ethnics." Many refugees have undergone victimization.

8. *Settlers vs. sojourners.* There is a huge movement of migrant workers (sojourners) around the world, yet family therapy continues to see them as immigrants (settlers). The distinction means, among other things, that sojourners maintain family and financial obligations to their countries of origin. For instance, in 1981 Pakistanis overseas sent home remittances comprising 9 percent of Pakistan's gross national product, financing 86 percent of its trade deficit (Sowell, 1996, p. 21).

9. *Indigenous peoples.* Throughout the Americas, in Arctic circumpolar nations, and in Australia and New Zealand, many subgroups of indigenous peoples have complex, sometimes tragic relationships to the mainstream cultures of their societies.

10. *Language issues.* Language issues are seriously underplayed; language barriers are rarely discussed and there has been little sophistication in the use of translators.

WHEN THE THERAPIST IS A STRANGER—
IDENTITY ISSUES, INSIDERS, OUTSIDERS

There is a near-silence on diversity among therapists and in the construction of the therapeutic system.

11. *Therapist's cultural identity.* Family therapy still has the culture of the therapist under wraps behind the one-way mirror, rather

than visible and active in front of the family: as a result, the therapist's cultural issues are missed.

12. *Therapist as a minority member*. There is no significant literature about what happens when the therapist is a minority member of society treating mainstream families or working with immigrant or minority families.

13. *Therapeutic system as an outsider*. What happens when both therapist and the family are cultural outsiders? There are exciting possibilities for advocacy, culture-brokering, and translation in such encounters that are rarely discussed.

14. *Insiders and outsiders*. There has been little discussion about how to deal with requests for a therapist with a specific background. In practice, there is often an unquestioned acceptance that families are better treated by someone from their own cultural community (insider) rather than someone who does not share the aspects of the family's culture that are used to label them as different (outsider).

EXPANDING THE CONTEXT FOR FAMILY THERAPY

All of this results in the unexamined assumption that the family is the exclusive locus of pathology for mental illness, relational problems, and other human predicaments, as well as the key arena for their resolution.

15. *Family as the exclusive locus for problems and solutions*. In failing to recognize differences among cultural communities, in assuming that their goals as minority members in society or as immigrants are to assimilate into the host society, in failing to examine therapist issues and the construction of the therapeutic system or model, family therapy has reframed all diversity issues as family problems. This is a conceptual problem: we cannot reduce problems from one level to another, even if it appears to make such problems more manageable and even if we do not have the tools to work on the appropriate conceptual level. Of course, it is very tempting to fit problems into the models we know and practice comfortably.

Just as family therapists provoked individual therapists with the fundamental question about who really has the problem in the family with the notion of the *identified patient or client*, cultural family therapy now needs to provoke the family field by asking, "Where is the locus of pathology?" Some critics challenge whether family therapy recognizes "the social nature of illness" (McLean, 1986) and argue that it is "a clinical paradigm which locates problems within families and hence avoids examining wider systems" (Treacher, 1986, p. 274). We should ask: what is/are the most useful context(s) for examining the predicaments of particular individuals and their families?

Using the model of levels of analysis, we need to know how we decide to focus on the individual (and on which aspects of the individual—biological, psychological, interpersonal), the family, social structures, or the larger culture. Sometimes, the pathology or problem may not be at a particular level, but rather in the lack of fit between levels. In order to make meaningful use of each of these levels, we need to make our models of family therapy comprehensive and flexible enough to encompass the observations from each level, rather than reframe everything into a narrow and rigid paradigm. To integrate cultural observations, we can use the above critique to construct a model of family therapy that is more culture-inclusive, sensitive, and responsive.

NEW SOCIAL REALITIES, NEW MODELS OF THERAPY

CHANGES IN SOCIETY AND THE HUMAN SCIENCES

Since I proposed my synthesis of family therapy and transcultural psychiatry (DiNicola, 1985b, 1985c) and presented my critique of family therapy's cultural analysis (DiNicola, 1990a), there have been a number of significant developments:

In society:

- Diversity issues have become much more prominent in most Western societies; bilingualism and translation are common social concerns (Edwards, 1994).
- Racism has become more clearly identified as a *systemic* problem in society and in health-care professions (D'Souza, 1992; Fernando, 1988).

- Professional discourses have become politicized; for example, there is discussion of the political implications of psychiatric diagnoses and of professional practices.
- There has been a greater emphasis on understanding patients' perspectives, issues of advocacy, rights, and empowerment by professionals.
- The self-help movement, represented by the formation of the World Alliance of the Mentally Ill (by representatives of patient, consumer, and self-help groups in many countries), has grown.

In the humanities:

- Postmodernism, born of the perpetual crisis of modernism, including the diverse demands of multicultural societies, emerged as the dominant social theory (Harvey, 1989), undermining the foundational philosophy of the Western tradition (Rorty, 1989).
- With "text" emerging as a ubiquitous metaphor in social thought (Geertz, 1983a), the field of semiotics (the study of signs and symbols) became the hot new social science, from literary and film theory, to narrative approaches in therapy (see Josselson, 1995).

In cultural studies:

- Transcultural psychiatry debates centered on the key themes of the universal and the particular, similarities across cultures versus differences and uniqueness, the "classic transcultural psychiatry" versus the "new cross-cultural psychiatry" (Kleinman, 1977).
- Pragmatically, much of the research in transcultural psychiatry focused more on clinical issues and introduced some valuable clinical ideas for diagnosis (on culture-bound syndromes, see Simons & Hughes, 1985; on PTSD, see Marsella et al., 1996; on cross-cultural diagnosis, see Westermeyer, 1987), interviewing (see Kleinman's work on mini-ethnographies and explanatory models of illness, 1988), and treatment (on self-mutilation, see Favazza, 1996; on clinical methods in transcultural psychiatry, see Okpaku, in press).
- "Cultural consultation is a collaborative effort" aimed at sup-

porting rather than undermining local authority and expertise, relying on others as equals (Kirmayer, 1995, p. 168).

- Medical anthropology and cross-cultural psychology have become more mainstream, visible in undergraduate programs and in medical and other professional curricula.
- Psychology and other social studies have turned even more to questions about the construction of the self, identity, autobiographical memory and family stories (Bruner, 1990; Gergen, 1991; Kotre, 1995; Shweder, 1991).
- Sex-role studies have significantly rewritten the postmodern social landscape (Gilligan, 1982; McDermott et al., 1983).

In the family therapy field:

- Attempts have been made to integrate individual and family therapy (Braverman, 1995; Feldman, 1992; Nichols, 1987).
- Increasing client-orientation is reflected in more *visible* techniques (open reflecting teams, instead of strategic messages from a hidden team) and a more collaborative stance (interviewing as a conversation; therapy as a dialogue).
- More emphasis has been placed on pragmatic issues (how to resolve problems, how to empower clients) and brief therapy approaches.
- Constructivism and social constructionism have become the dominant conceptual models of family therapy, eclipsing systems theory (see Hoffman, 1990).
- Narrative has emerged as a new perspective in family therapy (echoing cultural anthropology's reviews of its own work) (see Paré, 1995).

In the light of all this, there have been a number of calls for paradigm changes—throughout the social sciences and among clinicians. We will examine two—one from cultural studies and another from family therapy.

"PARADIGMS LOST"—CHANGES IN SOCIAL THEORY

This catalogue of social changes has had its reciprocal impact on social theory. In addition to the examples given in this chapter—Kleinman's (1977) call for the "new cross-cultural psychiatry," Fernando's (1988) socio-cultural psychiatry, and Paré's (1995) cultural/narrative family paradigm—there is Robinson's (1991) radical theory of translation as "somatics and dialogics," presented in Chapter 4. Here are three other related areas where new paradigms are being imagined.

1. *Anthropology.* In "Blurred Genres," a brilliant essay that prefigured its impact on therapy, cultural anthropologist Clifford Geertz (1983a) calls the text analogy "the broadest of recent refigurations of social theory" and "the most venturesome" (p. 30). In *Works and Lives* (1988), Geertz examines the "anthropologist as author," with rereadings of some of the key texts of ethnography.

2. *Psychology.* Jerome Bruner (1990) and Richard Shweder (1991) call for the establishment of a "cultural psychology." Bruner, in response to the mechanistic features of the information-processing approach to cognitive psychology, wants to reinject meaning and narrative into psychology, with a focus on culture. Shweder rejects cross-cultural psychology, psychological anthropology, ethnopsychology, and other universalist approaches to a general psychology, arguing for cultural psychology as a study of the ways mind and culture jointly make up each other (p. 73).

3. *Developmental studies.* Jaan Valsiner (1989) has conducted a trenchant critique of developmental psychology, calling for a "culture-inclusive developmental psychology." With Valsiner's work and others as a spring-board, I have called for a "transcultural child psychiatry" defined as "developmental questions about children's mental disorders in cultural context" (DiNicola, 1992, p. 40). The latter studies are integrated into Chapters 5 and 6.

SOCIO-CULTURAL PSYCHIATRY: "A RELEVANT VIEWPOINT FOR MULTICULTURAL SOCIETIES"

In his critical book on race and culture in psychiatry in Britain, Suman Fernando (1988) defines a new approach to these issues. In a key chapter, Fernando reviews my earlier claims for a synthesis of family therapy and transcultural psychiatry:

> although one may accept, with some reservations, DiNicola's view that some methods of analysis by Western family

therapy . . . are portable across cultures and that the central tenets of family therapy with large systems may be used
for cultural analysis, family therapy, as practised today in
Western Europe, cannot be a model for an effective practical
psychiatry that is sensitive to culture in a social context. (p.
104)

Fernando argues that psychiatry needs its own definition of its
social and cultural tasks—not one imported from anthropology or
family therapy. What Fernando thinks we need is:

a "*socio*-cultural psychiatry" that is sensitive to culture in a
broad sense while maintaining a practical, perhaps pragmatic, stance in insisting on being relevant and useful to
people that psychiatry is supposed to deal with. Socio-
cultural psychiatry is a means whereby psychiatrists, and
other health workers who use psychiatry in a multicultural
setting, can examine themselves, their institutional practices and their disciplines for social influences that produce
and perpetuate bias. (p. 104)

In Fernando's view, socio-cultural psychiatry would incorporate
sensitivity to cultural factors and extend psychiatry from individual
concerns to family and cultural group, as I have argued. But above
all, socio-cultural psychiatry is:

a viewpoint, as well as a way of working, that is relevant to
the needs of a multicultural society, taking in social realities
that affect cultural groups. (p. 104)

In his scholarly book on *Culture, Health and Illness*, Cecil Helman
(1994) writes: "The relation of *culture* to family dynamics is complex, and to some extent controversial" (p. 288). Helman echoes
some of the concerns voiced above about "the danger of stereotyp-
ing all Italian families," for example, in the "mini-ethnographies of
the family cultures of different ethnic groups in the USA" in the
volume by McGoldrick and her associates (1982). Helman also reg-
isters the corollary concern of "ignoring major differences *between*
families" based on other social and cultural variables (p. 299). He

also articulates something that concerns me deeply—and is always treated dismissively when I raise it—that "family-oriented ethnic groups are sometimes described as if their differences from the Anglo-Saxon family type (with its emphasis on individual, rather than family goals) were pathological by definition" (p. 288). I will take this up in Chapter 7 on the myth of independence.

A NEW STORY FOR FAMILY THERAPY:
"THE FAMILY-AS-CULTURE"

Bringing many of these threads together, David Paré (1995) calls for a new paradigm in family therapy, summed up in the following question and answer:

> What would a family therapy look like that made no pretense of being value-free, that included a temporal dimension, that included both persons and relations, that was contextual, that induced the reduction of power differentials between therapist and family, that hoped for, and promoted, the empowerment of families, that valued equality over authoritarianism, and that valued an education method as well as the therapeutic? (Erickson, 1988, p. 233)

Paré's answer is: "a therapy that views families as storying cultures" (1995, p. 14). The narrative metaphor, a textual reading of life that sees lived experience as a text, "places persons in interpretive communities" (Paré, 1995, p. 14). By offering a model of therapy as "sense-making," searching for meaning, Paré argues that systems theory is an outdated story. The conceptual model he offers in its place is social constructionist epistemology. On the other hand, the postmodern stance moves away from either/or constructions to both/and juxtapositions. In this spirit, Paré reassures us that there is no need to reject useful ideas from the systems era of family therapy (see p. 15). But what is the truth? Where do we find bedrock? There is no final truth, only "preferred meanings" (Paré, 1995), "edifying discourses" (Rorty, 1989), and the "stories we live by" (Howard, 1991). I think it is time to stop calling for new paradigms and turn to *syntagm*:

> Instead of bringing a working method with me into the session (paradigm), I try to capture a fresh, different dis-

course with every family, in every session (syntagm).
(DiNicola, 1993, p. 54)

There is no bedrock, only "final vocabularies," the irreducible
language we use to make sense of the world, according to Richard
Rorty (1989). When "stories go awry" (psychopathology, relational
problems, human predicaments), the task of therapy may be best
described as "story repair" (Howard, 1991). The best available tool
for story repair may be the articulation of a new story in new words:
what Michael White (1986) calls "redescription." As Paré aptly concludes: "by changing our meanings, we change our worlds" (1995,
p. 15).

And what is the new metaphor for families, if they are not best
seen as systems? In the "family-as-culture metaphor" (Paré, 1995),
families are interpretive communities, or storying cultures. In his
book on the "anthropologist as author," Clifford Geertz (1988) argues that we take anthropologists seriously due to their narrative
skills, convincing us that they have truly "been there," among
other people. Ethnography, he suggests, is a kind of writing. In
their book on "narrative therapy in the postmodern world," Parry
and Doan (1994) invite clients to become authors, telling the stories
of their own lives and recruiting an audience for their stories.

All the changes in society and in family theory that have
coalesced into the emergence of a new paradigm for family therapy—based on narrative metaphors and social constructionist approaches—"families as storying cultures"—come together with my
proposal for a synthesis of family therapy and cultural psychiatry.

HOUSEKEEPING IN THE
HOUSE OF FAMILY THERAPY

Before moving on to apply this new approach to families in therapy, though, we have some housekeeping chores to deal with,
cobwebs to clear. They can be represented by three straightforward
questions.

First question: *Is there an adequate language for human predicaments?*
Confusion reigns about family therapy's theory of what consti-

tute problems. Why are family therapists reluctant to deal with psychiatric diagnoses? Can such disorders simply be defined away by reframing them as relational disorders? Are they always family or relational problems? Are they always generated within the family? What about the role of individual factors (trauma, biology, genetics, personal choice)? What about the role of society and of culture? Are there differences between psychiatric disorders and what American social psychiatrist Harry Stack Sullivan called "problems in living"? It is time for family therapy to end its "bootstrap complex" and start paying attention to valid and reliable data established by social sciences (such as anthropology and sociology) and clinical investigators in medicine, psychiatry and psychology.

Answer: Multiple descriptions

Family therapy needs to give up its "bootstrap complex," seeking to create its own world. Being responsible for the care of others is too important a task for this. For this task, we need diverse vocabularies that enable multiple descriptions, explanatory models, and therapeutic idioms—what I call the postmodern language of therapy. Family therapy can make meaningful use of these concepts and distinctions from its allied disciplines:

- idioms of distress (medical anthropology) vs. therapeutic idioms (the clinical knowledge of health-care professions);
- signs and symptoms of disease (phenomenology of illness);
- complex, syndrome, disorder (medical diagnosis);
- disease vs. illness (medical sociology);
- diagnosis vs. predicament (explanation vs. understanding);
- clinical formulation (psychiatry) vs. client's explanatory model of illness (cross-cultural psychiatry).

Just as not all human problems are diseases, neither are they all relational problems. Making such distinctions will help to elucidate a fuller account of human problems. In focusing solely on the family, we run the risk of making families and their members shoulder the bigger burdens of social problems (poverty and racism, for example).

Gloria Perez: "The Many Faces of Self-Starvation"

I would like to illustrate this with reference to the predicament of a young woman in the mid-1990s. As director of an eating disorders program for children and adolescents, I work with such predicaments daily. And I know that no single approach can understand, let alone cure, eating disorders. Of the two dozen cases in this book, several of them involve eating disorders.

Gloria is a 17-year-old who restricts her food intake, has lost 25 percent of her body weight, avoids eating with other people, is socially withdrawn, has a depressed mood, feels controlled by her family, and feels fatigue that limits her social activities and her school work. Nonetheless, she adamantly continues to work out up to five hours a day on her gymnastics routine.[5]

To properly assess Gloria's predicament, we need a multidisciplinary team, which should include a physician and a psychiatrist, a psychologist, a family therapist, and a socio-cultural specialist (e.g., a medical anthropologist or a cultural psychologist/psychiatrist).

1. *Medical.* Gloria's weight loss may have medical consequences:

- Her weight loss is probably due to decreased intake coupled with increased exercise leading to her body taking energy from her fat stores.
- Her fatigue is likely part of her inadequate nutrition, not keeping up with her body's energy demands.
- Her menstrual periods have stopped for over a year, a consequence of her weight loss.

2. *Psychiatric.* Gloria's weight loss may cause or worsen psychiatric symptoms:

- Anxiety and depression are common overlapping problems with eating disorders.
- Dissociation and self-mutilation may also be associated features of eating disorders.

3. *Psychological.* Gloria's weight loss may have an impact on her thinking and her feelings:

- The "psychological engine" of Gloria's weight loss is probably based on cognitive distortions that lead her to misperceive herself as "fat" and generate a "drive for thinness."
- This may result in diminished social- and self-esteem.

4. *Family therapy*. Gloria's symptoms may lead her family to express their concerns with criticism, hostility, protectiveness, and guilt.

- Parent-child problems can occur due to the demands of caring for their sick daughter.

5. Social stigma can arise.

6. Gloria's own experience, though, may be best understood as her "idiom of distress"—a way of speaking through symptoms.

7. Whether this individual is at risk for this disorder at all depends overwhelmingly on two features that are both "above" and "below" the family—(a) living in a Western society of affluence, and (b) being female (see DiNicola, 1990b, 1990c; see Chapter 6).

The family's culture will shape its beliefs about how to define the foregoing problems, how and where to seek help, and what solutions are culturally sanctioned and acceptable to them. Let us imagine that Gloria's family are Seventh Day Adventists living in a small town in Southern Ontario or Cuban immigrants living in Miami who take part in Santeria, a syncretic religion which combines Caribbean and Latin American derivatives of Yoruba Vodoun from West Africa and Catholicism (see Migene Gonzalez-Wippler's *The Santeria Experience*, 1992, a scholarly first-person account of the fastest growing religion in the United States). These subcultures have belief systems that may put them on very different pathways in their search for solutions. In fact, we can outline a whole "cascade" of interlinked factors, events, and outcomes with reciprocal and circular feedback. A full elucidation of the sick person's predicament (see Taylor, 1985) requires an understanding of the clinical tools of medicine and family therapy, as well as the conceptual tools of medical anthropology and sociology used by cultural psychiatry.

Even in the routine work of family therapy, distinctions need to be made. It is important to ask of any family theory, what is its model of the relationship between family events and the emergence of individual problems? If this question isn't asked, then fuzzy thinking occurs and unspoken, perhaps unwarranted assumptions will prevail.

FAMILY THERAPY MODELS OF MENTAL DISORDER

In an overview of family therapy in child psychiatry, I identify three major models of mental disorders in family therapy (DiNicola, 1990e):

1. *Relational disorders.* Mental disorders as emergent from family process. In this view, mental disorders are redefined as relational disorders.

2. *Triggering events.* Family conflicts are triggering events for underlying or overarching risk factors. By "underlying" I mean individual vulnerability, whether biological or psychological. By "overarching" I mean social and cultural risk factors.

3. *Maladaptive responses.* Family process becomes distorted and distorting, growing around the problem or event, as a maladaptive response to it.

Second question: *Why, in the face of so much apparent consensus, are there so many contradictions in the family field?*
Answer: Therapeutic temperaments

People have different answers to this problem. But beyond looking at the reasons why one particular issue or another is discounted or misperceived, I believe many of the differences in the family field revolve around a tension that has been evident from the outset. There are two therapeutic temperaments among family therapists (DiNicola, 1990d): the *technocratic temperament,* which stresses the techniques of therapy, and the *phenomenological temperament,* whose main concern is family process. (This binary opposition of temperaments is related to an embedded pattern of Western social science. See my discussion in Chapter 4.)

The technocrats in family therapy tend to be oriented in the here and now, to believe in universals (such as family structure), and to seek objectivity. In their hands, family therapy has created an "invisible technology" every bit as formidable and mechanistic in its social impact as architecture or medicine. The communication theorist Neil Postman (1993) asserts that our culture has surrendered to technology, a condition he calls "technopoly." One of the goals of technopoly is "to solve, once and for all, the dilemma of subjectivity" (Postman, 1993, p. 158). In the search for objectivity, one subgroup of technocratic family therapists is almost exclusively concerned with measurement and with outcome. Despite the best intentions of these therapists, technopoly treats humanity itself as an object. Both history and culture get in the way of their objective, pragmatic, fix-it-now attitude. Again, as Postman warns: "Diversity, complexity, and ambiguity of judgment are enemies of technique" (1993, p. 158).

Technocrats are endlessley enamored of new techniques and paradigms and continually redefine themselves as their tools change (e.g., as structural family therapists, paradoxical therapists, systems consultants, co-editors of the family story). Meanwhile, the "family" is not always so prominent in their concerns. At their best, the Milan team's inventiveness—their construction of guidelines for interviews and their therapeutic rituals—was brilliantly technocratic. The solution-focused therapists are technocrats in phenomenological clothing—they sound so warm and caring, but under it all are their technical marvels like the "miracle question" (where's the miracle—in the client's ability to imagine new possibilities or in the therapist's clever reframings?).

The phenomenologists are more concerned with issues of meaning and interpretation. As opposed to the technocrats, phenomenologists explore subjectivity with "experience-near" approaches. This makes them more likely to be curious about the family's history and culture, even when they do not have special training or inclination to explore them. They are not so sure of their tools and resist defining their task and themselves in terms of techniques. They are more genuinely interested in the family per se. I would predict that they take on advocacy roles in society. They are open to integrative or eclectic approaches. Phenomenologists are not sure what they would "measure" in their work and are similarly puzzled by the meaning of "outcome." The work of therapists like

Virginia Satir and Carl Whitaker, not so easily defined by a method but by their willingness to step into the indefinable Heraclitan flux of family life, is what I have in mind by the description ''phenomenological.''

Like the insider and outsider positions I have described, these are not meant to be exclusive categories. I have applied them to the work of different members of the original Milan team (DiNicola, 1990d), and see parts of myself and my colleagues in each of them. Cultural family therapy, as I construct it through both family stories (phenomenology) and conceptual tools (technique), attempts an integration of these basic temperaments.

Third question: *Are Western models of family therapy portable across cultures?*
Answer: ''Different cultures, different rationalities''

With all this in hand—an understanding that family life has a larger social context, that families are the bearers of unique cultures, that there are different levels of adaptive behavior including cultural costume and camouflage; understanding the nature and difficulties of intercultural encounters, family therapy's limited or problematic cultural analysis, the need for multiple descriptions, and acknowledging different therapeutic temperaments—what are we to make of the claims of family therapy? Can they be exported to other societies or used with minority cultures in our own backyard?

There are three positions we can take in conducting models of Western family therapy across cultures.

1. *The universalist approach.* The application of family models of the host or dominant culture to families from immigrant or minority cultures without modifications. In this approach, family process is assumed to be ''universal,'' expressing itself everywhere in much the same way, making the techniques of family therapy exportable anywhere. This is problematic for two reasons.

First, our informed view leads us to see culture as part of ''mind,'' rather than as window-dressing on something that is supposedly more fundamental (such as biology or individual psychology). As cultures vary, so do mind, family process, and cultural identity—''different cultures, different rationalities'' (Marshall Sahlins, cited in Geertz, 1995, p. 6). Second, the notion that family process is universal has to be demonstrated rather assumed, a difficult task. Even if this assumption is granted, practical problems like translation (see Chapter 4) arise in meeting families from different cultures. In fact, ethnographies from several generations of cultural anthropology do not support the notion that family process is universal.

2. *The retrofit approach:* Family therapy models of the host or dominant culture are held to be cross-culturally valid but need to be adapted. This approach assumes that family process is universal but its local expression is variable; as a result, the techniques of family therapy may need to be tailored to specific cultures. I call this "the retrofit approach," which asks if there are specific tools for specific types of families, specific ethnic groups, cultures, social classes, etc.? This is what was attempted in books like *Ethnicity and Family Therapy*.

In this approach, the danger is of arbitrarily selecting one feature of a family or a culture and shaping therapy around that as though we have grasped what that family or culture is all about. The alternative is to work on some more general tools that affect your way of seeing. I see working across cultures as a special example of the larger problem of empathy, which is about resonating with other people. The more people are different from oneself, the greater the empathic leap.

3. *The social constructionist approach.* The validity of all models of family process and of family therapy needs to be examined both culturally and historically. The assumption in this approach is that family process is fundamentally "protean" (i.e., it has no intrinsic character) and that it has a "situated nature" (i.e., it is constructed socially and culturally in a specific place and evolves fluidly over time).

This fluidity is demonstrated by the incredibly difficult task of trying to define what we mean by *family* and by trying to define aspects of family life that hold across cultures and over time. In fact, it's hard to agree beyond a few observations of human biology: that infants and young children need adult care to survive and that no immediate or short-term advantages accrue to the caregivers, who must be supported by others, making the child-caregiver dyad the fundamental basis of the human family and culture. Sociologists (Berger & Berger, 1984) have observed that the mother-child dyad is a universal human image—what anthropologist Mary Douglas calls a "natural symbol" (Douglas, 1978). However, as Berger and Berger (1984, p. 187) note, "There is no male figure in this icon; the father of the child is absent" (p. 187). These few facts have been the basis for theories of the family as diverse as communism (see the work on the family by Karl Marx's collaborator, Engels, 1972) and sociobiology (Wilson, 1978).

Examples of the problems created by not understanding the culture that people bear have to do with how each family culture defines health and what health-seeking behavior is sanctioned by its culture. Common misperceptions about ethnic or immigrant groups in the West concern their patterns of health-seeking behavior, either about their underutilization of individual and family therapies or their higher rates of major psychiatric disorder and hospitalization for these disorders (these kinds of questions were once the core of "comparative psychiatry," see H. B. M. Murphy, 1982).

In principle, I take the social constructionist position, questioning the validity of the models of family process and of family therapy that I hold. My experience of consulting across cultures and languages has convinced me that family process is protean. This means that there is no intrinsic character to the experience of the family. The family's "presenting culture" (Seltzer & Seltzer, 1983) is constructed socially and culturally in specific places and, at least in health, evolves fluidly over time. Each society will have to make its own models, responsive to its cultural realities.

In practice, the context usually places me as a therapist somewhere between the second and third positions. That is, I am prepared to begin by radically redefining everything in my encounter with the family, but a shared world of experiences quickly puts me in the position of feeling that at least some parts of my "tool-kit" are familiar to the family culture in question, although readjustments may have to be made.

Chapter 3

THE PRESENTING CULTURE

A Context for Family Therapy

[F]amilies of all cultures have a tendency to select or emphasize from their culture's repertoire of customs and ceremonies those modes of behavior that fit their own style.

—Edwin Friedman,
"The Myth of the Shiksa"
(1982, p. 522)

*In this chapter, I review the "situated nature" of family life, expressed
through its history and geography. With its unique way of putting the
world together, each family can be met in terms of its "presenting culture." This forms the basis for a new way of looking at the adaptive
responses of individuals, families (familism and family myths), and cultural communities (masks or* cultural costume and camouflage, *the
second conceptual tool of CFT). The cultural uniqueness of each family
makes it crucial to examine intercultural encounters in therapy. Dominant
conceptions of cultures are identified, leading to a comprehensive definition
of culture. Intercultural encounters call for a culture-inclusive model of
family therapy. The roles of* insiders and outsiders, *the third conceptual
tool of CFT, are offered as ways to conduct such meetings.*

"MEETING STRANGERS"

Montreal in the mid-1980s. The four members of the Della Seta
family are in their first session. Within a short time, Silvano and

Lucia, the parental couple, begin arguing. Silvano blurts out that Lucia has never loved him. Lucia says she felt deceived because only after many months of courtship in Rome did Silvano tell her he is Jewish. By then, she was in love with him and agreed to get pregnant in order to convince his Jewish mother to allow him to marry a Catholic. His Jewishness is a complex but powerful presence in this family, which everyone except Lucia seems to share intensely. Although she never converted, her daughters see themselves as Jewish (Judaism is a matrilineal religion). Sarah, who is 22, feels "completely Jewish," in spite of being engaged to Mario, an Italian Catholic. Alessandra, the identified patient, who is 20 and likes to be called Sandra, feels "very Jewish" and pointedly says she wishes to marry a Jewish man. However, she once tried to go into a synagogue but was turned away because no one believed that she was Jewish!

What is going on here? Who are these people? How do you relate to them? As *Italians*? As a *Jewish* family? As *immigrants*? As part of the cultural mix of a cosmopolitan city? The answers to these questions depend on how you look at them (if you want to choose an identity for the Della Setas) or on what questions you would ask them (if you want to know how they define themselves). And the whole point of *cultural* family therapy is that just as you cannot negotiate therapy without knowing the family, you cannot know the family without knowing their "presenting culture." Before we can think about the meaning of the parents' argument or link the engagement of "completely Jewish" Sarah to a Catholic man with Lucia's ambivalence about marrying Silvano or hypothesize that they are in crisis over the imminent change in the household with Sarah about to marry, we need to know something about their cultural identities.

Besides some "obvious" answers—that they are culturally Italian with a Jewish religious identity, that they are Jewish Italians (these are different statements), or that they are a culturally complex family with an interfaith marriage—there are other layers. For one thing, although they were all born in Rome, the children have been raised in Montreal—how has that shaped their identities and affiliations? It may surprise readers who do not know Montreal that immigrants there are given a rather forced choice to ally themselves, largely because of spoken language, with one of the two dominant groups. So another identity choice for the Della Setas in the context of Montreal in the 1980s is: are they "anglophone" (English-speaking) or "francophone" (French-speaking)? Although this session was conducted in English, the therapist could have switched to French or Italian. Montreal is a bilingual city where daily life is lived in a mix of French and English. Immigrants like the Della Setas are often trilingual, adding their mother tongues to the language soup. We will revisit the Della Setas further on in this chapter.

Family life has a context: it has a history and a geography. To develop a family therapy that is genuinely based on the family's lived experience, with a full accounting of its *situated nature*, we must take into account two aspects that many schools of family therapy have either discounted or ignored: broadly conceived, these are *time* (or history) and *place* (or geography). Before we can play with these aspects of family experience and begin to grasp what memory and myth can do to transform them into its *presenting culture* or the stories of family life, we must admit them into our way of thinking about families. To understand what effects emigration has had on the Della Setas, to grasp how they respond to the cultural politics of Montreal, we must know their presenting culture—or cultures—since they may individually or as a family incorporate more than one. Understanding the history and geography of a family is clinically valuable in bridging the family's lived experience (its "historical truth," understood across time and place) and its presenting culture (its "narrative truth").

"People are trapped in history and history is trapped in them," wrote James Baldwin (1955, p. 163) about the Black experience in America. Family therapists, influenced by the turn away from the historical reconstructions of psychoanalytic psychotherapy in the 1950s, represented by behavior therapy on the one hand and strategic family therapy on the other, have often regarded the family only in the here and now. Families, however, crave continuity. "Each man speaks with his father's tongue," wrote Leonard Cohen, "Ask a man who he is and he names a race" (1963, p. 125). The obvious fact is that each family has it own history, quite apart from whatever history it shares with other social groups, institutions, or therapists. History matters; the therapist meeting a family shares neither the family's history nor its common identity forged by the places where the family members have lived and the shared symbols of nationality, religion, race, class, and gender.

Earlier in this century, Sigmund Freud (1924, p. 178) paraphrased Napoleon to coin a compact distillation of his psychosexual theory of development: "Anatomy is destiny." But perhaps Napoleon (who, after all, knew a great deal about the displacement of people from their homelands), uttered the broader truth: *"Geography is destiny."* Identity for families (as for nations) is bound up with place and the idiosyncratic, vernacular culture of daily life. Families live at once in worlds they themselves build, while being shaped by the larger culture of which they form a part. In this sense, we may meet families in terms of their "presenting culture." There is an increasing recognition that the family's construction of meaning, its myths and its memories, is bound up with, shaped by, and situated in the places where its members live and those they recall. This includes the places where we actually live and those that have a hold on our hearts and minds through shared memories and symbols. This mental geography, both literally and figuratively, "holds us in place."

These aspects—time and place—come together in the mythology of families and cultures, setting the stage for all our personal and communal stories. We can open a window onto these stories by listening to the aspirations and frustrations of both individuals and groups. Napoleon's aphorism acknowledges the aspirations of people who share a common land. James Baldwin's (1955) essays written in Europe grasped the reality that the "interracial drama acted out on the American continent has not only created a new black man, it has created a new white man, too" (p. 175). Before the reconstruction of their national dream in Israel, the Jewish people, who have undergone successive displacements and diasporas, expressed this wish in the saying, "Next year in Jerusalem!" Writing about his "palimpsest-country" with "no name of its own," Salman Rushdie (1983) described Pakistan (a name made up by Muslim Indian intellectuals in the West) as a "failure of the dreaming mind. . . . full of irreconcilable elements, midriffbaring immigrant saris versus demure, indigenous Sindhi shalwar-kurtas, Urdu versus Punjabi, now versus then: a miracle that went wrong" (p. 92).

FAMILIES AS UNIQUE CULTURES

Family therapists are beginning to see families as unique cultures and to recognize a compatibility in the structures and functions of the two systems, *family* and *culture*. The parallels or isomorphisms in the definitions of these systems, in their adaptive responses, in their shaping of, and claims on, the identity of the individual, offer a valuable bridge to the study of families and other cultures (DiNicola, 1985b, 1985c, 1986).

The developmental stream of family life is a powerful private world complete with its own expressive language, symbols, and rules. Family members are the bearers of both their own private and unique culture and the larger society in which they live. Accordingly, a family coming to therapy can be understood in terms of its "presenting culture" (Seltzer & Seltzer, 1983).

A useful definition of culture by anthropologist Clifford Geertz (1973a) has found wide acceptance:

> culture is best seen not as complexes of concrete behavior patterns . . . but as a set of control mechanisms—plans, recipes, rules, instructions (what computer engineers call "programs")—for the governing of behavior. (p. 44)

This definition of culture and its functions is deeply compatible with the functions of the family. Some societies have such a strong myth of a common culture that the differences within these societies and among their communities are "white-washed" away. A striking example is the myth of the United States as a melting pot, wherein people of diverse backgrounds become "Americans" like all others within a short period of time. As minorities in the U.S. became more confident in their self-image, moving "beyond the melting pot" (Glazer & Moynihan, 1963), this homogenizing metaphor has been replaced by images of the mosaic, tapestry, or rainbow, reflecting the culturally heterogeneous and resilient populations in North America.

After a generation of innovative research in the United States, ethnicity finally emerged as a therapeutic variable in the 1980s. The meaningful consideration of culture and ethnicity and the problems that are presented by immigrant or minority families awaited interpersonal or relational theories and therapies. The interpersonal theories of family therapy allow these broader contexts to be studied. A general rule of human communication is that "a phenomenon remains unexplainable as long as the range of observations is not

wide enough to include the context in which the phenomenon occurs" (Watzlawick et al., 1967, pp. 20–21). On this basis, Selvini
Palazzoli (1974/1963) argues that, "family therapy is the starting
point for the study of ever wider social units" (p. 241). The focus
on the family is a switch from the intrapsychic to the interpersonal,
in which, as Antonio Ferreira (1967) noted, "the functional unit of
behavior is not the individual but the relationship" (p. 186). We are
now ready for a fuller inclusion of culture in family therapy in the
1990s.

FAMILISM AND FAMILY MYTHS

The concept of familism is also helpful in building links between
family and culture. Edward Banfield (1958), an anthropologist,
used this term when arguing the notion that the family unit is
defended against outsiders even at the expense of conflict with
authorities. Familism has been used in similar ways in diverse
fields, including anthropology, sociology, and psychiatry. For example, in their discussion of Jewish families Fredda Herz and Elliott
Rosen (1982) state that familism, "a belief in the importance of the
family as a sacred institution, stems from the idea that it is a viola-
tion of God's law not to marry" (p. 365). The common ground in
definitions of familism is that the family is a natural group that
presents a united front to others. Antonio Ferreira (1963, 1964,
1967) demonstrated the survival value of familism, refining it further into the concept of the family myth.

According to Ferreira (1963), the family myth refers to:

> a series of well-integrated beliefs, myth-like, which mem-
> bers of the family entertain about each other and their rela-
> tionship . . . [that] is not only shared but actually promoted
> by all family members. (p. 55)

Family myths are the rules of relationships, embedded in every-
day actions and sayings. We can catch a glimpse of them through
the private clichés of family life: in a Portuguese immigrant family,
where the father withdraws to drink on his own in the basement
where the wine is kept, they say, "Father is doing the laundry"
(see Chapter 10). Despite their child's repeated school and social
failures, another family insisted he was bright and outgoing,

arguing, "The school system is at fault," which they repeated when therapists at successive institutions "failed" them. Echoing Geertz's (1973a) definition of culture, Ferreira (1967) argues that the family myth is, "in effect a blueprint of action . . . a set of programmed patterns and rituals with a definite economic value to the relationship" (p. 187). The common front that family members present gives life to the family myth, in return bestowing survival value to the myth:

> family members not only accept the family myth uncritically but often join forces to protect and ensure its continuance . . . everyone in the relationship [works] to keep the family myth intact, unchallenged, and unchallengeable. . . . the family myth functions very much like a *group defense* against threats to or alternations in the relationship. (Ferreira, 1967, p. 187)

Family myths are powerful organizing constructs for family relationships, with an import beyond their factual basis or their ability to capture the truth of the moment. They replicate themselves in family life—often across generations. In evolutionary biology, there is a concept describing units of cultural transmission, to grasp the enormous rate of human cultural evolution (in contrast to the very slow process of biological evolution). That concept, coined by biologist Richard Dawkins (1976), is the *meme*. Memes are replicators—ideas with a life of their own. We can recast Ferreira's concept of the family myth as a meme. As a meme, the "family myth" has two functions: (a) it describes how certain notions ("myths") are perpetuated in family life, and (b) by following those notions in various theories and therapies, it traces the evolution of the field of family therapy. The second function represents an intriguing new way to construct the history and development of the field of family therapy—by tracing its memes—from older memes such as "homeostasis" and "systems" to "games" and "dramas" to present-day memes, "the family as a text" and "family life as narrative."

In a key but neglected comment in his classic paper, Ferreira (1963) maintains that "the family myth is to the relationship what the defense is to the individual. The myth, like the defense, protects the system against the threat of disintegration and chaos" (p.

60). As with defense or adaptive mechanisms in the individual, family myths serve the function of being protective and useful; at the same time, they may also be used in the service of forgetting and denial. Mara Selvini Palazzoli (1972) outlines labeling processes that may take place in families and distort the perception of individuals within families. She identifies biological identifications among family members, which become powerful labels for identifying and prescribing behavior, as ''racism in the family.'' Wencke Seltzer (1988) sees such processes as destructive family myths.

A Destructive Family Myth: ''Racism in the Family''

Ottawa, late 1980s. Three generations of the Szabo family are in my office. The consultation began with concerns about their 15-year-old daughter, Julie. Soon, however, we expand the context to consider other family issues. Hélène, the mother, comes from a family where several generations of women have found partners outside their own cultural community, while maintaining their French-Canadian identity. She married Endre, who is a Hungarian immigrant. Talking about their marriage, they slip into social stereotypes of each other, as ''French'' and ''Hungarian,'' but struggle to break free of them. They have accepted my suggestion to invite their oldest daughter to join us today. Natalie is 24 and lives with her two-year-old daughter, Tiffany. The Szabos all dote on Tiffany, and the activity of the session centers around her needs. Julie is preoccupied for much of the session with her niece.

As we discuss Tiffany, I learn that her father is only peripherally involved in her life. When I ask why, Natalie blames it on her own father, who did not approve of her partner. ''My father's a racist,'' she adds. This is a well-worn tale among them. Endre does not react. His affection for Tiffany, his mixed-race grandchild, is obvious.

Dr. DiNicola: So your father is not a racist in the family, only for outsiders?

Natalie agrees that her father genuinely loves his grandchild.

Father: It's not about what he is, but who he is. He was never interested in Natalie or Tiffany.

Natalie: You made our relationship so difficult, that we couldn't stay together.

At this point, mother offers a different perspective.

Mother: Natalie, it's not just your father who acts like a racist. Why did you go out with a man that you knew would drive him crazy? It's not that he's different, it's that you just didn't care enough about him to bring him home. To let us meet him, get to know him.

Natalie is still, listening silently, playing with her daughter's tresses. Mother continues:

Sometimes, I think you just went out with him to get back at your father.

Natalie is upset; her father has tears in his eyes. There is an intense, undifferentiated emotion between them like something waiting to be carved from a block of stone. By speaking an unacknowledged family truth, mother seems to have broken the spell of a family myth.

I simply observe mother's courage in saying her truth about the relationship between Natalie and her father. After some moments of silence, I wonder how she came by her insight. In previous sessions, we had discussed Hélène's and Endre's families of origin. Going back to her family genogram, I point out that, like her own mother and sisters, Hélène had married outside the French community.

Mother: So you're saying that my daughter did the same thing I did?

Father: That's ridiculous.

Dr. DiNicola (addressing mother): No. What I am wondering is, is there some way to understand how these two people (*indicating Endre and Natalie*) who love each other so much have developed such a talent for keeping each at arm's length?

This family's therapy moved from the opening positions of ''racism in the family'' to a discussion of mother's notion that Natalie's partner choice was a message to her father. From there, it was rather easy to give this meaning across several generations of women in the family. It is not so much that the family's ideas about race changed (I don't think they did), but that they tried to stop using race as a way to distance and disqualify each other.

LEVELS OF ADAPTIVE BEHAVIOR: A NEW MODEL

These findings suggest a new conceptualization of adaptive interpersonal and social behavior, operating on three levels. The underlying assumption here is that there are different levels of functioning that are distinct and not reducible one to the other. Family therapy pioneer Lyman Wynne (1969) has suggested four: biology, psychology, social structure, and culture. I see these as levels for understanding and explaining "mind," progressing from individuals (understood biologically and psychologically), through families (as units of "mind" and as subcultures), to social structures (ethnic and other social groups), and culture. Based on this, a new model of levels of adaptive functioning can be proposed (DiNicola, 1985d): the adaptive mechanisms of the individual, family myths and rules, and cultural costume and camouflage.

In the individual, they are called defense mechanisms, as elaborated by Anna Freud (1946). In the family, Antonio Ferreira has identified them as family myths. On the cultural level, the conceptualization of the adaptive strategies of ethnic groups and cultural communities has eluded the cataloging of anthropology and transcultural psychiatry. Ferreira (1967) hinted at the relationship of family myth to "larger social myths, such as racial myths (the 'inferiority' of the Negro), national myths (the Irish 'temper'), religious myths ('mine is the only one true God'), and others" (p. 195). (In thinking about Ferreira's examples and his language, remember that he was writing thirty years ago.) One of the few successful attempts to make sense of such behavior patterns presenting on a community or cultural level has been by Edwin Friedman (1982), a family therapist who coined the clinically useful concepts of cultural costume and camouflage.

MASKS: CULTURAL COSTUME AND CAMOUFLAGE

The way individuals and families carry their culture is an important aspect of their functioning, one that offers valuable clues to the therapist. Learning to read these *masks* is the second conceptual tool of cultural family therapy. Following Geertz (1973a), culture may be thought of as the intergenerational transmission of a set of control mechanisms—plans, recipes, rules and instructions—that govern behavior. Friedman (1982) developed the concepts of cultural costume and camouflage to describe the way people express their ethnic identity; his use echoes Geertz's (1973a) notion that humans exist in society through the mediating variable of culture.

Each family, Friedman observed, draws its cultural costume from the available repertoire of their culture. Cultural costume is the particular set of recipes the individuals or families of a community employ to give meaning and shape to their experiences through shared ceremonies, rituals, and symbols. Like defense mechanisms and family myths, cultural costume can serve two functions. Used adaptively, cultural costume is protective, giving the community a meaningful program or set of recipes for behavior, allowing communication and understanding.

Under some circumstances, people become uncomfortable with their cultural costume, often in times of cultural change or migration. The old recipes do not seem to address the issues at hand; that is when culture-change syndromes emerge (DiNicola, 1985c, 1985d, 1990c; see Chapter 6). On the other hand, problems with the expression of cultural costume may reflect problems that are better understood on interpersonal or individual levels, rather than as cultural. When culture is invoked as a smokescreen to obscure individual states of mind or patterns of family interactions, cultural costume becomes camouflage. A good rule of thumb is to listen for clichés and stereotypes. It is as if the intolerance between communities becomes internalized.

Here are two examples. Caught between her own needs and her allegiance to her grown-up daughter, a widowed mother who cannot decide to remarry hides behind her community, saying, "Armenian women don't do that." Another woman, a Greek immigrant, resentful of her husband's deeper assimilation into the French-Canadian community of Montreal, camouflages her personal conflict as a cultural complaint that "French girls attract our best men." Conflicts within a relationship are mapped onto a handy and visible cultural label.

Sometimes, cultural camouflage can produce a kind of "linguistic Stockholm syndrome," where individuals or families accept the dominant or host culture's stereotypes of their own group. When cultural communities perceive this pattern of individuals "turning" on their group, they label them as "sell-outs" or "Uncle Toms." It's as if we are taken hostage by other people's perceptions of ourselves and come to believe them. "I'm an Irish lush," someone will say. When these stereotypes are used by members of a family toward each other, it can produce what Selvini Palazzoli (1972) calls "racism in the family." "Linguistic Stockholm syndrome" in one's own mind, "racism in the family," and "cultural camouflage in the community" are markers that stereotypes are masking relational issues, not just in the family but on the larger social screen of culture.

Paul Lake/Pablo Sanchez: "A Latin Temperament"

Paul is a ten-year-old boy who lives with his sister, Robin, and their mother, Rachel Lake, in the small town of Salterton, near Kingston, Ontario. Rachel brought Paul to a children's mental health center in the mid-1990s for a variety of problems. Paul suffered from nightmares, pronounced stuttering, and obsessive-compulsive disorder—all different manifestations of anxiety. In the first session, I also identified two other problems: racism in the family and a lack of positive images of the father or of Mexico.

Rachel clearly described racism in her extended family's attitudes towards Paul. Paul's father, Gabriel Sanchez, was Mexican. Rachel and the children had lived with Gabriel for a time in Mexico where they had learned Spanish. Some of Paul's cousins called him a "dirty Mexican" and other names. Although he was named Gabriel, after his father, when he first went to school in Canada the child would not respond to his given name. He was sullen and mute. When Rachel explored this with him, he said he did not like his name. He tried various names, such as Leonardo and Donatello from the popular "Ninja Turtles." Mom helped him select a more appropriate name and he eventually chose Paul. Surrounded by negative attitudes in his Canadian family towards his Mexican name and family, the child rejected them, opting to be less visible as "Paul."

When I asked Rachel about her feelings towards the father, it was clear that she was quite negative about him—they had all suffered from his substance abuse, neglect, and violence. In spite of this, I explored with Rachel the need for her children to know their father and to have some positive images of him and his culture. She was receptive to this, but did not know how to create such images. Rachel saw both of her children as having "a Latin temperament" like their father. This is a problem in cross-cultural perception; she could see Paul and his problems only through the mask of cultural camouflage.[1]

Both Rachel and her extended family were critical of Gabriel and generalized their understandable criticisms from the person to the culture. Some members of her family thought of him and his family—including Paul and Robin—as "dirty Mexicans." Rachel herself had milder but still stereotyped cross-cultural perceptions, such as attributing Paul's problems to his "Latin temperament." This was why I thought it valuable to identify some positive qualities in Gabriel, his family, and his culture. This is an intervention I often use with separated or divorced parents: finding positive qualities of the other parent for the children to identify with. It usually works. In Paul's case, it was a very effective intervention.

In the course of therapy, Paul learned from a letter from his Mexican grandparents that his father had died of medical complications of alcoholism. His grandparents also called him to discuss it with him and to offer their grandchildren financial support. His reaction was muted: he did not cry, but was sad and quiet for a few days. He was able to discuss it with his family and in therapy.

With her fears of Gabriel returning to stalk them allayed, Rachel was now able to actively pursue the issues I had identified in our first session. She could see the value of a connection for her children with Mexico and Gabriel's family: "This is part of his heritage that's blank." The Mexican grandparents called again on Paul's birthday, inviting him and Robin to visit them in Mexico. When they called him by their son's name, Gabriel, Paul firmly insisted that he was "Paul" now, not his father; he said he didn't mind if they called him "Pablo"—the Spanish version of his name. Although he calls himself Paul Lake, another very real identity is waiting for him to complete his story: Pablo Sanchez.

"It's kind of overwhelming," Rachel said about the changes that occurred in their lives. Stories change, evolve with unexpected turns, move into new directions. "One of the good things about the call from Mexico," Rachel said, "is that it's a reminder that he has cousins who are Mexican and they don't mind that he's Mexican—he can't get that here from his cousins in Canada." I silently noted her way of putting it—"they don't mind that he's Mexican"—and commented that for some members of his Canadian family it's acceptable that Paul is Mexican, but what his Mexican family could offer is a celebration of that fact, a comforting naturalness about it.

Rachel was upbeat: "It's better late than never. He's only 10. It just opens up a whole new perspective on his situation. We were so isolated. The whole other half of his life was hidden from him." Rachel began to review her life with Gabriel as well. The key for her was the sadness that Gabriel's mother felt. "She lost her son. She wants to see his face," referring to her son Paul, "it's all they have left of their son." She now began to recount more positive stories about first meeting Gabriel.

After several sessions (and some remarkable "external" events), Rachel describes their lives as transformed—"things are totally different." So far, we see Paul/Pablo largely through his mother's eyes, in terms of possibilities, the way adults understand children. As for Rachel, she looks radiant. Instead of "leftover life to kill" (in the words of Caitlin Thomas, 1957, the widow of the Welsh poet Dylan Thomas), she is beginning to live in the present, with "a new lease on life." This is not an "outcome," in the language of the research literature on family therapy, although I have no doubt that this was a very effective course of brief family therapy. More importantly, I had the unusual experience of observing, in the relatively short period of time of several months, the realization of the possibilities I had imagined for this boy in my very first session with his family.

"Outcome," with its sense of an endpoint or a finished product, is an unsatisfactory word because Paul is a growing child, whose story is still evolving. One day, perhaps, he will tell his own story in his words. Will it be like the story that Richard Rodriguez (1983) told in *Hunger of Memory*, making a choice to be part of mainstream American culture at the expense of his Mexican heritage? Or will it be more like *When Memory Comes*, the story told by Saul Friedlander (1980) about the Czech Jewish childhood that was ripped away from him by the Holocaust? Like the boy in this story, Friedlander, too, went through name changes—from ''Pavel'' as a Jewish boy in Prague, to ''Paul'' in hiding as a Christian in France, to ''Shaul'' in Israel, and finally to ''Saul'' as a professor of history at the University of Geneva. What's at stake here is not just identity as a summary of who and what we are—but how we live in the world, the symbols we respond to, the meanings we resonate with. Both of these men have triumphed over adversity. I have read their books closely and with profit. From Rodriguez I get a sense of argument, struggle, and overcoming by insisting on the right to tell your own story in your chosen language. Friedlander leaves me with very different emotions—those of reconnection, of reconstruction, and the emotional plenitude that comes from retelling history (one's own and that of others).

INTERCULTURAL ENCOUNTERS

Given the pluricultural nature of many Western societies and the movements of people within and among countries—migrations so large that the concept of ''global flows'' (Brown, 1983) was coined to deal with them—what models do we have for conducting therapy across cultures?[2] To answer this question, we need to review the epistemology of intercultural experience. Anthropologist Waud Kracke (1987) emphasizes the ''intercultural encounter as a psychological process'' (p. 62) and argues that we need models of intercultural encounters to understand the experience of confronting an alien culture. The outcome of the encounter is shaped, to some extent, by basic conceptions of the notion of culture, which may be positive or negative:

> negative conceptions of culture . . . stress the separation from one's own culture, [while] positive conceptions of culture . . . stress engagement with the other culture and a

process of integrating it . . . into one's own world view.
(p. 62)

Negative conceptions of intercultural encounters have been quite
dominant in the social sciences and among clinicians and have
shaped much research in transcultural psychiatry and clinical work
in psychiatry and family therapy. Such negative conceptions of
intercultural relations reflect a view of the other culture "as primarily of interest for its difference from us, or as essentially lacking
something we have" (Kracke, 1987, p. 78), rather than as a coherent
system. Three examples of dominant negative models are:

1. *Culture shock*: The encounter with a strange culture as a "self-
limiting crisis" or "dysadaptation syndrome" is perhaps the
most widespread and accepted model of the response to culture
change.
2. *Mourning*: Moving from one culture to another, people grieve
the loss of their known culture, while seeking "linking objects"
with the new one.
3. *Anxiety*: Immersion in a new culture triggers anxiety, resulting
from the open expression of themes customarily kept under
wraps in one's familiar culture.

More *positive conceptions* of the intercultural experience include:

1. *Resocialization through exploration* (see Kracke, 1987). Initial problems in a new culture induce a childlike period of exploration
and discovery, followed by "growing up in the culture" (resocialization).
2. *Key relationships* (see Kracke, 1987). Special relationships can
serve as models or keys in opening the doors in a new culture,
leading to the construction of a model of the larger society.
3. *Transitory identity*: Erik Erikson's (1960) notion that children
assume a "transitory identity" in response to the crises of uprootedness and loss of assigned or expected identity.

These are theoretical constructs. This book offers a different approach, encompassing the knowledge of models of intercultural
experience, by examining the family's adaptive cultural strategies

(DiNicola, 1992, in press) in a clinical setting. This approach reviews how families negotiate cultural change, which depends on how they carry their culture of origin, how they experience the host culture, and what models each of those cultures makes available to a particular family. Two examples of a family's adaptive cultural strategies are "creole cultures," which are syncretic blends of different cultures, and "double descriptions," where different cultures are expressed in different social settings.

DEFINING CULTURE

What overall concept of culture emerges from thinking about the encounter between cultures? Authoritative definitions of fundamentals are notoriously hard to come by, so we have to make do with some working definitions.

Many definitions of the concept of culture emphasize meaning, cognition, and the rules for generating and transmitting meaning, like the first definition we examined by Geertz (1973a). Another anthropologist, William Caudill, offered a conception of culture as a "shared cognitive map." In his view of culture, Waud Kracke (1987), whose work I have cited above, emphasizes meaning as a shared discourse, negotiated and shaped by the individuals who participate in it:

> Culture . . . is not just a shared template, but a set of symbols and meanings *in terms of which* individuals orient themselves to each other and to the world. Integration of meanings is not just at the cultural level, but at the individual level as well. The shared reality of discourse is a negotiated reality, not a static one defined communicably by the culture. (p. 79)

Others have emphasized cognition and ideation:

> Systems of shared ideas, systems of concepts and rules and meanings that underlie and are expressed in the way that human beings live. (Keesing, 1981, p. 8)

Cecil Helman (1994) synthesizes the anthropological literature:

> culture is a set of guidelines (both explicit and implicit) which individuals inherit as members of a particular soci-

ety, and which tells them how to *view* the world, how to experience it emotionally, and how to *behave* in it in relation to other people, to supernatural forces or gods, and to the natural environment. (p. 2)

Helman's view of culture brings him very close to family therapy's view of family life as contextual and processual. He emphasizes that culture is transmitted from generation to generation and that growing up is a form of *enculturation*, a process of slowly acquiring the cultural lens of our own society. Encounters with and immersions in other societies are understood as *acculturation*, a process of refocusing or changing cultural lenses.

For our purposes, in building a bridge between family and culture, we need to emphasize these elements in the foregoing models of cultures:

- Culture is transmitted from generation to generation, making the family the major vehicle of cultural transmission.
- Part of enculturation is embodiment, that is, culture is embodied in us: how we experience our bodies is a gift from our culture.
- Culture is not just an abstraction: cultural ideas, meanings, and rules are enacted by individuals and families.
- Culture is a set of programs for governing behavior, templates for shaping our thoughts, and guidelines for emotional experiences.

Other elements need to be added:

- There is broad agreement in the human sciences, from biology to evolutionary psychology and cognitive science, that cultural evolution is the major way in which human beings have survived and flourished since the biological emergence of *homo sapiens*; biology and culture each have units for their transmission; the unit of cultural transmission is the *meme*; what the *gene* is to biology, the *meme* is to culture (Dawkins, 1976).
- Anthropology, cross-cultural psychology, and transcultural psychiatry generally agree that living cultures (as opposed to the study of the Assyrians or Etruscans who have left the stage of

history, to use Arnold Toynbee's phrase) are not static, but fluid, dynamic, and evolving.

- Furthermore, living cultures are not "pure" and may be creole, hybrid, syncretic, contradictory, and multiple—all in the same society—to a greater or lesser extent.
- Not only are living cultures not pure, with their internal elements in a shifting flux, but cultures are in mutual contact, colliding, blending, or distancing themselves from each other.
- Lastly, we need to be mindful of the impact of cultural change on individuals and families, whether the change is occurring in their own society or is due to migration. (This is the major theme of Chapters 5 and 6.)

ROLES: INSIDERS AND OUTSIDERS

The perspectives of *insiders and outsiders* (Merton, 1973) offer a useful way to map the relationship between the therapist and the family culture (DiNicola, 1985c, 1986). Examining these *roles* constitutes the third conceptual tool for cultural family therapy. The therapist and the family can then move on to map the family's place in the culture in which they currently live. We all occupy both insider and outsider roles in different contexts; neither is superior, both may be transcended. It is a mistake to assume the insider perspective is best and to treat only people of one's own ethnic community. Sometimes families work from the assumption that outsiders are better, offering objective help. Therapists may occupy either role to good effect with families; the important thing is to recognize which perspective they have as well as the family's expectations, as the two vignettes below illustrate.

The insider position. As an insider, the therapist takes a position of shared common experience with the family. This is illustrated in a vignette from a later session with the Della Seta family, whom we met at the beginning of this chapter. This position requires detailed knowledge of their culture and some genuine identification with its rules and rituals. Even then, the therapist may have to relax the posture of therapeutic neutrality, allowing himself to be an empathic witness of their pain or an adaptive model for new solutions.

"A Familiar Stranger":
The Della Setas Define Being Jewish

In their sixth session, the Della Seta family is playful and pleasant after being congratulated on not having any family arguments for some time and for successfully getting Sandra to sleep on her own (instead of with her sister or parents). Sandra asks if I am Jewish. She observes that, "You seem to have a Jewish manner and expressions." Silvano flatly contradicts this, saying, "He is definitely not Jewish." A lively discussion ensues, addressing a number of key issues. One concerns to what extent the family is Italian and to what extent they are Jewish. They make it clear that the family identifies with both communities very strongly. Contrary to an earlier impression I had formed, mother says she wants her children to be Jewish and has the fantasy that Sandra, who is the standard-bearer for Jewishness since the death of her Jewish grandmother, will marry a Jewish man. There is a warm, close feeling among the Della Setas. The parents, Lucia and Silvano, are sitting together. The discussion of Jewishness is very important to Sandra, who is absorbing it like heat from a hearth.

In a previous session, we had explored ways for Sandra to have more positive interactions with her father. My suggestion was to initiate one of the Jewish rituals traditionally performed by women, such as lighting candles on Friday evening, the start of the Jewish sabbath. Sandra had done this, learning the *bracha*, prayer, in Hebrew, and felt very proud. But this is clearly the father's moment, an opportunity to assert his *Jewish* authenticity with his family. In order to highlight Silvano's knowledge of his own community, I ask him to explain how he came to such a confident conclusion about me. As he gives his explanation, the family validates Silvano as the carrier of Jewish tradition and knowledge. He concludes by pointing out how to tell from family names and towns of origin which Italians are Jewish. In the Middle Ages, Jews had settled in certain Italian towns, from which they took their names. As for their own family name, "Della Seta" refers to his family's long-standing association with the textile trade, *seta* being the Italian word for silk.

Sandra enjoyed this so much that she wanted it to go on. With great sensitivity to her family and to me, she continues to express curiosity about me. In the light of her father's explanation, she wonders if I am a convert and, without waiting for any confirmation, starts a string of associations about what my wife might be, whether we have raised our children as Jews, and so on. With these thoughts, the conversation moves on to Sarah's upcoming marriage to Mario and how he would become part of the family.

This encounter demonstrates the benefits and costs of the insider position in family therapy. I was prepared to use myself and my identity to facilitate a discussion about the meanings of being Italian and Jewish in this family. To do this, I had to relax my stance of neutrality and be open to direct questions about myself. While I think it is rude to refuse to answer clients' questions, in practice I rarely have to say very much about myself. And I cannot stress this enough: if you have not covered this ground for yourself, it may be unpleasantly provocative for you or unproductive for the family. You do not have to put yourself "inside" the family circle, but if you do, your personal disquiet and hesitations or incongruities with how you present yourself professionally will be greatly amplified. Be prepared.

This family's "conversation" with me was really just a way for them to stage a dialogue about their own identities. In the end, I wasn't really an insider for them at all—I was a familiar stranger. The family needed to keep me outside and felt more comfortable with me there. To paraphrase both Minuchin and the Talmud: they put "a fence around the Torah," drawing a boundary around the sacred circle of what was authentically Jewish for them. In therapeutic terms, I vacated a space in this family, which was more appropriately occupied by the father. This space has been called many things in family therapy—such as "the director of the family drama" (by Andolfi & Angelo, 1981) or the editor of the family narrative. In this family, the father finally became, in the best sense of a Jewish tradition, the family *rabino* or teacher.

The outsider position. As an outsider, the therapist can be explicit about his differences with or inequalities in relation to the family. One can either take the posture of an expert or a one-down position by acting as cultural outsider. In this way, the outsider comes either with professional expertise, despite his lack of detailed knowledge of the culture, or he is prepared to learn the family's culture. The role that the therapist assumes yields information about the family's own location in its community. In the following encounter, the therapist takes the outsider role with a Parsee family in Montreal.

Navroz Nariman: ''Elephant Boy''

Montreal, mid-1980s. Navroz Nariman was a 21-year-old youth admitted to an inpatient psychiatric unit following a suicide attempt. I was in charge of Navroz's ward treatment and brought his case to my family therapy supervisor for a family assessment. When we convened the family for a meeting, Farhad, the father, dominated the session with expressions of shock and guilt. As Parsee immigrants from Bombay (now Mumbai), India, the Narimans were tremendously hard-working and goal-oriented. I explored what their son's suicide attempt meant to them. Phiroza, his mother, said she was more shocked by the fact that he would attempt to hurt himself than that he kept things to himself, but father was clearly hurt by the implication that he had lost contact with his son. Pained by this thought, Farhad turned to his son to ask, ''Is there anything wrong at home?'' But Navroz adamantly defended the famly myth that all was well—''I told the doctors that my family life has nothing to do with it!'' Farhad then asked Navroz to promise not to do it again. I asked the family if this was father's way of getting to know his son again.

Trying to involve Navroz's 17-year-old brother, Burjis, in the conversation, we learned that Burjis was not so surprised by his brother's suicide attempt. Burjis said he was the black sheep who had always suffered by comparison with his brother, Navroz, who was better at everything. They had never really been brothers and did not communicate with each other unless it was absolutely necessary. Father interrupted to ask why this problem had not been brought to his attention. Burjis retreated from this barrage of questions, while Navroz tried to get the family off the hook by externalizing the problem as academic problems in his first year in computer science at McGill. Again, Navroz came to the rescue of the family myth. And again, father intervened. Farhad was very disappointed in Navroz's career choice; he wanted his son to study engineering, which was well regarded by his family in India. It was very important to him that his children should earn prestigious degrees to vindicate his hard work as an immigrant.

With this view of the family's dilemmas, we moved to a different role in the session as outsiders curious about their culture. We learned that Navroz came to Canada from Mumbai at the age of four. At school, other children called him "elephant boy" but he was quite sure that it had never bothered him. However, father, who is a very proud man, was indignant about how they were treated in Canada. We asked them to teach us about their way of life. The Narimans are Parsees from Mumbai. It is both a historical/cultural identity ("Parsee" refers to the province of Fars in ancient Persia) and a religious one (they are Zoroastrians, an ancient faith) for them. They saw themselves as standing apart from other communities—whether in Mumbai or Montreal. As they did not wish to assimilate, the parents themselves made their son a stranger in the outside world, where he was perceived as an "elephant boy."

They had attempted to preserve their Parsee lifestyle, including wearing a muslin shirt called a *sadra* with an attached cord called a *kusti*. In fact, Phiroza was much more knowledgeable and observant than father, while their sons only followed the traditions for the sake of their parents. Phiroza had experienced a series of losses—of her community, her mother, and her religion—and tried to reconnect to her life in Mumbai through religious observances. When her mother died in Mumbai, she could not attend the funeral in time, because in their faith the body must be buried within twenty-four hours. Farhad was much more caught up in being a success in Montreal.

In later sessions, we learned even more about their culture. During the course of therapy, Phiroza returned to India to attend her brother's wedding. Acting in her mother's place, she had the honor of giving her brother away to his bride. Phiroza had cherished this role and was very happy to return to India to see her family of origin again. As outsiders, we highlighted these important family experiences, asking about the details of the Zoroastrian wedding and other customs. We were an audience for their cultural uniqueness. From this position, we were able to make therapeutic connections.

After discussing the advantages of mother's absence—and return—Burjis said it would be nice if his parents could go away together. This led to a discussion of the advantages of family life and developing a separate life. An issue lurking in the background was whether Navroz was seen as healthy, whether the parents could safely leave him. In a major shift for the family, they could now see Navroz as well. Father was more willing to accept his son's career choices. And they all found more positive things in life in Canada. At this point, we had a wide-ranging discussion about different cultures. In a lovely moment, we all shared the feeling that back home for each of us—for the family and also for myself— one followed a culturally-sanctioned and satisfying way of life. Yet, away from home, in a new community, one was freer to make other, more personal choices. With my supervisor, I witnessed the Nariman family's Parsee world view from an outsider perspective. At the end, I was able to join them as an "insider," not as a Parsee, but as a fellow immigrant, gently opening space for a dialogue about new possibilities.

What prompted the family's shift? Three things. First, Navroz's suicide attempt had provoked a crisis and the family expressed willingness to open space for him. Second, mother's visit to India meaningfully reconnected her to her culture and family of origin, while cooling the hothouse atmosphere of the family in Montreal. Third, by playing with insider/outsider roles in therapy, we explored identity as a meaningful personal, family, and cultural construction rather than a factual given.

We may instructively compare the perspectives of insiders and outsiders in social relations with Umberto Eco's (1994) notions of the authors and readers of texts. They both concern points of view: you can adopt the point of view of each family member or that of the parental couple or the children. You can also adopt an "outsider" point of view. But what does "outside" mean? The narrator of a text may be a third person, "outside" the action described. Can a therapist be like a narrator? We can certainly write up our cases like narrators—but what about conducting therapy? While we must be careful not to adopt the false (and paternalistic) stance of the objective omniscient observer, any point of view can work in therapy. Many possible narrators/therapists can be imagined: unknowing, "broker," referee, coach, negotiator, arbiter, judge, insider and outsider. Each of these positions can be used, although always with planfulness and irony rather than commonsense. What's wrong with "commonsense"? Assuming you share "sensible" or "obvious" viewpoints can be misleading (you may not share them) or paternalistic (family members may feel you are imposing your views). The sensible thing to do in a given situation is part of the social stock of knowledge that each society gives its members. Hence, "commonsense" differs from place to place and time to time.

In each of the cases discussed above, I knowingly took one position—insider or outsider—but by playing with it, giving it a twist, I shifted my position from insider to outsider with the Della Seta family and from outsider to insider with the Nariman family. In one case, health meant that, after being provoked by my own blurred identity as Italian/Jewish, the Della Setas came to their own family definitions, which "included me out." In the other case, it was healthy for the Narimans to make a bridge with a fellow immigrant seeking meaning in a balance between historical and cultural continuity and the possibilities of a new society.

BY WAY OF A CONCLUSION: "THE ENIGMA OF ARRIVAL"[3]

Unlike science, social research never discovers anything new. It only rediscovers what people once were told and need to be retold again.

—Neil Postman (1993, p. 157)

Let's take stock of Part I. Chapter 1 offers an overview of the problems encountered in "meeting strangers"—my metaphor for working with families across cultures. I introduce my first conceptual tool of CFT, "spirals," which describes a collaborative way to conduct cultural interviews. Spiraling is demonstrated through several cultural consultations involving language translators.

In Chapter 2, I renew my call for a synthesis of family therapy and cultural psychiatry and review problems with family therapy's use of the concept of culture. To address such problems, we need a culture-inclusive model of family therapy. Unlike other attempts to include culture, the purpose of this book is not to provide ethnographies of any particular group (or an encyclopedia of such ethnographies). It is a meditation on the difficulties of trying to conduct therapy as part of intercultural encounters. The roles of insiders and outsiders are offered as a way to enter such meetings.

To prepare ourselves for a culture-responsive family therapy, I attend to a few housekeeping tasks—addressing the need for multiple descriptions of human predicaments, acknowledging two basic therapeutic temperaments (technocratic and phenomenological), and problems with the portability of Western family therapy models to other cultures.

After reviewing the situated nature of family life, expressed through its history and geography, Chapter 3 examines families as unique cultures. This forms the basis for a new way to look at the adaptive responses of individuals and families (familism and family myths) and cultural communities (cultural costume and camouflage). Examining cultural costume and camouflage as "masks" is my second conceptual tool for cultural family therapy. We then took a look at intercultural encounters, which led us to examine definitions of culture.

If we abandon our cherished paradigms, if every family is to have a fresh approach—a syntagm—will we be up to the task? My hopeful answer is yes! My maternal grandmother, Nunziata, who is 86 years old and living in Canada as I write, is an illiterate monolingual woman from the mountains of central Italy. I have never seen her at a loss for words, never lacking a recipe for how to respond to a situation—how to comfort a hurt child, how to sit by the bedside of a dying friend, how to celebrate the living or mourn the dead. She has never said, "I haven't read a book about that," or complained that Piaget or Freud are at odds with each other. This is not to say that I agree with everything she says and does—this is not a plea for "commonsense" or traditional wisdom—but rather that, in spite of her lack of a bookish model of life, she is fully and completely engaged in living. And I hope that here and there you will feel my grandmother present in my work.

If we sweep enough of the cobwebs away, and divest ourselves of the myths of our society, like the myth of independence (see Chapter 7), and give up our fascination with techniques and our claims to universal models, can we recapture the immediacy of experience of the phenomenologists (in philosophy and psychiatry and in family therapy) and the sure touch of our grandmothers?

Ironically, I had to read through many complex texts in a variety of fields to pose this question seriously. These included texts on postmodernism (Harvey, 1989), narrative (Paré, 1995), anti-foundational philosophy (Rorty, 1989), the philosophical critique of the "sources of the self" (Taylor, 1989), cultural psychology (Bruner, 1990; Shweder, 1991), language studies (Steiner, 1975), translation theory (Robinson, 1991), and autobiographical memory (Kotre, 1995). The enigma of arriving at this question is not only that there are no final answers, but that I found my grandmother sitting where I left her so many years ago.

Ah, but therein lies a tale . . .

Part II

ON THE THRESHOLD: LANGUAGE, IDENTITY, AND CULTURAL CHANGE

The sense of self . . . is not just based on the physical self but depends on meaning. Because meaning occurs only within a contextual network of relationships, it seems safe to conclude that *identity is a linguistic construction.*

—Roy F. Baumeister,
*Identity: Cultural Change and the
Struggle for Self* (1986, p. 15)

Chapter 4

BEYOND BABEL

Cultural and Therapeutic Translation

Civilization is the sum total of different cultures animated
by a common spiritual numerator, and its main vehicle—
speaking both metaphorically and literally—is translation.

—Joseph Brodsky,
"The Child of Civilization"
(1986, p. 139)

*A*spects *of language and culture in therapy are explored in this chapter.
Two images of communication are contrasted: the Tower of Babel as a
symbol of linguistic diversity and the Rosetta Stone as a symbol of unity
through translation. Translation is at the heart of intercultural encounters.
New ideas in translation theory, the somatics and dialogics of translation, are applied to therapy. After defining language translation, I introduce the fourth conceptual tool, codes, which encompasses cultural translation and* therapeuetic *translation. Cultural translation clarifies
clients' idioms of distress and explanatory models to understand their*
predicaments. Therapeutic translation *articulates clients' suffering in
therapeutic idioms. After a discussion of the epistemology of translation, I
explore clinical examples of working with language in therapy. The section
on* code-switching *illustrates the clinical value of following language
switches in therapy with bilingual/polyglot families with two vignettes.
"The Japanese Earthquake" is a detailed vignette of translation during a
cross-cultural consultation followed by practical guidelines for the use of
translators in therapy. The chapter ends with a discussion of the broader
problems with language and therapy, including skewed research on lan-*

111

guage and emotion in psychiatry and the tyrannical uses of language.
Finally, using language as the vehicle for narrative resources, we can
alleviate cultural impoverishment by helping other people find their own
voices.

TWO CONTRASTING IMAGES

According to the Book of Genesis, the Tower of Babel was a structure erected in the plain of Shinar to reach the heavens. For their
presumption, the Lord confused the builders' tongues, rendering
them unable to communicate with each other. The myth may have
developed to account for the diversity of human languages and was
probably inspired by the Babylonian *ziggurat*, a tower-like structure.
The word Babel, indicating the confusion of tongues, derives from
the Hebrew word *balal*, meaning to confuse or confound. The
Tower of Babel has become a symbol of human incomprehension,
especially across cultures.

The Rosetta Stone, an ancient Egyptian stone found in the town
of Rosetta (or Rashid) in 1799, contains an inscription in two languages and three scripts: Egyptian hieroglyphics at the top, de-
motic characters in the middle, and Greek on the bottom. This
stone gave us the key to the translation of hieroglyphics and
opened up the comprehension of a whole civilization. The Rosetta
Stone has accordingly become a symbol of translation and of access
into other cultures.

The Tower of Babel and the Rosetta Stone are two contrasting
images of human communication. One is the image of the problem
and the other the image of the solution. These two images represent the diversity and unity of humanity and reflect a tension in
transcultural psychiatry about whether cultures are better understood by grasping their local and *particular* distinctions or their
universal commonalities. Arthur Kleinman, an anthropologist and
psychiatrist at Harvard University, argues for the particular approach in what he called the "new cross-cultural psychiatry"
(Kleinman, 1977). This approach may be characterized by the saying, "When in Rome, do as the Romans do." It emphasizes personal experience and meaning with local specificity over Western
psychiatric categories (see Kleinman, 1988). In contrast, according
to Kleinman, the universal approach is associated with the "classic

transcultural psychiatry,'' founded at McGill University and associated with such pioneers as Eric Wittkower, H. B. M. Murphy, and Raymond Prince. The universal approach may be summed up in the saying, ''All roads lead to Rome.'' This view emphasizes ''comparative psychiatry'' (as H. B. M. Murphy describes it, 1982) and overarching categories of psychiatric disorders over ''local knowledge'' (to use Clifford Geertz's term, 1983c).

This characterization of approaches in transcultural psychiatry, however, creates a false dichotomy. Much of the work in transcultural psychiatry employs a richer, more subtle, and complex set of approaches and attitudes that interweaves the comparative methods of classic transcultural psychiatry with the newer cross-cultural psychiatry's search for local meanings. A more comprehensive, synthetic, and nondoctrinaire overview of a cultural approach to medicine and health care is offered by Cecil Helman (1994). For a sampling of the rich variety of clinical methods in transcultural psychiatry, see the volume edited by Samuel Okpaku (in press). To see cultural scholars at work on clinical problems, see the fascinating study of self-mutilation by cultural psychiatrist Armando Favazza (1996) and the multi-author text on ethnocultural aspects of posttraumatic stress disorder by cross-cultural psychologist Anthony Marsella and his associates (1996).

ANTHROPOLOGY AND TRANSLATION

All translation is only a somewhat provisional way of coming to terms with the foreignness of languages.

—Walter Benjamin (1968, p. 75)

Anthropology gets us right to the heart of the matter, to questions of meaning: ''What does this word, that action mean?'' ''What does such a kinship relationship mean to these people?'' By and large, cultural anthropology has not bypassed meaning (validity) for the sake of measurement (reliability), as much of academic psychiatry has done. Research in psychology and psychiatry has become so concerned with measurement that issues of meaning are now taken up almost solely by disciplines at the creative edge: represented by narrative approaches in psychotherapy (Schafer,

1992) and family therapy (Parry & Doan, 1994); the emerging cultural approaches in psychology (Bruner, 1990; Shweder, 1991; Valsiner, 1989); and the elucidation of "explanatory models" and "mini-ethnographies" of Kleinman's cross-cultural psychiatry (1988). Translation is at the heart of what anthropology is about: an encounter with another cultural tradition. And as I hope to demonstrate in this chapter, translation is also integral to the therapeutic encounter in family therapy.

Anthropologist Mary Douglas practices what Clifford Geertz (1973b, 1983c) calls "interpretive anthropology." In an essay about causal theories of behavior, Douglas (1975b) examines what we find obvious or "self-evident." She says that without challenging our tendency to see our own causal theories as self-evident, the only tool we have is translation from another culture into our own:

> The better the translation, the more successfully has our provincial logic been imposed on the native thought. So the consequence of good translation is to prevent any confrontation between alien thought systems. (Douglas, 1975b, p. 277)

Douglas reminds us of the two contrasting images of communication: the Rosetta Stone—"Translation flourishes where experience overlaps" (Douglas, 1975b, p. 277)—and the Tower of Babel—"But where there is no overlap, the attempt to translate fails. The challenge of a new meaning by which to test our own ideas is turned into a challenge to find a new expression for our old meanings" (Douglas, 1975b, p. 277). She illustrates this with examples from ethnographies: "The most baffling translations of foreign ideas are the shortest ones, presented out of context, as parts away from their wholes. The Bororo told [an anthropologist] they were parrots. . . . The Nuer say human twins are birds. . . . The Karam say the cassowary is their sister's child" (Douglas, 1975b, p. 279). These statements, Douglas suggests, are problematic for us, because we do not share the customs of these peoples. Interestingly, many of these puzzles about other cultures concern family relationships (see D'Andrade, 1989).

Clearly, Douglas is asserting that translation is fundamental to anthropology and to meeting people from other cultural traditions. As well as being central to anthropology, translation is a clinical tool and a metaphor for the encounter between clients and clinicians. Translation is a key metaphor for my work as a clinician, applying to both assessment (defining what a problem is) and therapy (finding solutions acceptable to the clients).

TRANSLATION THEORY

Ever since there has been more than one language, contact between people using languages has made language translation a necessity. A practical, mainstream definition of *language translation* is:

> the process of rendering a communication or message from one language (the source language) into the "closest natural equivalent" (Nida, 1959, p. 19) words and idioms of another language (the receptor or target language).

While this appears reasonable and acceptable for practical purposes, there are more recent, richer, and more daring definitions of the task. Douglas Robinson (1991) wants to explode the "structures of equivalence" that have dominated translation theory with two notions. The first is that translation is *somatic*: not primarily a cognitive task but an intuitive, gut-level sense of the "right" word or phrase. The second is that translation is *dialogic*: a variable, unpredictable interaction of the translator with the source-language writer (or speaker) and the target-language reader (or audience). Together, Robinson's notions argue for translation—for any communication—as an encounter and an embodiment of language. Robinson's (1991) paradigm shift calls for:

> a new way of understanding the use of words in human society, the use of words to bring people together, to make them feel good or bad or frightened or empowered, the use of words to bring about changes in bodies, bodies politic and psychologic, ideo- and idiosomatic. (p. 257)

Clearly, this is a view of translation as more than a practical tool or something secondary in communicative value to the source language. Robinson (1991) positions the translator as a full-fledged, *fully fleshed* human partner of the conversation between language users, visioning "Translation as conversation, as embodied dialogue . . . " (p. 257). I find his theory of translation a breath of fresh air because it raises the stakes of language as the vehicle for our humanity.

If we put the interpretive anthropology of Mary Douglas together with Douglas Robinson's theory of translation, we can arrive at an almost dizzying sense of what it means to communicate with other people. Douglas demonstrates that a real encounter between cultures and languages challenges our commonsense, what she calls "self-evidence." By positioning the translator in the space where the encounter is alien and strange, Robinson is saying that finding the right words is not primarily a cognitive task but a gut-level somatic reaction. He emphasizes somatic terms: "felt connections," "gut-level sense," and "embodied dialogue." Such work of meaning-making requires a human being as an intermediary, not a machine. As a translator, I feel that the great personal effort it takes to make meaning across languages and cultures endorses Robinson's striking conclusion:

> Through its insistence that we immerse ourselves in cross-cultural conversation, in the *felt* connections between people who speak different languages, translation can restore us to ourselves—to our full humanity. (p. 258)

The task of the translator is not to lull us asleep with "comfort words" we already know, but to waken us with new words for new experiences, as Franz Kafka urged—embodied words and texts that will serve as an axe for the "frozen sea within us." We need to accept the translator that Robinson offers us as "fully human" in order to expand our own sense of our humanity. The old canard of intercultural contact—"they are just like us"—accomplishes nothing but the diminution of other people. They, in fact, are often not like us. So what are they like? And what does that mean for us?

EMPATHY AS TRANSLATION

And there stand those stupid languages, helpless as two bridges that go over the same river side by side but are separated from each other by an abyss. It is a mere bagatelle, an accident, and yet it separates.

—Rainer Maria Rilke (1969)

Robinson's approach to translation as a human, bodily experience brings us to consider empathy in our meetings with other people. My understanding of empathy and how to conduct cross-cultural therapy is similar. We locate the other person's experience within our own. However, keeping in mind Alfred Korzybski's (1933) statement that "the map is not the territory," our empathy or resonance with other people is not the same thing as their own experience.

But what happens when we cannot—when there are no apparent parallels between ourselves and other people? We cannot resonate with experiences totally outside our own. What we can do is to try to enlarge our repertoires so that we learn to build bridges between what is genuinely our own and other, strange experiences. In therapy, this can be done implicitly by collaboratively creating a space where all involved can reveal something of themselves. Every participant in the encounter is offered a chance to work on the bridge. In guiding the family to share its vulnerability, therapists, too, can reveal some of their own vulnerablity to the family. If this is not attempted, the therapeutic situation can be all too much like Rilke's two bridges over the same river: side by side, each has a purpose, each one leads somewhere, but they do not meet. The bridge that the client and family cross is built on the words of their distress, structured by their explanatory models, built with the tools given them by their predicament. The therapist builds a bridge with the language of therapy.

In order for these bridges to meet, we must rely on translation of languages and culture, continually shuttling between familiar points of reference and the novel and strange points on the other side of Rilke's river. For this task, the traditional definition of translation will not do. Robinson's theory gets us closer to what we need. "Translation," in fact, may not be the best word for the concept I want to grasp. What I want to articulate is more like "word mapping." Let me give an analogy: there are cultures whose number concepts differ from those of classical mathematics, where they count, one, two, three, four, and many. As Jorge Luis Borges puts it in one of his anthropological tales, "infinity starts with the thumb.'' Does this mean that if they encounter more than four objects they cannot differentiate any more? Not quite: they do not differentiate with words, but they do in action. In trade, for example, they either exchange one for one, or make markers for each batch traded, effectively using multiples. They count large numbers by tally or correspondence. This kind of one-to-one mapping between my goods and yours, between my world and yours, may be more similar to what happens with the emotional experience we call ''empathy'' than reference to abstract terms invoking the inner world of the subjects, because the language of that inner world is like a dialect, expressing subjective, insider, experience-near terms.

This section has been written with metaphors and analogies. Two key metaphors arise commonly and, it seems, spontaneously in translation studies: bridges and maps. We will revisit these particular metaphors and the use of metaphor as a way of communicating and overcoming distress.

CULTURAL TRANSLATION

Cultural translation is the fundamental attitude and the most basic tool in cultural family therapy. As practiced by culturally informed mental health practitioners and in therapy, *intercultural communication and translation*, or *cultural translation (CT)* for short, is:

> the elucidation of an individual's or a family's idioms of distress, explanatory models of illness, and perceived predicaments using family members, culture brokers, and other informants when useful, and language translators when necessary, in a collaborative effort.

''*Idioms of distress*'' (IDs) is a concept used by medical anthropologists (Nichter, 1982) to identify the ways people express their dilemmas and their pain in their local language and folkways. ''For the anthropologist, the idiom is the symptom,'' says cross-cultural psychiatrist Arthur Kleinman (1988, p. 70).

''*Explanatory models of illness*'' (EMs) are what generate the client's answers to basic questions about their illness, such as: ''Why me?''

"Why now?" "What is wrong?" "How long will it last and how serious is it?" "What problems does it create for me?" "How do I get rid of the problem?" (Kleinman, 1988, p. 156).

"Predicament" is close to family therapy's notion of context:

> predicaments are painful social situations or circumstances, complex, unstable, morally charged and varying in their import in time and place. (Taylor, 1985, p. 130)

We find predicament through history-taking, where what we are seeking is context. The notion of predicament overlaps significantly with what family therapy means by such terms as *family process* and *context* (DiNicola, 1989). Indeed, Taylor says: "A fuller account of functioning within families, a family's manifestation of their predicament, is provided by 'family therapy'" (1985, p. 136). Stripped down, cultural translation is the effort to help people find words for their own pain in their own language.

THERAPEUTIC TRANSLATION

Once the therapist acknowledges that meeting families across cultures is always a cultural encounter and facilitates cultural translation for expressing their private predicaments expressed in vernacular language, the task is to move on to a translation of their distress into the more accessible, public language of therapy. *Therapeutic communication and translation*, or *therapeutic translation (TT)*, is:

> the process of rendering an individual's or a family's idioms of distress, explanatory models of illness, and perceived predicaments into therapeutic idioms.

Therapeutic idioms (TIs) are formal, systematized schemas of mental and relational disorders used by professionals to facilitate exchange. This captures not only formal diagnostic schemas such as *DSM-IV* (APA, 1994), but all the core concepts of each therapeutic approach. A large part of the process of becoming a professional consists of acquiring the TIs of one's field. If the language becomes too arcane and opaque, we stand the risk of being obscure or elitist, a charge that has been made against family therapy (Rakoff, 1984; Treacher, 1986).

In family therapy, TIs include classical concepts such as "scape-goating," "homeostasis," "family myth," and "enmeshment/disengagement"; interviewing guidelines such as "joining," "neutrality," and "circular questioning"[1]; and newer metaphors such as "therapy as a conversation and dialogue" and "the family as a storying culture" (Paré, 1995). Transcultural psychiatrists use the term "culture-bound syndromes" (CBS) (Simons & Hughes, 1985) to describe psychiatric disorders that emerge in some socio-cultural conditions but not in others. Medical anthropologists use terms like "idioms of distress" to try to grasp vernacular expressions of pain (Nichter, 1982); as *constructs* these terms are also part of the professional vocabulary of anthropology that is imported into clinical work. As an example of the second use of this term, Kleinman (1988) argues that vernacular expressions of predicaments are better understood through the anthropological "idioms of distress" construct than by the transcultural psychiatric term, CBS. Often, there are multiple descriptions of phenomena, expressed in competing TIs. Rather than argue for one description or another, I prefer to use them selectively as part of my "tool-kit" (Foucault, 1980) of frameworks and lenses.

Here are two examples of therapeutic translation, moving from the client's idioms of distress, through therapeutic idioms, to a new description of the clients' predicaments, from two prominent research-based therapeutic models.

"Unlovable" (Wilkes et al., 1994, p. 116)

Client ID: Jessica is a 15-year-old female adolescent whose key beliefs are that she is "no good," "unlovable," "ugly and fat," and that she "may as well die." After she was sexually abused at home, she was separated from her family and endured many relocations. Her parents separated and divorced and her relationship with her mother culminated in a "frank rejection." She perceived herself as "unlovable," believed she was being punished, and anticipated future rejections from everyone.

TI: Cognitive theory of depression.

TT: This model of therapy calls its TT a "cognitive formulation," which is "a written explanation of the problem, highlighting cognitive factors that are hypothesized to play a role in the development and/or maintenance of the adolescent's depression" (Wilkes et al., 1994, p. 115). A cognitive formulation of Jessica's predicament is: "Jessica's depression was . . . precipitated by her perceived rejection by her family of origin." She also believed her sexual abuse caused her parents' divorce. "As a result, Jessica felt guilty and worthless and had many self-deprecatory cognitions. . . . Her key assumptions [were that she] was the cause of her family's breakup and that she was . . . unlovable and unworthy" (Wilkes et al., 1994, p. 116). Although she was reluctant because she anticipated further rejection, Jessica attended cognitive group therapy, where she had a positive experience. This unexpected experience challenged her key assumption of being "unlovable."

"Drifting Apart" (Waring, 1988, pp. 89–92)

Client ID: After eight years of marriage, a couple is drifting apart and having bitter and frequent arguments. When asked their "theories of why they are drifting apart," the wife stated that after the birth of their second child she became bitter that he spent little time at home, became more temperamental, and stopped being a companion, leaving her lonely. His "theory" is that he became bored when his wife was preoccupied with the children and domestic life.

TI: Marital maladjustment due to lack of marital intimacy.

TT: "I suggested that their lack of intimacy was probably related to an inability to resolve differences of opinion which had been present during courtship and which both had observed and experienced in their families of origin" (Waring, 1988, p. 91). Waring offered them 10 sessions of marital therapy to enhance marital intimacy by facilitating cognitive self-disclosure.

Critics may point out that therapeutic idioms serve to shut out the client and the family with opaque language. For example, British psychologist Andy Treacher (1986) warned of the "danger of family therapy becoming a 'disabling profession' with the prime goal of protecting family therapists and their knowledge rather than protection of consumers and a sharing of knowledge" (p. 280). As

George Bernard Shaw (1911/1946) put it in his play, *The Doctor's Dilemma*, "All professions are conspiracies against the laity" (Act I, p. 115). This is a profound critique that goes beyond a concern with labels, to address whether the *conduct* of family therapy is accessible and visible. Here are several guidelines to achieve this:

1. Collaborate and negotiate (this goes much beyond informed choice) in order to grasp the client's predicament (ID).
2. Explain the therapist's theory of change (TI).
3. Reduce the gap between how therapists understand the family (TI) and how they convey (explain) their understanding to the family (TT).

For most North American clinicians and therapists, the two vignettes, "Unlovable" and "Drifting Apart," are self-evident, to use Douglas's term. But how would you translate the following well-documented idioms of distress into therapeutic terms?

> *Ataques de nervios* (attack of nerves) among Puerto Ricans is a folk complaint associated with headaches, trembling, palpitations, difficulty concentrating, insomnia, worries, and gastrointestinal symptoms.

> Among the Hopi, indigenous categories of sickness that are believed to affect their minds or spirits include: "worry sickness," "unhappiness," "heartbroken," "drunken like craziness with or without alcohol," and "disappointment, pouting."

These two examples are from Kleinman (1988), who has a research interest in the cross-cultural presentations of depression. The transcultural and medical anthropological literatures are filled with interesting perspectives and debates about idioms of distress or CBSs. Kleinman, having significantly expanded mainstream psychiatry's notion of depression through his cross-cultural research among Chinese, ironically has been criticized by Chinese psychiatrists for the use of the Western diagnosis of depression in his studies. Kleinman (1988) offers an overview of the sorts of idioms employed in traditional and in Western societies:

> In traditional societies, *religious and moral idioms of distress as well as bodily complaints* communicated what was amiss and shaped the social form of distress. . . . [I]n contemporary Western society . . . such idioms are being superseded by *psychological idioms ranging from a general language of stress to more specific existential and affective expressions*. These newer idioms convey discontinuities in one's social world not as sin, chest pain, or oppression by the forces of evil, but rather in a language of intrapsychic angst, personal demoralization, and often self-defeating, morbidly introspective hopelessness. (p. 70, emphasis added)

Together, these two tools—cultural and therapeutic translation—offer a double description of each family's experience: the family members' own private language for their pain and a more public, more accessible therapeutic language. This process of double description in family and therapeutic languages also underscores that CFT is a collaborative effort among family members and therapists.

THE EPISTEMOLOGY OF TRANSLATION

Cultural and therapeutic translation have a common epistemological issue: there is a binary opposition of constructs that require translation from one to the other. Cultural anthropologist Clifford Geertz (1983a) outlines some of these binary pairs: "inside" versus "outside" or "first person" versus "third person" descriptions; "phenomenological" versus "objectivist" or "cognitive" versus "behavioral" theories; "emic" versus "etic" analyses (see Table 4.1). All of these pairs are of interest and value in understanding other people; indeed, they all address the issue of whether one can understand other people on their own terms (inside, first person, phenomenological, cognitive, emic) or translate them into other accounts (outside, objectivist, third person, behavioral, etic). As I noted earlier, this tension is reflected in Arthur Kleinman's (1977) contrast of "universal" versus "particular" approaches in cultural research in psychiatry. Kleinman (1988) and Roland Littlewood (1990), who are both anthropologists/psychiatrists, oppose "contexts to categories."

Geertz grasps the essence of these binary pairs with psychoanalyst Heinz Kohut's distinction of "experience-near" versus "expe-

Table 4.1. Binary Opposition of Constructs in Cultural Studies

CONCEPTS

Experience-near	Experience-distant

DESCRIPTIONS

Inside	Outside
First-person	Third-person

THEORIES

Phenomenological	Objectivist
Cognitive	Behavioral

CULTURAL ANALYSES

Emic	Etic

LANGUAGES

Vernacular	Standard

CULTURAL PSYCHIATRIC APPROACHES

Particular	Universal
Context	Category

THERAPEUTIC TEMPERAMENTS

Phenomenological	Technocratic

PROFESSIONAL MODELS

Connotative	Denotative
Meaning-centered	Syndrome-centered

rience-distant'' concepts. An experience-near concept is generated ''naturally and effortlessly'' to describe oneself and is ''readily understood when similarly applied by others'' (Geertz, 1983a, p. 57). Such concepts are expressed in the immediacy of local language (dialect, vernacular). An experience-distant concept is employed by specialists for "scientific, philosophical, or practical aims" (Geertz, 1983a, p. 57). These latter concepts are expressed in a more widespread idiom (such as standard national or scientific languages) and have the remoteness of abstraction.

There is yet another layer in these distinctions—they contrast client and professional idioms. In family therapy, I believe this opposition is expressed in two sharply contrasted therapeutic temperaments: the "phenomenological" and the "technocratic" (see Chapter 2). In professional discourses, these contrasts reflect an underlying tension about meaning-centered versus syndrome-centered definitions of medical and psychiatric problems (cf. Kirmayer, 1989). The medical model is *denotative*: it indicates distress and names syndromes and diseases. Social sciences like medical anthropology (e.g., Littlewood & Lipsedge, 1989; Lock & Gordon, 1988; Young, 1980) and medical sociology (e.g., the labeling theory of Scheff, 1975; the work on illness behavior by Mechanic, 1982; and research on the social origins of depression by Brown and Harris, 1978) are *connotative*: reading symptoms for their meanings, they expand the context within which disease and distress are understood. But just as the social sciences have voiced critiques of the medical model, there are pitfalls in the connotative approach to distress and disease when metaphors become reified (what I call "metaphor as illness," see DiNicola, 1988b) or when nosology is replaced by cultural attributions using explanatory models ("illness as explanation").

WORKING WITH LANGUAGE IN THERAPY

Culture and syntax, the cultural matrix which syntax maps, holds us in place.

—George Steiner (1975, p. 465)

Concepts from cultural anthropology and transcultural psychiatry are useful for cultural translation across cultures. However, cultural knowledge alone is not enough for therapeutic work, which is aimed at change: the alleviation of a family's pain and suffering. As Mara Selvini Palazzoli (1986a) wrote in response to my overview of family therapy and transcultural psychiatry (DiNicola, 1985b, 1985c):

no tribe ever asked an anthropologist "Come and change us"; neither has any state asked such a thing of a sociologist. But a family therapist is asked exactly that. Consequently, the therapist is authorized by his clients to make changes. (p. 85)

"Authorization," meaning to give authority, to endorse, or to empower, has a fascinating history based on the Latin, *auctor*, a narrative notion meaning the "author, originator" of a story. If clients invite therapists to be the "authors" (understood collaboratively as co-authoring and co-editing) of their stories, therapeutic translation must be more than journalism as reportage and anthropology as ethnography, reaching for a healing transformation of troubling experiences.

George Steiner (1975) has written a penetrating book, *After Babel*, about language and translation. The heart of his insight may be stated for our purposes very simply—if language maps experience, then communication is always a kind of translation. Each particular language maps the experience of that community in a way that reveals its history and traditions. Using translation in therapy must be done with the same care that we exercise with a family's expression of affect or pain. Or to put it more directly, it is the same uncertainty that accompanies the leap from a subjective report of pain to a known clinical entity. Two aspects of language in therapy arise from the multilingual situation—the problems of language switching and the problems of translation.

CODE-SWITCHING

Sociolinguists call switches from one language to another "code-switching" (see Crystal, 1987; DiNicola, 1985a). Following code-switching in therapy with bilingual or polyglot families can reveal fundamental details about their affective and cognitive states. By doing so, the therapist may construct a map of affects and other aspects of a family system in a systematic and objective way. This allows the therapist to draw a functional map of the languages of affect analogous to the structural map that neuroscientists construct when mapping language sites by electrical stimulation of the brain. Such research indicates that in the bilingual brain the two languages show differential localization—they occupy overlapping but distinct areas of cortex (Ojemann & Whitaker, 1978). De Zulueta's

(1984) comprehensive review of the psychiatric aspects of bilingualism puts this research and other issues raised here in perspective for the reader encountering language issues for the first time.

Two clinical vignettes about families with an anorexic member illustrate two different functions that can be mapped by attending to code-switching. In the first vignette, "Mother's Space," language switches serve as boundary markers. They help to answer the question, "Who is heard?" As a boundary marker, code-switching enacts in words the alliances, coalitions, disqualifications, and exclusions that occur among family members.

Vignette: "Mother's Space"

Montreal in the mid-80s. The Karasimos family are Greek immigrants with a 19-year-old only child, Chrissoula, a daughter with juvenile arthritis since age eight and chronic anorexia nervosa for four years. Sessions were conducted in English. No one on the consulting team knew how to speak Greek. Father and the IP spoke English well. Mother's grasp of English varied in the following way: she could follow the therapist's statements about dates for meetings but became lost when asked to discuss her own perceptions of family events. At this point, she would turn to her daughter. When daughter was blocked as a translator and her husband was asked to translate, she would literally brush him aside and plow into her answer, making the best of her command of English. This pattern was seen repeatedly. While her daughter was prized as a confidante (to the point that they slept together), the husband's skill in translating and, more generally, his role as husband and father were disqualified. These code-switches made clear the structural positions of each family member and the need for therapy to begin with structural-strategic maneuvers aimed at realigning the boundaries in a more functional way. A dramatic weight gain followed the first session, which was maintained throughout the course of therapy. Helping Chrissoula move out of mother's space (bedroom and kitchen) was followed by modest improvements in her food rituals and some activities with friends outside the home.

In the second vignette, "A Private Language," code-switching helps in the localization of affect. It helps answer the question, "What is heard?" Listening closely for which topics produced code-switches proved a useful tool to map out sensitive topics, with whom they could be shared, and who was excluded.

Vignette: "A Private Language"

Montreal in the mid-80s. The Pasquinis are an Italian immigrant family with two daughters: Rosa, a bright, attractive, and successful 20-year-old university student, and Luisa, the identified patient, a 15-year-old who had become anorexic and withdrawn. The anorexic behavior became overt following the sister's graduation from college, informal engagment, and a celebrated trip to Italy won on scholarship. Therapy was conducted in Italian since the parents spoke very little English or French. The daughters understood Italian but preferred to respond in English. When affectively laden topics were touched on, the siblings invariably switched to English, ostensibly to express themselves better. However, when the therapist offered to translate, their qualifiers confirmed their reluctance to explore their feelings with their parents.

A tight bond between the two sisters was sealed by English, their "private" language, which they could share with strangers but not with their parents, dedicated immigrant parents who had made sacrifices for their children. The new values, tastes, and criticisms that adolescents inevitably unearth were kept hidden from them. By being "dutiful daughters" in "Italian" and rather bright, outgoing teens in "English," they had the best of both worlds for a time. The older sister's strides outside the home threatened this balance; the client, the most reactive family member, went on a hunger strike of protest. This configuration of generational differences between parents and children in acculturation is a common one among immigrant families.

These two families have much in common as immigrants, as the bearers of foreign and not yet integrated cultures, and as families organized around interactions that allow the anorexic family game to emerge. Yet they also show important differences: in one case the therapist shared the two languages and cultures of the Italian family, accepting the role of insider. With the Greek family, excluded from their "mother tongue," he used the role of outsider to learn their cultural and idiosyncratic family rules and rituals.

Nonetheless, something was learned about the use of each language; language communicated above all a family process. The observing team felt that the therapist was more at ease, more cognizant of the direction of therapy, and more perceptive of and responsive to the Greek family whose mother tongue he did not share. Working with two language channels has advantages in the richness of the content, which, however, may distract the therapist from the pattern of interactions.

TRANSLATION IN THERAPY

Translation is the second aspect of therapy with polyglot families and therapists. Steiner (1975) starts by exploring the "indeterminacy of translation" and ends by exulting in the diversity of languages and the varied experiences they map. The following vignette highlights what Steiner (1975) calls the "indeterminacy of translation." In searching for an equivalent, the translator employs what Robinson calls the "somatics of translation"—embodied meanings. But the consultant takes this to another level with a metaphoric transformation of the family's experience.

Vignette: "The Japanese Earthquake"

Rome, 1987. A Japanese family therapist, Tazuko Shibusawa, acts as consultant to Dr. Maurizio Andolfi for a session with the Brissa family he has been treating in Rome. To enhance Shibusawa's role as a consultant, Andolfi speaks only English in the session. I act as Italian-English translator. Andolfi now has the experience I had in my consultation with the Savelli family in Rome (see Chapter 1, "The Berlin Wall"). Andolfi restricts himself to communicating in English in the session while understanding both. This has the very clear effect of creating space for Shibusawa as a consultant, since Andolfi is not communicating in Italian. By speaking in English, he is less directly available to the family. It also creates space for Andolfi, giving him a meta-position in the session. This is confirmed at the end when Shibusawa offers a different view of the family and Andolfi acknowledges that this opens a new approach for the therapy.

For me, being a translator is a very different experience from being a consultant. My role is to follow and translate the dialogue among family members, consultant (Shibusawa), and therapist (Andolfi). To do so, I have to give more attention to language than to therapeutic process, being careful not to get caught up in it or become part of the consultation. I have to be as faithful as possible, given my skills, to the intended meanings in both languages. Meanwhile, the exaggerations, distortions, and other playful and therapeutic meta-communications that are going on (and which I, as a therapist, am aware of) are very distracting. Through translation, I try to convey the words as intended, with or without irony, as the speaker intends, but without any irony I experience within myself during the process.

Present in the session are the Brissa couple and their two children, Giovanna, 22, and Dario, 20, who both live at home. At the outset, the father, Signor Brissa, says that they initially came to therapy because "my wife had doubts about our relationship." As Shibusawa tries to clarify this, he is evasive, finally deferring to his wife, who says, cryptically: "The existence of another woman." Although this refers to events of three years ago, they are still dealing with it. In the exchanges below, keep in mind that both therapist and consultant only spoke in English and the family only spoke in Italian. I had to translate each statement, which gives the session an unusual rhythm and pace.

Consultant (to Signora Brissa): You were saying this was affecting the whole family. How was it affecting the family?

(TRANSLATION INTO ITALIAN)

Signora Brissa: Terremoto, terremoto!

Translator: An earthquake, an earthquake!

Consultant: In what way?

(TRANSLATION)

Signora Brissa (translation): This was a very big crisis for her. She started to look around to see who this person was and started to involve the children.

Consultant: Did they believe her, support her?

(TRANSLATION)

Signora Brissa (translation): They supported her emotionally, but since it was a private thing between the two of them, she feels that even now they don't believe . . .

Dario (translation): He says he definitely doesn't believe this.

Giovanna (translation): She also doesn't believe it.

Signora Brissa (translation): The wife said she saw with her own eyes . . . he came home in a car that wasn't a colleague's . . .

Notice that in the exchanges spoken in or translated into English, we are sometimes speaking about the family members in the third person, not as though they are absent, but as if we are offering them reflections. What this takes away in "immediacy," we gain in "reflectivity."

There are many ways to use translation in therapy. For immediacy in therapy, a different approach can be taken: clients and therapist face each other, speaking in the first and second person ("me and you"). Immediacy was created with the Shami family in the session I called "Two Old Men" in Chapter 1, where the grandfather and I are seated face to face and we speak to each other in Arabic and English, through a translator. By "immediacy," I mean a process that creates intimacy and rapport, enhanced by attending to paraverbal (tone of voice and rate of speech, for example) and nonverbal (hand gestures and body posture, for example) communication and direct eye contact. "Reflectivity," a more cognitive process, is enhanced by speaking in the third person (even about oneself), by downplaying nonverbal aspects of communication, and by sending messages through other parties.

Consultant: When you said "earthquake," I can see how it must have been an upheaval and very, very difficult for everybody.

(IN TRANSLATING THIS, I STRUGGLE WITH THE WORD "UPHEAVAL" IN ITAL-IAN, TRYING "HOUSEBREAKING," WHICH AT LEAST REFLECTS THE FAMILY PRO-CESS. EVERYONE LAUGHS AND HELPS ME OUT, AND WE FIND AN EQUIVALENT WORD, "SHOCK.")

In Japan, there are many, many earthquakes all the time . . .

(PAUSE FOR TRANSLATION)

And sometimes when the earthquake stops, you can't tell if it's completely stopped. Sometimes you're waiting to see if it'll go like this again (*flapping hand up and down*) . . .

(TRANSLATION)

And sometimes it's still and you know it's over . . .

(TRANSLATION)

Signora Brissa (*nodding in agreement; translation*): It's a very good analogy, she feels you've understood her.
Consultant: She feels the earthquake is over.

(TRANSLATION)

Signora Brissa (*translation*): I think so.
Consultant: They experienced the earthquake, too. (*indicating the children*)

(TRANSLATION)

Sometimes after the earthquake is over, your heart is still beating very quickly . . .

(TRANSLATION)

Dario (*translation*): The fear is there.
Consultant: So for you, the earthquake continues . . .

(TRANSLATION)

Dario (*translation*): The fear is there that it will start all over again. . . . He doesn't know if it's just a pause or a definitive end, a completion to this problem. . . .
Consultant: What are you afraid of?

(TRANSLATION)

Dario (*translation*): That my parents would break up . . . if there would be a real reason that we could understand, that we could see . . . the tragedy becomes even bigger . . .
Consultant: So the earthquake can hit a volcano, and explode . . .

(TRANSLATION)

The metaphor for this session and for this family's experience is that they are living in an earthquake zone. There are three crucial points about the use of metaphors in therapy. First, to work, using metaphors requires a collaborative context. Shibusawa drew the metaphor out of Signora Brissa's own description of her experience, rather than introducing something out of the blue. Although it is possible and powerful to introduce fresh, even startling metaphors to describe a family's predicament, such an intervention requires a correspondingly greater level of therapeutic confidence and family trust. Second, metaphors need to be relevant to everyone present. In my view, Shibusawa's metaphor works because it is a systemic metaphor. Everyone in the family is living with the earthquake. Shibusawa transforms it into a systemic metaphor about how families build their own worlds. At this point in the session, Shibusawa (as consultant) turns to Andolfi (as therapist) to give her reflections.

Consultant (to therapist): What I'm seeing is that there was this earthquake and it seems like it's still shaky . . .

(PAUSE FOR TRANSLATION)

Therapist (nodding in agreement): Ah-hah . . .
Consultant: And it's left them (pointing to the children) with a lot of fear . . .
Therapist: Yeah . . .

(TRANSLATION)

Consultant: And them (pointing to the parents) with a crack that still hasn't healed.

(PAUSE FOR TRANSLATION)

Are we seeing a crack that's still opening or is it closing?

(DEMONSTRATING THE ACTION WITH HER HANDS)
(TRANSLATION)

Or, are there many, many more cracks?

(TRANSLATION)

Therapist: I think the earthquake has been moving from the territory of the parents to the territory of the children.

(TRANSLATION)

This exchange highlights the third crucial point about metaphors in family therapy. Shibusawa created a context for the session with the earthquake metaphor, based on Signora Brissa's own description. From there, she has drawn out the systemic implications with each family member. Andolfi draws this out further by talking about the different territories of parents and children. This extension is based on a structural family therapy idiom of generational boundaries. This two-stage therapeutic tag-team or relay is called *metalepsis* in the study of "tropes" (turns of phrase)—which are the tools for conveying and shaping communication (Robinson, 1991). In family therapy, *metalepsis* means drawing out the systemic implications of metaphors. This is what gives metaphors their energy in therapy, not some arresting or appealing image. They give the session a propulsive force, opening up new territory for exploration. Given this new energy, Andolfi pursues the possibility of more age-appropriate, less fearful lives for Giovanna and Dario.

Therapist (translation): The risk that I see is that she has to jump from not being an adolescent to becoming a "pseudo-adult."
Consultant: How old is she?

  (TRANSLATION)

Giovanna (translation): Twenty-two.
Therapist: In this country, twenty-two is still considered an adolescent . . .
Signora Brissa (translation): She agrees.
Giovanna (translation): At my age, I don't feel complete . . .
Therapist: They are preschool children. The idea to be adults is so hard as to be dangerous . . .

  (TRANSLATION)

  They are three-and-a-half and five-and-a-half. *(indicates their ages by holding his hand out to these imagined heights of children)*

  (TRANSLATION)

Consultant: I have a different feeling about it: they have some adult parts that the parents don't recognize.
Therapist: If your idea is right we would have to see them in a different context, maybe with their friends.

Consultant: I think that the earthquake is not an earthquake that destroys. . . .

(TRANSLATION)

It's to let the roots loosen a little bit to let them grow. Sometimes the earth gets packed too tight. You shake things up a little bit and new things can grow.

(TRANSLATION)

Therapist: I think we can "fire" these two. *(indicating the children)*

(TRANSLATION)

Giovanna: Yea! *(waving her arms in victory)*
Therapist: We want to see how they can grow.

(TRANSLATION)

My own experience of the session, which still resonates with me after a decade, taught me three things. First, it demonstrates that participating in therapy, even with an apparently "technical" or "neutral" role as a translator, engages you as a whole person. Second, my own somatic responses to the emotions of the session were a useful guide to its meanings. Where words led me astray, emotions spoke eloquently. Third, by speaking in another language through a translator, the therapist allowed the consultant with her different culture to create a new context for this session. The cultural differences between the therapist and the consultant required the therapist to articulate his assumptions about generational boundaries and Italian cultural expectations for young people. And the therapist also heard the consultant's different cultural ideas about the possibility that families can survive earthquakes, even use them to grow.

GUIDELINES FOR THE USE OF TRANSLATORS

The interpreter has the unenviable task of being the go-between and helping two strangers get to know each other.

—Hitesh Raval (1996, p. 33)

Anyone who works with more than one language can appreciate the Italian proverb, *Traduttore, traditore,* a pun on the similarity of the words for "translator" and "traitor." Jay Lappin (1983), starting with this caution, makes an argument against the use of translators in family therapy. Carlos Sluzki (1984), who practices with bilingual families (Spanish and English), applies the same caution when recommending how to use translators effectively. Hitesh Raval (1996), a clinical psychologist and family therapist working in London's richly multicultural environment, offers an informed model of the "therapist-interpreter-client (TIC) triad" as a three-way relationship for conducting cross-cultural therapy based on his research with Bangladeshi families. So here we have a spectrum of opinion from the rejection of translators in therapy (Lappin), to their cautious use (Sluzki), to warmly embracing them as colleagues in the therapeutic task (Raval).

Translation has been a central aspect of my daily experience—learning new languages, translating for my family as a child in a new country, friends translating for me in my sojourns in other places. Translating some of the Italian texts of Mara Selvini Palazzoli (e.g., 1986) and of Maurizio Andolfi and his colleagues (e.g., 1989) and having my own work translated into other languages (e.g., DiNicola, 1995a) have expanded my respect for the necessity and difficulty of translation. As the above vignette illustrates, I have worked as a translator in therapy and have used translators across many languages, including sign language and telephone translation with hearing-impaired clients. These guidelines are based on my own experiences and my review of the literature (see DiNicola, 1986, 1994).

Some variables to keep in mind are:

- the difference between translation and interpretation;
- the different roles of translator, culture broker/community worker, link worker, and advocate (see Raval, 1996);
- who is the conductor of therapy (this can get fuzzy);
- the relationship between the therapist and the translator: allies or adversaries, co-therapists or colleagues;
- the impact of having another person in the room: alliances, identifications, and roles;
- the impact on the session of double-coding: lingering vs. haste;

- who has clinical responsibility for the session;
- choosing the language of therapy (not so obvious; you can *experience the session* in their language, with your words translated for them; or you can *conduct the session* in your language, with their words translated for you);
- choosing a translator: yourself (if you have the skills), a professional translator, a co-therapist (with the requisite language skills), a culture broker, a family member;
- how to use language and translation to create *immediacy* or enhance *reflectivity*.

PROFESSIONAL TRANSLATORS

The use of professional translators introduces a *medium* between the therapist and the family. This may be used constructively to enhance *reflectivity* and distance. In this reflective approach, the therapist is not replaced by the family's more immediate experience with a culture broker or link worker. "Therapy" and "community linking" or "culture brokering" are distinct processes, but often there is temptation to blend them.

1. When using professional translators, you need to be clear about the therapeutic process and who is guiding it. Negotiate this in advance. Be careful about proceeding if this cannot be agreed upon. The therapist should not allow the translator to take over.
2. Therapist and family members should face and speak directly to each other; the translator should sit to the side between therapist and family. There should not be direct exchanges between the family and the professional translator.
3. Firmly insist that all exchanges between therapist and the family are translated fully, without editorial comment from the professional translator.

FAMILY MEMBERS AS TRANSLATORS

1. Choosing to use family members as translators creates *immediacy* in the therapeutic experience. It is not directly within your control as a therapist, so you have to work through one or more family members.
2. When using family members as translators, it is futile to try

to keep them out of the family process. The therapist should be aware of their involvement in the process. You may or may not decide to make them part of the therapeutic process as a co-therapist, but this should be a collaborative therapeutic choice, not left entirely in their hands or unknown to you.

COMMUNITY MEMBERS AS TRANSLATORS

When using a member from the family's own community or culture, the issue of their involvement in both family and the therapeutic processes is very important.

1. Clarify their role in advance through negotiation. Is this person only translating, or does he or she also have another role? Other possible roles include (see Raval, 1996):
   - culture broker/community worker (interpreting a family's culture in their social setting),
   - link worker (supporting clients to make informed choices about services based on an understanding of their needs),
   - advocate (negotiating on behalf of a family in light of identified concerns for a particular community).
2. Considerations include:
   - ethics (nonprofessional outsiders will learn a great deal about the predicament of the family),
   - cultural expertise (the translator may understand the language but not the nuances of the culture, including idioms of distress and explanatory models of illness),
   - differences (similarities in language and culture may mask other differences, such as religion and social class),
   - mental health expertise (capacity to deal with potentially disturbing symptoms and stay focused on the task).

TRANSLATORS VS. INTERPRETERS

Many of the above issues are captured by differences in the connotations of the words, "interpreters" and "translators." "Interpreting" is a a hermeneutic process, an act of understanding, an act of "making meaning" in Jerome Bruner's term (rather than receiving accepted meanings). Interpreting examines communicative intent as much as the communication itself (think of interpreting a film, a poem, or a psychoanalytic interpretation). As such, interpreting is the role of the therapist or consultant (as in "interpreting experience"). "Translating" is a dialogic process, facilitating a conversation between two parties (as in "translating words"). While you may not endorse this distinction, it has practical implications when conducting therapy. The literature on translation is necessarily saturated with the personal experiences and values of the writers. Look for those personal values. Do not gloss over differences. Do not try to do what you are not comfortable with or go beyond your expertise. Do not let other people's expertise guide you without careful reflection about how to proceed. Finally, there can be only *guidelines* for translation. There cannot be a cookbook for translation in therapy any more than there could be one for therapy itself.

WHEN WORDS FALL SHORT

And will they come to me, these metaphors?

—*Il Postino*

In the Italian film, *Il Postino*,[2] the simple village postman Mario meets the exiled Chilean poet Pablo Neruda. Struck by an image in one of Neruda's poems about being tired of existence, Mario says to him: "That happened to me too. Except, until now, I didn't know how to say it." When Mario learns about metaphors, he asks Neruda if he will be able to invent metaphors too. An emphasis on language, on the narrative resources represented by storytelling, on code-switching as a window on family processes, on explanatory models of illness, on cultural and therapeutic translation, offers new perspectives on relational problems and how to work with them.

These powerful tools, however, are not always available. All too often, people do not have a full grasp of their language. Of course, this may be because they have migrated from other language communities. But it may also be a problem in their capacities to express themselves well or meaningfully in their own tongues. Let me be clear about this: this does not reflect any intrinsic deficits of a particular language or culture, but rather the ability of a community to transmit its cultural resources to its members or the barriers that impede individuals from learning or using them. In other words, under some circumstances words fall short because a culture does not transmit from one generation to the next tools to foster the expression and creative development of its communal stories and symbols. In some northern Canadian Native communities, for example, a combination of factors, such as forced relocation and education in the language and stories of mainstream Canadian society, has led to the disruption of traditional ways so that young people are neither well prepared to live in the ways of their ancestors nor to integrate into the southern mainstream of Canada. This form of narrative impoverishment is illustrated in the story of River Running (told in Chapter 5), who was raised in a Cree village but migrated with his family to southern Ontario where he was ill-prepared to live.

LANGUAGE, AFFECT, AND CULTURE

The section on "code-switching" from one language to another during family sessions demonstrated that the choice of language spoken in bilingual or polyglot families is a rich source of information about family interactions and emotions. However, code-switching has simple operational markers: whether the family members speak one language or the other. We still do not know how language taps affect. And we know too little about how culture shapes and interacts with language and affect. The little research on language and emotion that is being done in relation to psychopathology is skewed and inconsistent. Three examples stand out: (1) research on alexithymia and *pensée opératoire*; (2) the work on expressed emotion (EE) and psychiatric disorders, such as schizophrenia; and (3) Julian Leff's cultural hierarchy of emotional expressiveness.

1. *Alexithymia.* American psychiatrist Peter Sifneos (1972) coined the term alexithymia (meaning literally in Greek, "no words for moods") to denote a cognitive-affective deficit in the experience and expression of emotion in people with psychosomatic disorders. It is similar to the French term *pensée opératoire* (concrete thinking). While the work that is presented here connotes above all a respect for the family culture, including its own language of affect, idioms

of distress, explanatory models, and preferred solutions, the concept of alexithymia proposes a distinction that is closer to the discourses of castes, classes, and races. It is a concept whose assumptions are more easily shared than proven; this is demonstrated by the fact that it is described by different clinicians and researchers with "remarkable consistency" (Taylor, 1984) despite controversy and confusion as to what it actually describes or taps when applied as a research instrument.

Faced with the narrow range of patients who are amenable to individual psychotherapy, the concept of alexithymia may fulfill a useful face-saving function for psychotherapists who have not been able to extend their methods beyond the so-called "psychologically minded" middle class of urbanized Western industrial societies (Krystal, 1982). The concept of alexithymia is a paternalistic prejudice in scientific garb; the underlying notion is that people cannot think for themselves, do not feel what they should, and cannot relate the meaning of their existence.

2. *Expressed emotion.* This is another culture-bound concept which can be reliably described but cannot be validly defined (Kuipers, 1979).[3] The Social Psychiatry Research Unit of the Institute of Psychiatry in London created an important research tool with an index of "expressed emotion" (EE) in families with a schizophrenic member. The positive point to be made is that EE is the first paradigm for family research with both clinical appeal and testable hypotheses since the "double-blind hypothesis" was introduced by Gregory Bateson in the 1950s (Bateson et al., 1956).

The overall EE measure consists of ratings on five principal scales: *criticism, hostility, overinvolvement, warmth,* and *positive remarks.* There are specific criteria for each scale based on relatives' observable behaviors in relation to the patient. Raters score mostly verbal behavior, including vocal aspects such as rate, volume, and tone. Families who score above certain cut-offs are rated as high in EE. Another crucial aspect is the patient's length of exposure to the family environment. Patients who spend at least 35 hours per week with their high EE relatives are at greater risk for relapse.

EE is important for research in family therapy because (1) it has testable hypotheses, (2) it deals with interactional aspects of family life, and (3) it concerns the schizophrenias whose comprehensive management (not to say cure) is beyond the foreseeable domain of psychopharmacology. EE is of further relevance to social and transcultural psychiatry because (4) it focuses on social interactions in families rather than biological features, and (5) it reopens the investigation of possible differences related to such variables as culture and social class, the intercultural distribution of schizophrenic disorders, and the differences in outcome between industrialized and Third World nations.

A positive comment about the EE index is that it is not just another paper-and-pencil test but a sample of real life. It is an interactive measure. From the beginning of the family therapy movement, clinicians have been stressing the importance of the process of family interactions as compared to static definitions of inherent qualities. In EE, we have something that approaches the family environment as a process. However, its appeal as a clinical construct has reified this measure of a *process* into a *thing*.

I would like to see this research move further into the area of interactive tests. One promising technique is the experience sampling method (ESM), which is a "research procedure for studying what people do, feel, and think during their daily lives" (Larson & Csikszentmihalyi, 1983). Because it is a self-report measure, sampling experience throughout the day and across different contexts, the ESM can reach further into the minute-by-minute experience of individuals and families than even participant observation. Focusing on what happens in the family may produce better information about what, if anything, in the environment of schizophrenic patients leads to relapse and the deterioration of social skills.

However, there is something naive and worrisome about the ideas at the heart of the EE index. The dichotomous categories low EE (good) and high EE (bad) are stereotypes of real behavior (Hatfield, 1987). In cross-cultural studies on EE conducted in North India (Leff et al., 1987; Wig et al., 1987a, 1987b), the research team of British and Indian psychiatrists mentioned how the Western emphasis on individuality has led to introspectiveness and "the untrammelled expression of emotion" in the West. This description is value-loaded: it suggests that low EE is desirable, at least in British society, because it is associated with better outcome for schizophrenics there. But how can this Western notion be applied in North India? This is never made clear, in part because the researchers do not explore Indian experiences and idioms of distress but rather attempt to apply British notions there.

The central problem with EE is that it may be reliable and predictive but not valid, even in the West. In fact, after much research, we still have no reason to dispute the assessment of a member of the EE research group that "it is still impossible to say what exactly the measure is reflecting" (Kuipers, 1979, p. 241). "Reliability-validity" is the Janus-faced demon of modern psychiatry. If something is measurable—it may be reliable, even predictive, but it may not be valid. Witness: *DSM-IV* (APA, 1994). If it is meaningful or sensible—it may have face validity, but its reliability is in question. Witness: clinical judgment.

Part of the appeal of anthropology and transcultural psychiatry is that they plunge one right into the heart of the matter, addressing questions of meaning (validity). Measurement issues (reliability) are secondary to meaning. I associate reliability with measurement because that is just how it is defined and tested. As used in the social sciences, reliability is a technical construct, what Neil Postman calls an "invisible technology" (1993). I associate validity (which strictly means whether something is what it purports to be) with meaning. Reliability can *never* resolve issues of meaning, but serious attention to validity may begin to address the meaninglessness of our constructs. At some deep level, validity and meaning overlap. Any first year college student can run a reliability test; posing meaningful questions can be beyond the grasp of even accomplished teachers. We currently have a reliable rather than a valid approach to psychiatric diagnosis because reliability issues are easier and within our grasp. As Ludwig Wittgenstein (1958) rudely reminded us:

> The existence of the experimental method makes us think we have the means of solving the problems which trouble us; though problem and method pass one another by. (p. 232)

Cultural and therapeutic translation get us closer to meaningful descriptions in psychiatry and family therapy. Putting the experience sampling method (ESM) and cultural and therapeutic translation (CTT) together, we can build a more powerful approach to the experiential world of schizophrenic patients and their families; ESM provides better measures of daily experience, and CTT provides a more subjective language of the individual's illness and the family's experience of it.

3. *Cultural hierarchy of emotional expressiveness.* The most absurd spinoff of the colonialist myth that other people are emotionally inexpressive is British psychiatrist Julian Leff's (1977, 1981) proposition of an *affective hierarchy of languages,* suggesting that some languages and cultures are more developed in the differentiation of emotions and the range of words to express them. Leff (1986) argues that:

> over time there has been a shift in focus from the bodily expression of distress to its communication through language, with a consequent progressive differentiation of the vocabulary of emotion. This historical process has occurred unevenly, so that in many cultures today emotional distress is still communicated through a rich variety of somatic symbols. (p. 33)

To support this, Leff invokes the "disappearance of conversion hysteria" in Western cultures, despite its persistence as a "common form of neurosis in the Third World" (p. 33). This is a very debatable assertion. For one thing, the notion of "hysteria" has been highly criticized for its cultural and gender bias. For another, the phenomenon Leff refers to as "conversion hysteria" (a form of paralysis) has been compellingly constructed in very different terms by Canadian medical historian Edward Shorter (1992) as operative in contemporary Western societies, having undergone a shift from "paralysis to fatigue" (chronic fatigue syndrome).

Contrary to Leff's view, "Every language grants us eloquence when it is time to cry for help," according to Laurence Kirmayer (1984, p. 159), a transcultural psychiatrist who conducts research on psychosomatic disorders. And this very diversity expands the human situation. Writing in the simple voice of his own people, the peasants of central Italy, Ignazio Silone (1949) said in the preface of his novel, *Fontamara,* "We give to each person the right to tell his own story in his own way." Steiner (1975) has put this accurately and poignantly:

> Through language, we construct what I have called "altern-
> ities of being." To the extent that every individual speaker
> uses an idiolect, the problem of Babel is quite simply, that
> of human individuation. . . . To a greater or lesser degree,
> every language offers its own reading of life. To move be-
> tween languages, to translate . . . is to experience the al-
> most bewildering bias of the human spirit towards freedom.
> (p. 473)

The relation between language and emotion may be approached from an anthropological perspective or as an issue in the sociology of knowledge. Taking the first two examples as anthropological data, we might conclude that according to indigenous psychiatric theories, in the United States and France bottling up emotion will make the body sick (alexithymia, *pensée opératoire*), while in Britain expressing emotion will make the mind of another person crazy (EE). In one theory (EE), emotions are dangerous and should be calmed. In the other (alexithymia), emotions are to be explored and venting them is the key to therapy. The third example, Leff's notion of a cultural hierarchy of emotional expressiveness is both absurd and dangerous as post-colonial chauvinism. We can use Steiner (1975) again for an apt rebuttal: "No men inhabit a 'middle king-dom,' all are each other's guests" (p. 116).

Furthermore, the study of language has its own scientists in an-thropology (D'Andrade, 1989; Douglas, 1975a, 1975b), cognitive science (Pinker, 1994), linguistics (Crystal, 1987), psychology (Ed-wards, 1994), and sociology and sociolinguistics (Bernstein, see Douglas, 1975a). However, psychiatric researchers have hardly bothered to connect their work with other research on language (an exception is Kuipers' critical review of expressed emotion, 1979). If they had, what might they have found? For example, the work of British sociologist Basil Bernstein on language as a "code" and his dichotomy of restricted and elaborated codes is clinically appeal-ing.[4] This may well have relevance to the expression of emotion in different social contexts and to notions about low EE and high EE families. Is it possible that a nurturing family is perceived as intrusive (high EE) because patients or researchers are not using the same code as the family? The clinical applications of sociolinguistics to family therapy need to be explored further.

LINGUISTIC TYRANNY AND
NARRATIVE IMPOVERISHMENT

There are other reasons why individuals, families, and sometimes whole groups cannot give words to their predicaments. And why they may need our help to find a voice.

1. *Linguistic tyranny.* Sadly, while language is a vehicle for narrative innovations in revisioning the future, language is also one of the main instruments of tyranny. Through ideology, language is the first victim of dictatorship and oppression. Remember the cautionary tale of Pygmalion. In George Bernard Shaw's (1916/1940) version, Henry Higgins, a professor of phonetics, gives Eliza Doolittle, a working-class Cockney woman, a language "makeover." Liza undergoes a kind of linguistic "Stockholm syndrome"—taken hostage by circumstances in another culture, caste, or class, people sometimes become enamored of the language of their masters. To assimilate, to find acceptance, they speak only the words of the dominant culture.

In his autobiography, Richard Rodriguez (1983) poignantly narrates the shift from the intimate private world of his family, communicating in Spanish, to the public world represented by a decision (really a demand) to speak only English. For Rodriguez, this led to a turn away from the narrative resources available in his Mexican heritage. He is critical of bilingual education in the United States, yet the opening lines of his memoir suggest that he has retaliated against the imposition of English on his growing mind: "I have taken Caliban's advice. I have stolen their books" (Rodriguez, 1983, p. 3).

I will return to Rodriguez's memoir, which is moving in its passion and forthrightness, later. It is one man's story of how to deal with a plural identity. He chooses to see himself as an American who speaks English. He acknowledges that he is uncomfortable in Spanish and with his Mexican heritage. Before using Rodriguez's book as a model for a pluricultural society, we should listen to the stories of other people who are able to draw on their full repertoire of cultural narratives.

Language is a living thing, getting its life through its speakers. The attempt to impose one way of speaking (represented by education and class in the stories of Liza and Rodriguez) on another is a diminishment of what Steiner calls "alternities of being," expressed in language communities. This has echoes in current dilemmas: the debates over bilingualism in public schools in the United States, Canada's official bilingualism (while in Quebec, language laws give primacy to French in public life), and bilingualism in Ireland and Wales (see Edwards, 1994). I am not advocating either/ or solutions: neither suppression of these vibrant forms of communication nor giving them privilege over more commonly shared forms of expression (standard English or French). In fact, in much of the world, people are *diglossic*—speaking their own local dialect or vernacular and the national or standard language. Examples include Black English in the U.S., *joual* in Quebec, and *créole* in Haiti.

My concern is that, when faced with distress, people need the comforting familiarity of their own language to express themselves. Any host society that treats its immigrants with contempt toward their preferred way of speaking can only add to their distress. Any national majority that restricts public discourse to approved or official languages is practicing linguistic tyranny. This is done at every level, not just by governments. It is practiced by agencies and health care centers which do not provide translation services to sizable, known populations of immigrants and minorities. It is present in encounters where therapists are ignorant of, indifferent to, or actively hostile toward the language of their clients or the limitations of their expressive skills.

2. *Narrative impoverishment.* In their work on narrative aspects of development and autobiographical memory, Jerome Bruner and Carol Feldman discuss the narrative resources that children draw from their families and their cultures (Cayley, 1995). But circumstances may constrain and diminish what some families and groups can impart, leading to a narrative impoverishment of their children. Carol Feldman gives the example of "children who emigrate from one language/literacy/narrative culture to another at a key age may

end up not knowing the literary products in the first language, and never really learning them in the next language either'' (cited in Cayley, 1995, p. 17).

Let me give a historical example. Anthropologists use the term ''empty rituals'' to describe actions that people perform but cannot explain. Examples include lighting sabbath candles and placing stones on graves by the *conversos* and *marranos* of the Iberian peninsula. They are descendents of Jews who were forcibly converted during the Inquisition but secretly retained the rituals of Judaism. After centuries of secret activity, however, many have lost any meaningful understanding of the Jewish basis for these actions and come up ''empty'' when asked to explain their rituals. Imagine an entire way of life filled with such actions and no meaningful belief system to support them.

Under other circumstances, people do not have the opportunity to develop their stories. For these reasons, Richard Rorty (1989) wrote on ''other voices'':

> So victims of cruelty, people who are suffering, do not have much in the way of a language. That is why there is no such thing as the ''voice of the oppressed'' or the ''language of the victims.'' The language the victims once used is not working anymore, and they are suffering too much to put new words together. So the job of putting their situation into language is going to have to be done for them by somebody else. (p. 94)

How can we do this? With cultural family therapy, our approach is first to elucidate their idioms of distress and explanatory models of illness by understanding their ''presenting culture.'' What we are after here is what Rorty (1989) calls the person's, the family's, the group's ''final vocabulary'': ''Those words are as far as he can go with language'' (Rorty, 1989, p. 73).

CONCLUSION

[A] human being performs an act of translation, in the full sense of the word, when receiving a speech-message from any other human being. In short: *inside or between languages, human communication equals translation.*

—George Steiner
(1975, p. 47, italics in original)

Translation is a metaphor for communication and relationships. What translation, code-switching, and working with culture teach me as a transcultural psychiatrist is that the Tower of Babel is an appropriate image for the diversity of cultures and the family's experience within them. What I have learned from conducting cultural family therapy is that there is no single Rosetta Stone for translating the experience of all families or all cultures. Understanding each unique family and its culture requires many such translations and many different tools ("When in Rome, do as the Romans do"). Translation is so fundamental that it has become the key metaphor for my clinical work. "Meeting strangers" always means a process of word- and world-mapping following the code-switches of language, of making comparisons, of perceiving cultural costume and camouflage, and above all, of translating.

Finally, family therapy, too, is more than words. The cultural family therapist becomes involved in a family process and a cultural encounter. As was evident in the treatment of the two immigrant families with an anorexic daughter, language is a tool in the perception of interactional patterns and affective states. Attending to the details of both family process and cultural costume, the therapist can come to know each family as the unique result of these factors. Furthermore, as the two cases demonstrate, the therapist can work effectively as either insider or outsider, in terms of culture, language, or working style. Even language problems can be used effectively by asking for repetitions and clarifications when significant patterns emerge. Language is only one expressive channel, given to the same uncertainties of interpretation as other aspects of the cultures that families bear. All therapy is a form of translation—of language, of culture, and of family process.

Chapter 5

CHANGELINGS

Children and Families in Cultural Transition

> . . . a harbinger of a multipolar and multicultural world,
> where no single philosophy, no single belief, no single solu-
> tion, can shunt aside the extreme wealth of mankind's cul-
> tural heritage. Our future depends on the enlarged freedom
> for the multiracial and the polycultural to express itself in a
> world of shifting, decaying and emerging power centres.
>
> —Carlos Fuentes,
> "Words Apart" (1989, p. 248)

In this chapter, I bring together the themes of this book so far—that individuals need to be understood in the context of their families and that families need to be understood in the context of culture. Identity is formed within and through the contexts of family and culture. The royal road for understanding "mind," "self," and "identity" is in the "presenting culture" of children and their families. This is examined and illustrated through the special problems of children undergoing cultural change, whom I call "changelings." These issues are explored in five stories of migrant children and their families and the issues for identity and adaptation that emerge while working with them in therapy. The fifth conceptual tool of CFT is the negotiation of cultural strategies that children and families use for adaptation and acculturation.

CULTURAL CHANGE

changeling *noun* **1** *archaic:* one that wavers; **2** *obsolete:* a fraudulent substitute surreptitiously left in place of a valued object or personage

150

adjective **1** *archaic*: wavering, inconstant; **2** markedly altered from an original or native condition

—*Webster's Dictionary* (1966)

Children and their families who are in cultural transition present a complex but rewarding task for the family therapist (Nann, 1982). The complexity arises from the simultaneous flux and interplay of several variables (Bullrich, 1989; Rakoff, 1981; Westermeyer, 1991):

1. the family's migration from one society to another,
2. the children's growth and development,
3. their encounter with a new culture,
4. the differential rates of adaptation among family members,
5. the diverse cultural definitions of interpersonal and mental problems and of culturally sanctioned solutions that shape help-seeking behavior.

What makes the task rewarding is the opportunity to work with people who are usually motivated to open and to enter new doors of experience, who are willing to instruct their providers about their cultures of origin and to explore together newly adaptive approaches to living. This is an optimistic view. I hope to demonstrate the reasons for my optimism in spite of the negative evidence of the available transcultural literature. Much of the transcultural psychiatric literature concentrates on problems:

- the potentially disorienting effects of migration (see Beiser, 1989; Nann, 1982; Pfister-Ammende, 1973),
- the difficulties of getting immigrants to mainstream health care services or the underrepresentation of certain cultural communities in mental health services (see Beiser, 1989; Murphy, 1973),
- the linguistic, economic, and social barriers encountered by both immigrants and providers in negotiating mental health care (Kleinman, 1988; Westermeyer, 1991).

There are both pragmatic and epistemological objections to this negative view of cultural transition. Pragmatically, this literature deals with migration under the most difficult circumstances: waves of mass migration in earlier eras (e.g., the Irish in nineteenth-century U.S.A.), mass economic migration (e.g., *Gastarbeiter* or "guest workers" in post-war Germany), and war refugees and torture victims (e.g., Argentinians and Chileans; see Allodi, 1989). It must also be noted that such accounts are as revealing about the limitations of health care delivery systems in host countries as about the cultural communities they hope to serve (Westermeyer, 1991). Furthermore, clinicians tend to report problems. There are few systematic studies of the experience of migration and cultural change among people who do not have identified medical or psychiatric problems.

Epistemologically, transcultural research on migration has been shaped by negative conceptions of the transcultural encounter rather than more positive conceptions that are available or can be constructed (see my exploration of this theme in Chapter 3; cf. Kracke, 1987). Cultural family therapy offers an opportunity to explore cultural encounters to construct new metaphors for child development (see Valsiner, 1989) and family experience and new tools for working with children and their families (see DiNicola, 1992, in press). Constructing new metaphors requires a reworking of our notions of culture, family, and child development. In Chapter 3, we examined ways to look at culture and family. This chapter draws on the work being done on transcultural aspects of child psychiatry (Canino, 1988; Canino & Spurlock, 1994; DiNicola, 1992, 1996, in press; Earls & Eisenberg, 1991; Grizenko et al., 1992; McDermott, 1991; Vargas & Koss-Chioino, 1992) and transcultural aspects of family therapy (DiNicola, 1985b, 1985c, 1986, 1994; Falicov, 1983; Seltzer, 1988; Sorel, 1990; Tseng & Hsu, 1991) that are useful in the practice of cultural family therapy.

Erik Erikson (1960) described a "transitory identity" that children assume in response to the crises of uprootedness and loss of assigned or expected identity. Due to the cross-currents of change in the lives of children crossing cultures, we can view them as "changelings"—an update on the fairy-tale notion of a strange child left in place of a family's own valued child. The notion of changelings not only *denotes* the children undergoing change, but *connotes* something about the family and cultural myths grounding that change. In postmodern society, the changeling is the child whose life is altered from her original condition in her native place. Sometimes, the child's life is changed by reason of her rapid acculturation to a new society or culture (see review by Berry et al.,

1987), putting the child at odds with the slower pace of adaptation of her parents or older siblings (see the stories of Samya Shami in Chapters 1 and 9 and Luisa Pasquini in Chapter 4). The ultimate changelings, in this sense, may be the children who are involved in intercultural or interracial adoption, an issue of increasing relevance and the subject of controversy (Cederblad, 1981; Green, 1983).

"LOOKING ACROSS AT GROWING UP": MIGRANT CHILDREN AND THEIR FAMILIES

I would like to illustrate these issues by examining the psychiatric problems of five young people and their families from cultural communities outside the Canadian mainstream—an exercise that anthropologist Charles Super (1980) calls "looking across at growing up." Each story illustrates different ways in which culture affects the inner experience, the family mythology, and the cultural construction of children's mental disorders.

These stories are about children and adolescents whose families moved across cultures as migrants. The cultural experience extended into and became a part of their therapeutic encounters with me. At times, this was helpful and healing; at other times, intercultural differences were a barrier. Parallel stories could be told about children and adolescents who experience cultural dislocation without moving. This is occurring among some Native groups in Canada whose subcultures are rapidly changing under their feet. The change is so great that the cultural continuity of entire families and communities is at stake. The devastating results for identity have created an epidemic of suicides among young Native people in some Northern Canadian communities (Gotowiec & Beiser, 1993–94). Similar intergenerational problems have been described in the rapidly changing societies in the Middle East (El-Islam, 1983; El-Islam et al., 1986).

Thami Kumalo: "The Story of an African Harlequin"

What else was he but a divided child?

—Derek Walcott (1986, p. 183)

Presenting culture. Ottawa, early 1990s. Thami Kumalo is an 11-year-old boy from Africa. His parents were born in Soweto, South Africa; his mother from the Xhosa tribe, his father a Zulu. The parents later emigrated to Swaziland, where father died of natural causes. Thami and his five siblings are being raised by their mother, Elizabeth. At the age of nine years, Thami witnessed the destruction of his home and the abduction of his mother by South African security forces. Elizabeth Kumalo was held for over two months in solitary confinement, where political demands were made to which she did not acquiesce. Within months of her release and return to Swaziland, mother fled in fear to Canada with her children.

Thami was brought to me because of a parent-child problem. I chose to work with him through his family (in family therapy) and to meet his family through him (he was my portal of entry into their world). In the first session, he was taciturn and terse, but willing to draw. He drew a harlequin figure, half orange, half purple, with red hair ''like mine,'' Thami said. The two sides of the figure were mismatched not only in color but in size and shape. For example, the pupils of the large staring eyes have markedly different sizes. To me, the drawing talks about differences, about trying to fit in and not making it. Of course, my perceptions and interpretations are literally ''colored'' by living in largely white European and North American cities. Thami, however, comes from a different world: what does a symbol like the harlequin, derived from *arlecchino*, a character in the Italian *commedia dell'arte* of the 1500s, mean to an African child? What has color come to mean for this boy?

In response to my questions (I do not know if he would have put it this way on his own), this is what Thami told me: the figure he calls George is from a tribe of people who are all of mixed colors—purple and orange. They live in a world where other people are different (e.g., some are green and blue, red and yellow) but they are all friends and they all get along, he said pointedly. I find it hard to put my own questions aside—why does the drawing have the English name George? Although Thami's parents both had European names, Thami and his siblings all have African names.

Do the two different colors and the English name state a perception of difference and a wish on Thami's part to bridge that difference? Is the difference about his parents who came from two

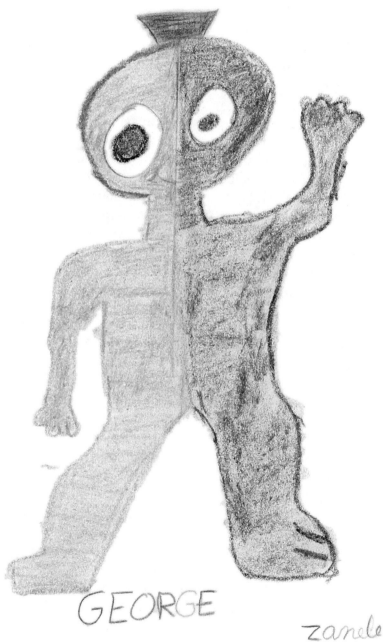

GEORGE

zanele

diverse tribes of southern Africans? Is the raised arm the militant salute of the African National Congress? Or is the difference represented in the harlequin about being a Black African in a largely White Canadian city? I am not sure if I can grasp the correct interpretation.

Cultural family therapy. There are several threads I can follow with Thami and his family:

1. Listen to Thami's story so that we can get to know each other's worlds. Together, we can map out a common language of perception and communication. That implies a mindful process, conducted over a number of sessions, perhaps in different settings, including his home. As Arthur Kleinman (1988) suggests, clients are more likely to tell their story in their own way (what he calls explanatory models) when they are on their own ground.

2. Ask Elizabeth about the African cultural context of her family life. For example, what does it mean in Africa when a Xhosa marries a Zulu? Perhaps the mother would not expect a Canadian psychiatrist to be familiar with these aspects of her life and might even be embarrassed to mention such parochial matters. Would Xhosa/Zulu intermarriage generate conflict, either at the time of their marriage or subsequently, given the social changes that have occurred in South Africa? And what of their children? How would children integrate the two backgrounds? Would Thami be, as Caribbean poet Derek Walcott asks in one of his most powerful poems, "a divided child"?

3. Chart the family's entry into Canadian society and how they negotiate their cultural encounters. Watch for differential rates of acculturation of the family members and the conflict this may generate. Facilitate their search for elements in their presenting culture that will help them in their new culture.

My construction of Thami's experience is the product of my cultural translation of his experience. This brings me much closer to the child's experiences across cultures, because my process of translation attempts to reconstruct his journey—not objectively but through my subjective effort to reach him. Thami's story and his drawing of the orange and purple harlequin illustrate therapy as a cultural bridge.

Alicia Edmunds: "A Caribbean Cordelia"

Presenting problem. Ottawa, late 1980s. Alicia Edmunds was a 15-year-old Black Jamaican adolescent brought to my attention by the Children's Aid Society because of the violence she directed toward her sister Grace. The family also identified serious parent-child, marital and family problems.

The violent incident occurred when Alicia and her 16-year-old sister, Grace, were at home alone. During an argument, Alicia grabbed a knife and threatened her sister with it, lightly grazing Grace's face. The police were called in and the parents were contacted. The parents came home to face this situation with the police at their home and Alicia charged for attacking Grace. The Children's Aid Society became involved because of protection issues and Alicia was referred by the agency for a psychiatric assessment. Questioning revealed that over several months Alicia had become increasingly sullen and withdrawn, angry at home, and failing at school. The violent exchange with her sister seemed to be the culmination of her family and social frustrations rather than a pattern of conduct disturbance.

Presenting family culture. The father, Gregory, was a well-educated, older Black man from Kingston, Jamaica, where he had held a government position. Marion, the mother, was a much younger, uneducated Black woman from a rural Jamaican mountain town. In Jamaica, the parents had a "morganatic marriage," that is, a socially sanctioned arrangement between two people of different "castes" without a conventional marriage. This arrangement gave Gregory the children he had always wanted and an attractive, constantly available younger partner. Marion received financial and practical support to maintain a house for herself and her children, where Gregory visited regularly and sometimes lived. They both agreed that in Jamaica she had free reign over the house and children and that he was a financially generous but busy and uninvolved father. This predicament of the Jamaican family is captured in Mary de Chesnay's (1986) description of the "paradox of normalcy." Using de Chesnay's analysis, Alicia's father, as part of the ruling class, adopted a Eurocentric patriarchal family model, whereas her lower-class mother established a matrifocal family.

When political changes in Jamaica made Gregory's social position untenable, the couple opted to marry in order to immigrate to Canada. In Jamaica, Marion had free reign over her daughters and her house, where the father was essentially a visitor. In their new country, however, the social rules supporting their couple relationship no longer worked and the family became extremely dysfunctional. Here, they suddenly had to accommodate to a new arrangement: living together as married partners and sharing the parenting of their daughters. The patriarchal style of the father came into jarring conflict with the matrifocal home of the three females. In Jamaica, Gregory's lifestyle of seeing numerous women was socially accepted (or so he said) and made possible by having two different homes. This arrangement gave him the narcissistic gratification he sought, whereas living together under one roof made it impossible. Confined to one relationship and now parenting his daughters for the first time, Gregory chafed at the restrictions in his marriage and demanded loyalty and obedience from his daughters. After a few years, with the age difference and the rigidly hierarchical relationship he demanded from his wife, Marion became more and more like a third daughter.

Cultural family therapy. During our first session, the two sisters, Alicia and Grace, and their mother, Marion, sat quietly while Gregory explained why they had been sent to see me. The father told the story in great detail, patiently and deliberately. In my attempts to join with all the family members, I posed questions or comments to other family members, asked for confirmation of details, and tried to get parts of the story from the perspectives of the mother and the sisters.

Father would listen attentively to my questions, then plow doggedly on, adding more details to his account or embellishing what others said. Within minutes, a pattern was set: Alicia and Grace occasionally managed to complete a statement of their own, but Marion was effectively silenced by her husband. I couldn't be sure about the feelings of the women in the family, but father was clearly angry about the problems within the family and ashamed by the involvement of outsiders—police, the children's agency, and psychiatrists.

Noting this, I decided to move away from the presenting problem and work with the presenting culture. Due to Gregory's evident anguish and shame and his dominant presence in the interview so far, I sensed that he would place me as an "outsider" to his world. My first cultural intervention, therefore, was to adopt an outsider position. I expressed curiosity about Jamaica, noting that with my roots in Europe and North America, I had never had the opportunity to live or work there.

Gregory launched into an informative and lively discussion of Jamaica, drawing a map of the island, decribing his home town of Kingston and the mountains where Marion came from, and touching on the changing politics of the country. Again, I gently tried to draw Marion and the sisters into this exchange, with moderate success. So far, my approach had worked: there were more family interactions, less tension, and even some smiles and laughter as they described Jamaica and their home there. I now felt closer to Gregory, whom I perceived as working hard to be agreeable and helpful. I was genuinely fascinated by his culture but I could also sense the pain of dislocation he must be feeling in going from being a political mandarin in Jamaica to a mid-level civil servant in Canada.

The clinical issues I faced in this first session included: How could I help Alicia tell her own story with her family present? Given an unbalanced family, how could I join the family as a whole? Should I align with the father who asserted himself or side with the others whose voices weren't being heard? "Spiraling" is one of the first process issues in conducting family sessions. It was a problem from the outset with Alicia's family, as her father took charge and wanted me to fall in line with the rule of obedience that he obviously imposed on his family.

I decided to meet the family *through the father*. I thought it futile to create a space for Alicia if this would heighten tensions in the family. After their experience with the police and the Children's Aid Society, I wanted to establish my therapeutic credibility by working with the family as an ally rather than as an authority.

Practically, what I did is to continue obtaining the history from the father, taking notes of his account, occasionally checking details with other family members. The others looked like they were pinned to their seats, helpless and hopeless. In a sense, I never succeeded in working with the family as a whole. What I did have was a series of shifting alliances with different members of the family. I was able to engage Gregory as a person and, later, to work with Marion and the girls. What did not occur was their working together as a family.

If I had to do it again, I would consider two courses of action:

1. While continuing to work alone, I could discuss my predicament openly with the family. Many clinicians handle such situations by separating different tasks, seeing the parents (together or individually) to discuss marital issues and seeing the children separately.

2. Expand my therapeutic resources by bringing in a consultant (see Andolfi & Haber, 1994). I could bring in a family therapy consultant to identify and help manage the complexities. We could speak to the conflicting parts of the family system with a "reflecting team" that would voice the different concerns of various family members. When I experienced the control issues with Gregory, I could have sought a cultural consultant to inform me about Jamaican culture and families or to comment on the transcultural encounter between the family and me.

The parental couple. As therapy progressed, Marion's voice strengthened. I supported her in subtle ways, and gradually her daughters validated her right to tell her own story. Gregory's response was angry and dramatic.

He arrived at what was to be his last session stating with great ceremony that he had something to say. Ignoring the issues that had brought them into therapy, he complained that I had questioned whether he understood a word, treating him "like a boy in second form" (junior high school). In the previous session when Gregory was discussing relationships with different women in his life, Marion asked him about a letter she found from a woman which mentioned "eating a mango." From the looks they exchanged, I understood that this had a sexual meaning. Gregory launched into a pedantic explanation about mangos and then added, "I am dissembling." I suppose it was a kind of wink from one man to another, but it caught me off-guard. Surprised, I asked him, "I don't understand. Do you mean you're not telling the truth?" Initially, Gregory may have been annoyed at my ignorance, but after the session he apparently experienced my question as a narcissistic injury, which he resolved by rejecting me as a therapist.

But there is a greater systemic truth to his distress: the more damaging injury was coming from his wife, who was questioning their life together. My hypothesis that he externalized the threat from the family system to the therapeutic system is supported by the words he used to end the session: "I must admit you have done one thing, which is to make this family 'circle the wagons.' You have made me realize that I must take things into my own hands as I should have done all along." He never returned. "Circling the wagons" turned out to be Gregory's protest against intruders, not a commitment to his family. Marion responded to my offer of help for a time and the relationships with her daughters greatly improved with her separation from her husband.

Alicia. A colleague has commented that Alicia gets lost in the description of the mother and father. This is astute: Alicia was lost in the fog of confused family relationships. Later, when the parents' marital problems were more openly identified, Alicia's own dilemmas became clearer. The real issue is that Alicia got lost in the family move from Jamaica to Canada when the parental relationship was redefined. It is often true in troubled families that children are either ignored or recruited into dysfunctional roles. Children can be neglected when they are caught in triangles among other family members with stronger voices. Children can also develop psychiatric symptoms in an effort to resolve marital, family, or social problems and when they take on developmentally (e.g., adult) or structurally (e.g., parental) inappropriate roles.

Alicia's personal experience is complex. Although she was the identifed patient, having threatened her sister with a knife, she felt that more often she was herself the victim of emotional and physical abuse within the family. Alicia felt she had been her father's favorite and was puzzled and distressed by his anger towards her. After her father's exit from therapy, when the family problems were explored in marital, family, and cultural terms, Alicia quickly experienced relief. Her relationships to her mother and sister improved dramatically with father's emotional withdrawal from therapy and became stabilized when he left the home.

The family. Experience with family therapy teaches that changing family alliances can create family tragedies. In this family, the changes were brought on by the combination of transcultural change from Jamaica to Canada, by the changing needs for self-definition that adolescence brought to the daughters, and by the mother's increasing realization that her morganatic marriage had given her too little. Mother's acculturation to Canada meant that she wanted more within her marriage, but to her husband this became an unbearable lien against the limited sources of his self-esteem. In structural family therapy terms, the family system regained the stable structure that had worked in Jamaica with a return to a matrifocal family.

A transcultural interpretation. "Cordelia" is a metaphoric reference to Shakespeare's tragedy of King Lear, an aged and increasingly demented king who poses what appears to be a rhetorical question to his three daughters about how much each one loves him so that he can divide his kingdom among them. Lear's tragedy is in being taken seriously (by Cordelia) and in being unmasked by a serious response to a rhetorical question (see philosopher Stanley Cavell's interpretation of *King Lear*; Cavell, 1976). Alicia's father treated his much younger wife as a daughter and he acted very much like Lear in narcissistically gauging the love of three "daughters" (actually, his wife and two daughters) by the fateful yardstick of obedience and obeisance. This put him profoundly at odds (as he partly recognized) with the mainstream values of Canadian society.

In cultural terms, the parents could not adapt their marriage and family structure in ways that are culturally viable in mainstream Canadian society. Some family therapists suggest an acculturation model for migrants using the notion of two homes, where the task is a constant integration of the old home into the new home (Turner, 1991). The individuals in this Jamaican family were attempting this integration in different ways and at different rates, with the result that the family as a whole could not achieve a workable balance between the old home and the new home. When the family reverted to its previous Jamaican structure, the therapy had to be renegotiated with them to deal with individual issues (especially the mother's and Alicia's) and with dyadic relationships (mother-daughter, sibling).

This family has tragic dimensions because Gregory does love his wife and daughters and desperately needs their approval and affection, but he undermines his own needs by his overbearing behavior. Alicia takes her father very seriously and responds truthfully about her own and the family's distress. Like Cordelia, she is the father's favorite, and she pays a price for being truthful. Father feels betrayed by Alicia's "switch" from her privileged status as favorite daughter to "whistleblower." During the investigation into her own violent behavior, Alicia revealed all the troubled relationships within the family. This was a blow to the father's narcissism and his need for approval and control, coming as the most obvious and overt of a series of challenges he perceived. As a result of these events in Canada, the father began to experience Alicia as a stranger, a changeling he no longer recognized and could not accept. Although Gregory needed her affection, he could not accept her because his narcissism had made him increasingly rigid and incapable of changing.

The story of King Lear is finally the story of failed alliances, as the King recklessly mistrusts, mistreats, and abandons all his loyal allies. Alicia's father similarly seems incapable of alliances and of reaching out for help. When it is offered to him, his paranoid view of the world leaves him stranded on an empty island of his own making. This is the way narcissists end: by burning all the bridges to other human beings behind them. In a sadly parallel process, for Gregory this led to a stalemate of therapy and the dissolution of his marriage.

Musa Noor: "A Train of Traumas"

Presenting problem. Ottawa, early 1990s. Musa was a 10-year-old boy, a Somali refugee, with the presenting complaint of bedwetting. Musa sat in my office drawing Ninja Turtles just as any other Canadian boy would. The difference was in the details: vivid and realistic pictures of bombs exploding and bodies strewn in their wake. He explained one picture, in English, as "planes dropping bombs on my country."

Musa's father had worked for the president of his country and had been able to provide well for his family. However, when civil war broke out, Musa's father was accused of plotting against the government and tortured. Musa's mother said that her husband could no longer recognize her or their children. They escaped with their lives and little else, leaving family and friends behind. Musa and his family experienced many cruelties and privations during their escape from Somalia and in a refugee camp in Ethiopia.

At his new home in Canada, Musa lived with his mother and four siblings in subsidized housing near train tracks. At night, he was awakened by the nearby trains, which the mother believed caused his bedwetting. When the child awoke, he related nightmares to his mother, who had her own terrifying memories to contend with. From the noise of the train to bedwetting and nightmares, and to memories of their civil war, for this family one trauma summons another in a train of traumas.

One could tease out the individual components in this train of traumas: the bedwetting was diagnosed as functional enuresis, secondary type—regressive behavior caused by war trauma and now triggered by the noise of the train in the night (Garfinkel et al., 1990). Since enuresis occurs during nondreaming sleep, the nightmares were probably flashbacks that occurred after Musa was awakened in the night and understood as dreams. The child waking up fearfully in the night was in turn a disturbing trigger for the mother's own traumatic memories, although during the day she appeared remarkably poised. Over the months that we worked with them, the mother's poise was better described as a combination of a survivor's coping strategy and post-traumatic numbing. The components of this train of traumas add up in each case—both mother and child—to symptoms of PTSD.

Treatment with Musa and his mother was aimed first at explaining his bedwetting and then symptom relief. Two months' treatment with an antidepressant cured the enuresis. As the work shifted to the family and to mother's personal issues, I consulted with a French-speaking female social worker who joined as cotherapist. Gently, over time, while focusing on concrete issues like bedwetting, housing, and other practical needs, we were able to develop a working relationship with Musa's mother, who taught us much about Somali culture.

Musa's mother: "Moulting a layer of culture." Musa's mother, Nima, was raised as a Muslim. She had married very young to an ambitious Catholic man. Nima explained to us that 90% of Somalis are Muslims, but when Muslim women marry outside the faith they tend to adopt the other faith. Although she did not convert, she agreed to raise the children as Catholics. She went with her husband to Marseilles, France, where he pursued an education for several years. As a result, she spoke French fluently. Our family sessions (child, mother, and therapists) were quite complex, as there was no single language we all had in common. Mother and child communicated in Somali, while we conversed with the child in English and with the mother in French.

As a result of marrying young and going abroad, Nima managed to avoid "female circumcision" (clitoridectomy, or excision of the clitoris). However, she did undergo a form of "infibulation" (so-called "Pharaonic circumcision"—sewing up of most of the vulva leaving only a small opening for the passing of fluids, in her case without any excision). She told us that several young Canadian doctors who examined her had obviously never encountered women from North Africa, as they were shocked by the scars across her vulva from the sutures. It took extraordinary courage for her to refuse to take part in the ritual mutilation of clitoridectomy. In refusing this ritual as a child, she was distancing herself from a fundamental part of her own culture, jealously guarding what Alice Walker (1992) poetically describes as "the secret of joy." This courage, so evident in her childhood, is also the key to her resilience in adapting to Canada.[1]

As we treated Nima's depression and other symptoms of PTSD, this intelligent woman, who had survived the ordeal of civil war, entered a rapid process of culture shock and acculturation. She spoke at great length about the freedom of women in Canada, which contrasted with the stories of her upbringing, her arranged marriage and forced infibulation, and the ruses she had to use to avoid a clitoridectomy. She was "moulting a layer of culture." We witnessed her going through a rejection of her culture of origin, mostly aimed at men in Somalia/Ethiopia and how they had treated her. This became concrete when she sought a divorce from her husband, who was a chronic patient at a psychiatric hospital. I was concerned that in rejecting her culture of origin so vehemently and so quickly she would create a great void in her life. But she was propelled forward by the clarity of the experiences from which she wanted to distance herself. And this was a source of resilience for her.

The therapeutic process shifted from Musa to his family, from individual symptoms to the complex predicament described as PTSD and, finally, from clinical psychiatry to a cultural encounter. Both Musa and his mother were like changelings: their world was in rapid flux. Constant new adaptations and adjustments were required. The flux was not only in their new world but perhaps even more profoundly in their redefinitions of the one they had left.

Jasmine Prasad: "Culture as a Dirty Window"

Ottawa, late 1980s. Jasmine Prasad is a 15-year-old adolescent referred by a community agency. The presenting complaint concerned behavior problems at her group home and at school. Jasmine comes from Guyana, where her family was well-off and her father was politically prominent. When her father was murdered, the family lost its center, and her large nuclear family started to drift to other countries, so that she has siblings all over North America—in the U.S. and Canada. She came to Ottawa with her mother, who later left her with Jasmine's older sister. The sister became abusive to her; it was noticed at school and the children's agency stepped in, placing her in a group home. The agency sought psychiatric help when the placement was breaking down.

I did what child psychiatrists do: took a detailed history over several clinical interviews, conducted a mental status exam, administered rating scales, and sent her for further diagnostic psychological tests (all these diagnostic attempts have fundamental problems of both validity and reliability across cultures). I considered starting her on antidepressant medication for her depression complicated by a variety of losses: bereavement over her father, abandonment by her mother, abuse from her sister, and the loss of her homeland, her home, and her culture. She had witnessed the beating of her father, which led to his death, and now exhibited sequelae typical of PTSD: nightmares, anxiety, depression, and a numbed response to her social world.

Her social worker was active, supportive, warm, deeply interested in her, and spent a disproportionate amount of time with her despite a heavy caseload. After a couple of sessions with Jasmine, I asked to meet her sister. This was vetoed by her social worker; furthermore, the sister had refused to attend. I then asked to meet with her mother, who lived in Toronto, but she could not afford to come to Ottawa. As a last resort, I asked Jasmine to bring her foster-mother or a friend. She sadly stated that she didn't have any friends close enough to come and became very upset by my request to meet her foster-mother. She nonetheless acceded to my meeting her.

When the foster-mother came to the interview, I met an efficient group home manager who lectured at Jasmine for most of the session. I could make nothing of it.

As the weeks went by and she lost more and more weight despite her treatment, I suspected an eating disorder. As I questioned her about her eating habits, I learned she wasn't eating! Why not? She didn't like the food at the group home!

I have not mentioned Jasmine's ethnic or racial background. Jasmine is of East Indian descent.[2] The group home mother was a Black woman from the West Indies. The agency had thought that in placing this young woman of "color" with a Black group home mom, they had made an inspired match. Nothing could be further from the truth. Jasmine liked neither this Black woman nor the food she cooked. The Blacks with whom she had contact in her own country were mostly servants in her lavish home. She was never asked what she would think of living in this group home. In fact, it was assumed that she shared our view of herself as a cultural and racial "outsider" to our society. In this view, immigrants are homogenized as undifferentiated "others." Since they are not "us," they are naively assumed to have some kind of solidarity among themselves.

I arranged some practical interventions. First, she was given some money to buy her own food, for which we located grocery shops that sold the foodstuffs of her culture. Within a week, she started gaining weight. After several weeks, she was transferred to a new group home, and we spent a lot of time on a project where she wrote out her family and cultural history. When she had called herself "Indian," her workers had assumed she meant Amerindian, rather than East Indian. She joined a church group with people from her own country and faith. And finally, she was transferred to Toronto, where her mother and other siblings live and where there is a sizable community from her home country.

For this case, one had to be a child psychiatrist, know about depression and conduct disorders, and know how to manage PTSD. But all of these skills could not elucidate her predicament, that is, place this particular person with her specific problems in context. To do that, one had to know how culture interacts with all of this to produce Jasmine, a unique person with a highly individual problem. That is what transcultural child psychiatry is about in the clinic: the elucidation of the child's predicament. Jasmine's story illustrates what people generally expect to hear about ethnic misperceptions—that culture is sometimes like a "dirty window," obstructing our view of the other side.

River Running: "A White Boy Who Thought He Was Cree"

> There is no chart of his movement through
> the borrowed forest,
> A place so alien that all he could do with it
> was pretend it was his own
>
> —Gwendolyn MacEwen,
> *Grey Owl's Poem* (1987, p. 72)

Ottawa, mid-80s. River Running is an 11-year-old boy raised by his White parents in Northern Canada where they were the only White family in a Cree Indian village. Mother taught school and father ran the village store. The family was *in the village but not part of it*: it was not so much a racial issue as one of rank and power. As the operator of the only store, father was in a position to affect the lives of all the other families through his financial decisions about credit.

River grew up with Indian children and was socialized into Cree folkways and values. This seemed to work for River and his four younger brothers in Cree country, but when they moved to a southern Canadian city they had problems. River stood out as odd. Identified problems included urinating in the garden or on the playground. The parents explained that their child's behavior simply reflected the way he was raised in the Cree village. They could not appreciate the extent to which this put River at odds with others, as they themselves could not succeed in becoming part of the social mainstream. They rigidly maintained a combative attitude to the educational and therapeutic systems that offered help. Mother had left a convent to become a teacher in the Canadian North. Father, an intelligent man who could be a character study for Henry David Thoreau, left his small fishing village where he did not fit in and similarly gave up his university studies because he felt alienated there. The two parents met and married in the North and together maintained their apartness from their cultures of origin. They had five children and eventually decided to leave because of their unsuccessful integration into Cree village life.

This family's predicament has two components: (a) their cultural drift into and out of another cultural tradition, and (b) the social isolation of the parents both before and after their Cree sojourn. Their "apartness" blocked such adaptive strategies as the "double description" often observed in immigrant families, where the children adopt two parallel identities—the family's cultural identity at home and the host culture's mainstream identity outside the home. River's parents could not create a home identity with any clarity because they were both refugees from other Canadian subcultures. By default, if not by design, River identified with what surrounded him everywhere (except at home): Cree culture.

"The Grey Owl Syndrome." By going to Cree country, what were River's parents looking for? There is in Canada a long-standing desire, discernible both in the history of European settlement and in our fiction, which Margaret Atwood (1995), Canada's pre-eminent chronicler of our fictional landscape, calls "The Grey Owl Syndrome":

> that curious phenomenon, the desire among non-Natives to turn themselves into Natives; a desire that becomes entwined with a version of wilderness itself . . . as the repository of salvation and new life. (p. 35)

The "syndrome" is named for an actual individual, a European who convincingly became a Native known as Grey Owl. What is instructive about Grey Owl is not that he was a counterfeit, but that he was so genuine in his chosen identity. Grey Owl is not so much the embodiment of modernism's "identity crisis"—there is no evidence that it was conflictual for him—as an anticipation of a postmodernist liquidity of identity. Gwendolyn MacEwen (1987) wrote a wonderful poem, "Grey Owl's Poem," articulating his situation for us.

Cultural ambivalence. In choosing to live among the Cree, was the Running couple moving towards or away from something? This is not something they could give words to, expressing only ambivalence. As for their children, what could they do but respond to the world they grew up in? River and his siblings could not comfortably adopt the strategy of double description that some of the other children in this book did. Because their parents tried to leave their culture behind, there was no "ground" for them at home. And because they were not well accepted into Cree life, there was no "figure" either. Where, then, could River turn?

Another "cultural strategy of adaptation" (my fifth conceptual of CFT—discussed later in this chapter) is to construct a kind of "créole culture" through syncretic accretions of cultural elements. This was difficult for River, as his parents were the only White people in the village; moreover, this solution would have been maladaptive for the children, since it would make them stand out rather than blend in. Above all, River's family is not culturally adaptive: for them, Cree and other Canadian cultures are separate and unbridgeable. The parents were unsuccessful at "going native," as the British used to say in India. They could not even become "bridges" between two worlds. They had lost their way, wandering in no-man's-land, and no longer had any home to return to. In Atwood's (1995) reading of MacEwen's poem, Grey Owl is "a quester in search of himself," expressing a "tragic but necessary duality," which leaves him "alien both to his original homeland and to his adopted space" (p. 58).

They had given their child a name that echoed Heraclitus—"You can't step into the same river twice"—a predicament that was true for the whole family. This was evident in their isolation when they moved to Ottawa. River and his brothers are at risk for culture-change syndromes like selective mutism because of their cultural ambivalence and isolation.[3]

River's story illustrates that culture is not only an added layer over psychology—a layer that sometimes interferes like a "dirty window" as in Jasmine's story (see Kirmayer, 1989). Culture is part of our psychological make-up—providing the extra-genetic programs or recipes (Geertz, 1973a) for the construction of the self. Culture may be understood as what German philosopher Martin Heidegger called "being-in-the-world"—persons and culture are bound together like a snail to its shell, the figure *is* the ground. This is perhaps most evident in childhood, when the cultural influences are more discernible, and is thrown into the greatest relief when cultural programs or recipes conflict, as in intercultural marriages or immigrant families. In River's story, the main cultural problem is not a dirty window that obstructs our view of the other person, nor can therapy easily be based on building bridges between worlds. (In fact, therapy was unsuccessful on several levels—individual, marital, and family—and they all dropped out. The reason is simple: they did not and would not collaborate. They could be pleasant and affable, but demanded that the school—and the rest of the world—adapt to their ways of being.) No, for River the cultural recipe for living a life is flawed because the recipe calls for ingredients that are not available to him, a condition that Jerome Bruner and Carol Feldman call "narrative impoverishment" (Cayley, 1995). Another way to put it is that River is going hungry because he has the ingredients for one meal but the recipe for quite another. Cultural ambivalence can lead to psychological starvation.

"IMAGINARY HOMELANDS": CULTURAL PROCESSES OF MIGRATIONS

Many cultural issues can be identified among these cultural changelings. Let's call this territory "imaginary homelands," as an homage to Salman Rushdie (1991a) who has explored it in brilliantly inventive novels like *Midnight's Children* (1991b) about migrations and cultural dislocations. To start with, we can examine the reasons for migration and how the host country and new culture are imagined. It is helpful to understand each family's attitudes towards their starting points and how the native country and culture of origin are defined and redefined throughout the processes of migration and acculturation.

THE REAL SOCIAL CONTEXTS OF MIGRATIONS

Just like the negative conceptions of intercultural encounters which were discussed in Chapter 3, there are traps to avoid when asking questions about migration. This territory is filled with two kinds of traps—reductionistic thinking and a systematic failure to grasp the real social context of migrations:

1. Reducing complex problems to a simpler, more manageable level: for example, trying to explain migration due to individual psychological issues, which can be in the service of a family myth that denies family-level problems. Another example would be reducing larger social and cultural problems to the family level. An otherwise fascinating psychoanalytic study of migration and exile (Grinberg & Grinberg, 1989) is marred by just this sort of reductionism in looking at "emigrability" and "fitness for emigration," suggesting that there are two categories of emigrants. While these may be interesting speculations after the fact, in the luxury and safety of therapy, even a superficial acquaintance with the history and sociology of migrations reveals that economic factors and regional traditions account for "chain migrations" that overwhelm such putative individual inclinations (see Thomas Sowell's masterly study of migrations and cultures, 1996).

2. Failure to identify the real social context of the family's predicament—poverty, discrimination, racism, and all the traumatic contexts that are tragically common—disasters, atrocities, war, and political torture. When these circumstances are identified, there may be a parallel failure to grasp the meaning, the impact, and the long-term consequences of trauma. There are an estimated 19 million refugees worldwide (Weiner, cited by Sowell, 1996). These are not just adult migrant workers but children and families fleeing everything from persecution and civil war to natural disasters. There is almost no family therapy literature on posttraumatic stress disorder (PTSD), despite its documented impact on children and families (see DiNicola, 1996b). That is not just a gap, but a systematic failure of the field.

The best antidote for this kind of reductionism is to actually talk to migrants. Where to start? Almost any large city has an immigrant aid center, often in need of volunteers. To place such experiences in context, I recommend reading the kind of history and sociology that has a broad sweep—Thomas Sowell (1996), Theodore Zeldin (1995), and Edward Said (1994). Especially for readers who are allergic to the topic, I recommend a sickening dose of books on the history of war and its frightening human impact—Paul Fussell (1991) will serve nicely for newcomers. A personal anecdote: I spent several years as a young man working with Holocaust survivors, immersing myself in all aspects of the literature on the Holocaust. It was a transformative experience, shaping my career choices and my clinical work.

The first four stories all concern children and families caught in political or wartime atrocities: Alicia's father was ousted by a change of government in Jamaica, taking his family with him. When Gregory sought political asylum in Canada, he did not bargain on changing his family life. Both Musa's and Jasmine's fathers were tortured or murdered for political reasons. Moving to Canada allowed Musa's mother to make choices that she was aware of as a child, so her acculturation was self-propelled and satisfying. Jasmine's mother seemed much more distressed, creating a terrible void in Jasmine's life. Thami's mother was systematically terrorized and fled Africa in fear. The adults in each of these families were grateful for the safety and security provided by life in Canada and thus had rather positive images of Canadian society. This was not the case for the Running family, who, despite living in their native land, were simply not at home in the world. As a result, there were few positive images to build on.

Just as important to the construction of a therapeutic system is the cultural "fit" between the family and their therapist. While I am different in many ways from all these families—in terms of culture, religion, race, class and ethnicity—it was possible to find points of possible joining. This was attempted by a combination of insider and outsider positions with each family.

Differential rates of acculturation. Looking at the differential rates of acculturation among family members is instructive. Rapid culture change within a society can lead to differential rates of adaptation among family members (El-Islam, 1983; El-Islam et al., 1986) and differential rates of acculturation when families move across cultures. Children commonly adopt the cultural values of the host or dominant culture at a pace and in a way that threatens the internal cohesion of their families. In Alicia's family, this was doubly threatening, in that both the children and the mother challenged the father's dominant role. Not surprisingly, Alicia's family could not withstand this double challenge and a breakup ensued.

Insiders and outsiders. In each case, culture was explicitly brought to therapy by the families themselves. Their experiences revealed the dominant metaphors for culture, for migrants, and for diversity in their cultures of origin and in the host culture. Attending to these parameters was not an academic exercise in the treatment of these families; rather, it allowed us to map out the boundaries between the immigrant family and the host culture. I have suggested that the perspectives of ''insiders and outsiders'' (DiNicola, 1986) usefully capture a lot of information and help to predict how the encounter of different cultural values is resolved.

The language of insiders and outsiders reveals where the family and the host culture position each other and, in turn, where the therapist is placed in his transcultural encounter with the family. To Alicia's father, I was potentially an intruder from an alien culture. Although this alien role was given to me by the father, I was able to negotiate a more positive role in interactions with the other family members. To them, I was a welcome outsider, a teacher about a world they wanted to enter. This became true for Alicia's mother. To most of these children and their families, I was an outsider. Ironically, it was only with River's family, whose culture of origin I ostensibly knew best, that therapy was unsuccessful. In fact, with the parents' cultural ambivalence and the children's narrative impoverishment, posing questions about where and how they fit seemed to amplify their predicament.

Culture-bound developmental myths. The cultural issues that arise from the family crises of the two Jamaican adolescents, Alicia and Grace, include whether ''adolescent turmoil'' is a universal developmental stage or limited to certain cultures. In Canada, as in most Western societies, adolescent turmoil has become enshrined in folklore and in developmental psychology and child psychiatry (see

Rutter et al., 1976). Is adolescent turmoil inevitable for Alicia and Grace, who were raised in Jamaica?

An anthropological review of 186 societies outside of the industrial West (Schlegel & Barry, 1991) confirmed the view of "adolescence as a social stage in all human societies" (p. 198). This thorough review of available research did not, however, find in traditional societies the turmoil that is supposed to characterize adolescence in Western society, nor does such turmoil seem to characterize adolescence in modernizing societies outside the West. "Adolescent turmoil" seems to be a Western myth about adolescent development. Only when such beliefs are challenged do they become obvious as myths, as outdated pedagogical myths attest: "children should be seen and not heard" and "spare the rod, spoil the child."

Cultural clash. Both cases reveal how difficult and powerful the clash of values can be when one cultural tradition encounters another. For Alicia's mother, Marion, the clash was in the therapeutic encounter, as she was herself rejecting some aspects of her culture of origin. The clash occurred among members of the family; only when Marion sought an ally outside her family did it hamper my therapeutic alliance with the family: to take the sting out of his wife's complaints, Gregory tried to disqualify me as a therapist.

Cultural strategies for adaptation. Exploring a family's "cultural strategies for adaptation" (DiNicola, 1992) is my fifth conceptual tool of cultural family therapy. These cultural strategies can be examined in various ways, modeled on Kracke's (1987) analysis of negative and positive conceptions of intercultural encounters. Using these ideas, we can examine how families negotiate cultural change, which depends on how they carry their culture of origin, how they experience the host culture, and what models each of those cultures makes available to that particular family. This was explored in River Running's story, earlier in this chapter. If cultures provide a smorgasbord of choices, the subculture of the family, its class, caste, religion, and attitudes, will determine its adaptive style. One adaptive style is to develop a "créole culture" (DiNicola, 1992)—a local blend of two or more cultures created through the layer-by-layer build-up of cultural elements, much like the syncretic religions of Brazil and the Caribbeans. When this strategy is not possible in the face of cultural differences, family members sometimes employ "double description" (White, 1986). Within the family culture, members endorse one set of cultural values, while outside the family they experiment with and adopt another. This is more workable as a family strategy than as an individual one, since it exposes the individual to loyalty conflicts within the family (DiNicola, 1986).

We can call the overall process of adaptation *acculturation*, which spans the spectrum from *assimilation* or total immersion into the host culture (like the American image of the "melting pot") to *estrangement* or total separation (like the former South African policy of "apartheid"). In the families presented here, Nima, Musa's mother, underwent something very close to assimilation (adapting rapidly to Canadian society, but retaining aspects of her cultural identity), while Gregory, Alicia's father, felt estranged or alienated from Canadian society and from his own family as they assimilated Canadian cultural values.

The models that families or groups use for their adaptation to another culture are commonly misunderstood and themselves engender powerful reactions. For example, Orthodox Jews are widely misperceived as rejecting modern life, whereas Orthodoxy was the response of Eastern European Jewry to *Haskalah* or the Enlightenment (Kaplan, 1990). In historical terms, Orthodoxy was a modern answer to the question of how to maintain Jewish identity in a world that was letting down the barriers to Jews.

Culture and metaphor. Metaphor is a particularly rich vein to mine in therapeutic work across cultures. For one thing, families commonly refer to practices and beliefs that may be outside the therapist's experience or knowledge. As a result, cultural experiences have to be conveyed in new words and images for the therapist. This building of a common bank of images and metaphors is the task of cultural translation, which helps to build the therapeutic relationship. And by modeling a willingness to understand the family's culture, the therapist enhances the family's capacity to understand other cultures in fresh and less threatening terms. The therapeutic encounter itself can also be rendered metaphorically. I find it helpful to give family sessions a name; also, some families are more understandable when compared to families in myth, literature, and films. Myths and great literature distill common dilemmas and perceptions about human experience. Used accurately and appropriately, metaphors about families convey greater systemic truths about our experience of them than even detailed session transcriptions or videotapes (cf. DiNicola, 1994). During my work with Alicia's family, the metaphors of a great, proud but flawed King Lear and a bewildered, innocent Cordelia allowed me to see the father's pain and the daughter's pathos. As in Shakespeare's tragedy, Alicia's family grew and changed a great deal, but not in time to keep the family together.

Culture and identity. All of these factors together have a formative impact on the child's identity. The working assumption of child psychiatrists and social scientists has been that when the cultural background is in flux, the child's core identity is less "grounded," as expressed in Erik Erikson's (1960) notion of a "transitory identity" in children who are uprooted. But with so many immigrants around the world—a recent estimate puts it at 100 million (Weiner, cited by Sowell, 1996)—change and flux are so common as to become normative in many parts of the world. If this creates crises of identity, we had better get used to them as a persistent feature.

Seeing migration as a crisis is a modernist view—grounded in the notion that identity can only be rooted in one's native geography and history. As important as these are to understanding these attachments, postmodern society demands larger attachments—at once more complex, multiple, and overlappping. As such transitoriness becomes more normative, the child as a cultural changeling will have more positive connotations. For example, bicultural children may develop a personal synthesis of world-views reflecting the different cultures they have lived in to form a "third culture": "This is an international population that has loosened its ties to a home country but does not become totally integrated into the host country" (Werkman, 1978). Such children develop a sense of *who* rather than *where* they are. In the words of a young American who grew up abroad, "you breathe a sigh of despair mixed with relief and set out toward a native country you know you must create for yourself, inside" (Werkman, 1978). Third culture children—or changelings—with an ironic sense of themselves may identify more with each other, regardless of cultural background, than with monocultural children who accept their affiliations and identities with little or no reflection.

These themes are closely tied to the themes of the next chapter, which deals with "Threshold Therapy"—a synonym for cultural family therapy when conducted with children and their families in cultural transition. I will draw some conclusions for the study of changelings and other liminal people at the end of the Chapter 6.

Chapter 6

THRESHOLD THERAPY

Liminal People and Transitional States

The attributes of liminality or of liminal *personae* ("threshold people") are necessarily ambiguous, since this condition and these persons elude or slip through the network of classifications that normally locate states and positions in cultural space. Liminal entities are neither here nor there; they are betwixt and between the positions assigned and arrayed by law, custom, convention, and ceremonial. As such, their ambiguous and indeterminate attributes are expressed by a rich variety of symbols in the many societies that ritualize social and cultural transitions.

> —Victor Turner,
> *The Ritual Process*
> (1969, p. 95)

*I*n the previous chapter, I discussed the problems associated with cultural change. Because these issues are not merely isolated special cases, nor necessarily transient reactions, in this chapter I call for a study of liminal people and transitional states. Following a review of the relationship between culture and mental illness, culture-change syndromes are defined and illustrated with two stories of children with selective mutism. When it is applied to working with children and families undergoing cultural change and to studying liminal people and transitional states, cultural family therapy may be described as threshold therapy. Conclusions are drawn from the relational and cultural study of development and of mind.

179

CROSSING OVER

> The whole notion of crossing over, of moving from one iden-
> tity to another, is extremely important to me, being as I am—
> as we all are—a sort of hybrid.
>
> —Edward Said in conversation with Salman Rushdie
> (Rushdie, 1991a, p. 182)

Both family therapy and psychiatry can profit from the systematic
study of what anthropologist Victor Turner (1969) called liminal
people and transitional states. In Chapter 2, I reviewed the problems of viewing families across cultures with "static snapshots."
The limitations of this petrified view of culture become critical when
we meet families living through cultural change. And we are most
likely to need cultural family therapy when people are at the threshold of new worlds, in crisis, or at nodal points of the family life
cycle. Clinicians have tended to focus on the problems that people
import with them from other places, or to treat their predicaments
as a transitional state, a prelude to a more settled experience. We
need to study these predicaments because, although many people
move into the cultural mainstream through acculturation and other
adaptations, troubling aspects of their predicaments may persist.
For example, study of trauma and its aftermath has led to the development of the enormously useful concept of posttraumatic stress
disorder (PTSD). While disasters and other traumatic experiences
are often time-limited, they cast a long shadow over the lives of the
victims.

The goals of studying liminal people and transitional states are:

1. to identify the conditions of cultural change,
2. to study its impact on children ("changelings") and the family
   life cycle (see Chapter 5),
3. to catalog patterns of adaptation to cultural change,
4. to recognize psychiatric disorders that emerge under conditions
   of cultural change,
5. to construct models of identity formation and change.

In his work on identity and cultural change, social psychologist Roy
Baumeister (1986) observes that social scientists have used the term
"identity" in two ways—individually defined (by traditional West-

ern psychology) and socially defined (by sociology and anthropology). He calls these two aspects of identity the "outer context" and the "inner self." I believe, however, that we have moved beyond this dichotomy. To start with, family therapy represents an alternative to this formulation by constructing family experience as a bridge between what Baumeister calls inner and outer worlds. Supporting this are such new paradigms as culture-inclusive developmental psychology (Valsiner, 1989) and transcultural child psychiatry (DiNicola, 1992). Even more exciting is the call for a cultural psychology (Bruner, 1990; Shweder, 1991)—a different kind of general psychology which erases the boundary between individual and culture, making culture integral to identity formation. The declaration of a paradigm shift in family therapy to viewing families as storying cultures strengthens family therapy's claim to be a bridge between the individual and society. But just as culture-inclusive developmental psychology is a step toward a more general cultural psychology, family therapy needs to make the leap to a more general cultural family therapy.

CULTURE AND MENTAL ILLNESS

Transcultural psychiatry studies the relationship between culture and psychiatric disorders or mental illness. I have argued (DiNicola, 1990a, 1990b) that there is a *necessary connection* between culture and a number of specific psychiatric disorders. *Connection* is offered as a neutral term to describe this relationship. Let's use anorexia nervosa as an example. How are we to conceive of the connection between anorexia nervosa and culture? Is culture (1) a *cause*, (2) a *trigger*, or (3) a kind of social address or *envelope* where anorexia nervosa emerges? However we conceive of the connection between culture and mental illness, this connection must be included in any comprehensive interpretation of anorexia nervosa.

1. The strong version of this connection is that culture acts as a *cause* by providing a blueprint for anorexia nervosa; Susie Orbach's (1986) feminist hypothesis of anorexia nervosa as a "hunger strike" makes just this claim.
2. A more moderate version holds that specific cultural factors

trigger the illness, which is determined by many factors (including family interactions, cognitive schemas, or biological predisposition). Culture change can trigger the emergence of anorexia nervosa in adolescent girls from immigrant families living in highly industrialized Western societies; I view such cases as evidence of anorexia nervosa as a ''culture-change syndrome.''

3. The weak version is that culture is an *envelope* for the emergence of psychiatric disorders; in this version, culture is a specific socio-cultural address, container, or envelope for the expression of the illness. The specificity of the socio-cultural address or envelope is what is indicated in situating anorexia nervosa as a ''culture-bound syndrome'' of technologically developed, industrialized nations.[1]

CULTURE-REACTIVE SYNDROMES

Mental illnesses that have a marked geographic distribution, an affinity for certain socio-cultural circumstances, or an association with specific ethnocultural communities have an enduring appeal for anthropologists and transcultural psychiatrists (see Simons & Hughes, 1985). Numerous conceptual approaches have been offered to map this territory, including anthropologist George Devereux's (1980) notion of *ethnic disorder*. The most commonly used term is *culture-bound syndrome* (CBS), coined by Chinese transcultural psychiatrist Yap Pow-Meng (1974) in the 1960s. The term was refined by Raymond Prince (1985), a Canadian transcultural psychiatrist at McGill University, in this way:

> A CBS is defined as a collection of signs and symptoms of disease (not including notions of cause) which is restricted to a limited number of cultures primarily by reason of certain of their psychosocial features. (p. 201)

CBSs in our own backyard. Until recently, CBS was a category for exotic presentations in Western psychiatry. However, the notion of CBSs can be turned on its head and applied to the predicament of individuals and families in Western societies. Along with other transcultural psychiatrists (e.g., Littlewood & Lipsedge, 1986, 1987), I maintain that there are CBSs of the West, uncommon in other areas of the world. Invoking anthropologist Clyde Kluck-holn's idea that every culture has its "pet" mental disorders, Schwartz and associates (1985) expressed the concern that "eating disorders are becoming the pet mental disturbances of affluent cul-tures in general" (p. 96). In this view, anorexia nervosa is a CBS of the West.

Elsewhere, I have made a detailed argument (DiNicola, 1990b, 1990c) for understanding self-starvation as *anorexia multiforme*, a chameleon-like experience whose core meaning is defined by its cultural context. In its modern guise, anorexia nervosa is in large part a CBS of the affluent West. Anorexia nervosa also occurs as a culture-change syndrome among adolescents from cultures with a very low risk for eating disorders (e.g., Pakistan) who migrate to Western countries where the cultural drive for thinness and the social modeling of dieting and disordered eating is widespread (e.g., England).

CULTURE-CHANGE SYNDROMES

I use "culture-reactive syndromes" as a more general term, to dif-ferentiate CBSs from culture-change syndromes (DiNicola, 1985b). Culture-change syndromes (CCSs) are defined as specific problems arising during times of cultural stress and change that express a cultural conflict. CCSs are experienced by liminal people and arise during transitional states of their lives, but they may persist well beyond the period of actual change. The heuristic value of the con-cept of culture-change syndromes is that it draws attention to the problems associated with culture change, whether it comes as a result of migration or of living in a society undergoing rapid cultural change.

Again, the perspectives of insiders and outsiders is relevant. While negotiating new roles is difficult and stressful under each of these kinds of change, the circumstances differ in significant ways, including the attributions that people make about their experiences. When migrant families move between cultures, a host of factors determines whether they will experience *liminality*—being at the threshold of new experiences with many possibilities as potential insiders—or *marginality*—being at the periphery of society, outsid-ers with no perceived entrance into mainstream. These two terms are an elaboration of anthropologist Victor Turner's (1969) notion of "threshold people." When it is applied to working with migrants, to studying culture change, liminal people, and transitional states, cultural family therapy may be thought of as "threshold therapy."

TORN BETWEEN TWO CULTURES

Threshold people, moving between societies or caught in cultural changes in their own society, experience cultural conflict. A very fine rendering of the experience of being torn between two cultures is Richard Rodriguez's autobiography *Hunger of Memory* (1983). Rodriguez painfully dissects the different ways in which he was cut off from his Mexican roots (what he calls the "private world" of his Mexican immigrant family summed up by *tú*—the familiar Spanish address for "you") while growing up in California. Later, he was ironically segregated from the American mainstream that had become his identity (the "public world" of achievement represented by *usted*—the more formal Spanish address for "you") by being designated a "minority" in graduate school and for faculty hiring.

   Closer to home for clinicians is the story of the celebrated Quebec poet Émile Nelligan (1879–1941), who was committed to a mental asylum. The son of an Irish father and a French mother, Nelligan's story has been constructed as a Quebec "nationalist" symbol in the opera by Michel Tremblay and André Gagnon (Tremblay, 1990). In a critical scene, Nelligan's mother Émilie defines the family dilemma to David, his father:

> An English father. A French mother. The children forced to choose between their father and their mother. A family torn in two from the beginning, destined to fail. You tried to raise Émile in English, my poor David, but he switched to French as soon as you went out the door. Is it for that that you want to punish him? Is it the poet that you want to lock up in an instition or an unworthy son of Ireland? Your son, a *French* poet! A French poet! (Tremblay, 1990, Act I, scene 4, p. 44, my translation)

Caught in this impossible bind between the two stubborn solitudes of his parents, Émile turns to poetry for his brief moments of joy and of life:

I write! I write and the world changes!

I write and everything becomes beautiful! Everything becomes beautiful! My pain of living, my fear, everything gets blurred! I fly over Laval Street, I fly over Montreal, I am a stream of water that brings life! But who wants me? Who wants my joy? Who wants my pain? (Tremblay, 1990, Act I, scene 5, p. 47, my translation)

When his poetic passion could no longer contain the ambivalence, Émile became desperate and ill. The operatic reconstruction of his illness by Tremblay and Gagnon conflates psychiatry and politics. But there is another possibility, which is neither French nor English, neither psychiatry nor politics. That is the possibility of listening to Émile's own story, the story found in his poetry.

In a detailed monograph on transcultural child psychiatry, I described examples of culture-reactive syndromes that affect children and families (DiNicola, 1992). I also identified "culture-reactive constructs" of children's illnesses, illustrated by examples of "selective child attachment" in cultures as diverse as Brazil and Nigeria. Finally, I outlined many other child and family phenomena that vary across cultures, including parenting styles.[2]

SELECTIVE MUTISM

An illustration of how culture change can trigger relational distress is an unusual problem called selective mutism, also known as elective mutism. A startling and tragic case of selective mutism as a culture-change syndrome is illustrated by England's infamous "silent twins" (Wallace, 1986). June and Jennifer Gibbons are identical Black twins born in Barbados and raised in England. They refused to talk to others although they shared a rich fantasy life between themselves. They were eventually placed at Broadmoor, an English hospital for the criminally insane, after sprees of drug-taking, sex, and arson while they were adolescents.

Selective mutism is a relatively rare behavior pattern in children who possess age-appropriate speech but choose to remain silent, speaking only to self-selected persons, usually a small circle of family members, relatives, or close friends. It expresses a family conflict. This is a generally accepted definition. To this must be added the themes of alienation and isolation: the mutist child is isolated within the family, the parents are alienated from each other and the family is often socially and culturally isolated as immigrants within a ghetto.

Based on this larger view, a socio-cultural hypothesis for the emergence of selective mutism has been advanced (Goll, 1980). According to a study in Denmark and Greenland by Danish psychiatrist Knud Goll, two main factors are required: (1) a *society* that produces and maintains outsiders and outsider groups, and (2) the *ghetto family*, that is, a family with very little confidence in society (p. 145). This hypothesis is supported by the greatly increased incidence of selective mutism among immigrants. A review of the epidemiology of selective mutism reveals that the largest single risk factor is migration. Canadian child psychiatrists Susan Bradley and Leon Sloman (1975) found a ten-fold increase in the prevalence of selective mutism among immigrants as compared to English-speaking families in Toronto. Integrating these clinical and research data, I have proposed (DiNicola, 1985b, 1986) that selective mutism can be understood best as a culture-change syndrome.

There are serious gaps in research. Here are two examples: a major epidemiological study on selective mutism in London by Robert Wilkins (1985) purposely excluded immigrants, while other researchers (Kolvin & Fundudis, 1981) have seen immigration as a confounding factor. The evidence, in fact, points to cultural dislocation as a *central* and possibly *causative* factor. This demonstrates two things: first, that culture is critical to understanding psychiatric disorders; and second, that when cultural context is discounted as a "dirty window," we confound our grasp of psychiatric problems.

Rita Lomano: "An Acoustic Mask"

> Every completely unknown language is a kind of acoustic mask; as soon as one learns it, it becomes a *face*, understandable and soon familiar.
>
> —Elias Canetti (1962, p. 376)

Montreal, in the mid-80s. A consultation with Dr. Maurizio Andolfi. Rita Lomano was a 12-year-old girl with two siblings, both boys, seven and five years old. The parents were in their mid-thirties. Her three identified symptoms were selective mutism, enuresis, and a refusal to be photographed. What was immediately fascinating and ironic was the fact that two of her symptoms bore direct relation to the consultation, with the workshop audience watching and listening on an audiovisual monitor in another room. We did not find out to what extent she objected to being videotaped, but the communication problem was magnified by the context.

The nuclear family members, who were all present, all spoke Italian, and the mother spoke no English or French. Before he even met the family, Andolfi and the workshop audience were confronted with a problem that mirrors the family's predicament: whether to speak in their common (but to many in the audience a private and inaccessible) language or to speak in one of the public languages (of the audience and the host community, including school and therapy). Compounding the irony was the fact that here was a consultant from the family's own country of origin who was sharing their dilemma because of the different languages (English and French) of the host community.

As Andolfi was puzzling this out, the audience offered suggestions. One of the most interesting alternatives, suggested by Andolfi, was for him to communicate with the family in a "neutral" foreign language through an interpreter. Andolfi's idea is certainly creative and has been used in an experimental treatment of schizophrenics. Michael Simpson (1978) reported the work of Matulis in an article called, "The language least emotional to me," where he demonstrated that teaching a new language to patients allows them to explore experiences without the affective loading which may burden the mother tongue. Of the 23 patients who underwent this new twist to the "talking cure," several who had been unintelligible began to talk coherently in German. Even more impressive was the linguistic and social achievements of two men who had been mute for many years.

Andolfi ultimately chose a more workable route—he asked Rita to choose the language for the consultation. He made his offer in both English and Italian. The girl remained mute. After some 15 minutes, Andolfi left the family members to make the decision on their own. During his absence we watched the family on the monitor (with their knowledge and permission); someone in the audience came up with the idea of having Rita write her choice on paper. Andolfi returned to offer this, and after another lapse with considerable pressure from the family, Rita wrote out her choice. There was another emotional struggle as Andolfi held out his hand for the paper and the girl refused to give it to him until more family pressure was exerted.

The rest of the interview confirmed the fundamental dilemma posed by the family's acoustic mask. As Andolfi said, "The girl chose English—Italy is to be denied a reality. It is no coincidence that language was a problem in terms of which culture to join." The mother had never consented to leave Italy and consequently never really lived in Canada, expressing this by *not* speaking the languages (English or French) of her new country. The daughter, who had a somber, spinsterish manner (her hair was tied back in a bun and she dressed in dark clothes with a sweater that covered her like a shawl) joined the mother in her lifeless existence. This was a striking example of the axiom in systems theory that it is impossible not to communicate in an interpersonal situation (Watzlawick et al., 1967)—even a mute response speaks volumes.

I believe that by putting control in the girl's hands, Andolfi allowed her to drop her acoustic mask. She eventually did speak a little, but he did not reach the mother, whom he described to the audience as "the kind of person who lives so that you don't. She has to keep thinking and acting like she is living in a desert in her own life." Andolfi's final message to the family was the kind of prescription which is so close to the truth that one cannot finally decide whether it is a blunt fact or a provocative paradox. Turning to the girl, he gave her a warning: "Be careful, don't move too fast, you are in a very dangerous situation which is life and death for you. You are in a grave." Bateson (Wilden, 1972) described this kind of message as a "metaphor which is meant." In a neat, symmetrical move, written on the paper where the girl had written "English," Andolfi handed her a message as the consultation was concluding. Joining her in her refusal to choose between Italy and Canada, Andolfi amplified her predicament to absurdity with one word: "Japanese."

Pina D'Angelo: "Mum's the Word"

Montreal, mid-80s. A family in therapy. Pina D'Angelo was a six-year-old only child who had been mute at school for over six months. Mother was an expressive, expansive woman, who was born in Italy, had migrated with her family to Argentina at age six and later to Canada at age twelve. She was comfortable and at home in the multicultural environment of Montreal, where she wanted to stay. She was being treated for bipolar mood disorder, which was well managed. The father was a quiet, soulful man who was anxious and withdrawn. Although he felt at home nowhere, he wanted to return to his native Italy. He worked quietly as a back-room tailor: "I go to work, say hello in the morning, and then not another word until the evening when I say goodbye." In a pattern typical of selective mutist families (Meyers, 1984), the family had become socially and culturally isolated, and the parents argued over staying in Canada or returning to Italy. Confused by the emotional distance between her parents, their polarized styles, and their divided loyalties, Pina did not know where to turn or to whom to be loyal. She opted out of this impossible choice by barely socializing or speaking outside the nuclear family, that is, by becoming selectively mute.

German psychiatrist and family therapist Helm Stierlin's group (1986) emphasizes the need for neutrality in such cases, but other therapists choose to focus on one member of the family, such as a parent (Andolfi et al., 1983). In Pina's family, which is the parent to reach in therapy? Passive parents like Pina's father are harder to reach and work with in family therapy, as they also *feel and act like victims*. In this case, I worked with the father to help him come out of his shell and become more effective as a parent for Pina and as a buffer for his charming but overwhelming wife. Clinical work with families with mood disorder shows that interactions become polarized into extremes. With her extroverted interpersonal style, which occasionally spilled into a full-blown manic episode, Pina's mother occupied one extreme, while the father's more introverted style counterbalanced the family environment.

My therapeutic goal in their family therapy was to create a space for the two quiet people in the family, Pina and her father. After this, there was more opportunity to work with the mother in the sessions without squashing the others. By bringing these unspoken conflicts out into the open, Pina and her father gradually found a voice in the family and beyond.

FAMILY ROLES IN MUTIST FAMILIES

Knud Goll (1980) elaborates four special roles in the families of selective mutists:

1. the *selective mutist* as the identified patient;
2. the *mutist model*, a family member who is imitated by the mutist's use of "stubborn silence as a strong weapon";
3. the *symbiotic partner* joins the mutist in an unhappy relationship, which is mutually depriving of growth; the two partners cling closely in a pact that obviates change: "If you are not careful with me, I will get sick. If I get sick, we will both get sick, and we cannot even think of the dreadful things that might happen then—let us stay together and be careful" (Goll, 1980, p. 145);
4. the *ghetto leader* is the head of the family, which has a marginal position in society.

It is remarkable how closely the two families fit these roles. In Rita's story, the mother served two roles: as "mutist model" and "symbiotic partner." Andolfi unmasked the pact between Rita and her mother in terms very similar to Goll's hypothesis. In Pina's story, it is the father who acts as "mutist model" and "symbiotic partner." Our understanding of father's role in siding with Pina is improved by considering the impact of mood disorders on family interactions. Pina's father is too passive to be considered the "ghetto leader" of this family. A better example of this role is the father in the Running family described in Chapter 5—Mr. Running was defiantly at odds with his social world.

CONCLUSION:
"NEW MAPS OF DEVELOPMENT, NEW MODELS OF MIND"

> Mental health is a condition of being "at home with one's family and with the future."
>
> —Erik Erikson (quoted in Nann, 1982, p. 142)

Here, I draw together some insights from working with changelings (the subject of Chapter 5) and other liminal people, such as the selective mute children discussed in this chapter. There are several conceptual and experiential barriers to the use of cultural family therapy for children with mental illness. These troubled children may seem strangers to us because they are from different places (culture), because they have disturbing and alienating experiences (mental disorder), or because the world of their childhood has become unfathomable to us as adults (development).

Nonetheless, cultural family therapy with children can be a rich opportunity to construct new metaphors for child development and family experience and new tools for working with children and their families (see DiNicola, 1985a, 1985b, 1985c, 1986, 1992, 1993). This may require a reassessment of our notions of culture, child development, and family. These are four key propositions for dealing with children as cultural changelings:

1. *Culture is integral to identity.* Culture is one of the integral sources of the self. "Identity" is formed within and through the contexts of family and culture. As clinicians, we seek "mind" through context and relationship. The "self" we seek is culturally constructed and socially distributed. The royal road to understanding "mind," "self," and "identity" is the "presenting cultures" of children and their families. Culture should not be construed as a "dirty window" obscuring supposedly more fundamental biological or psychological variables, nor to "break the ice" in clinical work as a prelude for diagnosis and treatment. Cultural variables are relevant throughout all the traditional phases of clinical work.

2. *Familism is normative.* The family is the significant living context for examining the definitions and experiences of stages of life. The evolving family is the key context for therapeutic interventions aimed at redefining "ages and stages" and for adapting to new social and cultural realities. Cultural family therapy is a model for conducting family work with children across cultures.

3. *Child development is contingent and contextual.* This key concept for transcultural work with children means that childhood and adolescence are social, cultural, and historical constructs. Each society's experience of young people is deeply informed by its prevailing beliefs. The cultural embeddedness of developmental beliefs is of-

ten more evident when looking across at other societies. Westerners seem to find reports of suicides over academic achievement
among Japanese schoolchildren tragic but absurd, while only comparative studies and the more recent efforts of specialists will dis-
abuse Westerners of the notion of "adolescent turmoil," which has
the effect of denying or even normalizing the social epidemic of
suicidal behavior among Western youth. Developmental psychologist Jaan Valsiner's (1989) culture-inclusive developmental psychology and transcultural child psychiatry together offer a powerful
new paradigm to integrate culture and children's development.

4. *Cultural change is global.* The worldwide prevalence of children
and their families undergoing cultural change needs to be recognized as an embedded feature of global cultural interpenetration. If
we take cultural psychology seriously as a general psychology
(Bruner, 1990; Shweder, 1991) and cultural family therapy as a
more comprehensive approach to family therapy, cultural change
is not merely a transient phase but a profound and ongoing reorien-
tation of identity. "Identity, too," Canadian transcultural psychiatrist Laurence Kirmayer observes in a recent essay, "has become
intercultural" (1995, p. 167). We should, accordingly, recognize the
potentially traumatic and persistent impact of cultural change on
children's mental health. By doing so, we can identify culture-
change syndromes such as anorexia nervosa and selective mutism.

Taken together, culture-inclusive developmental psychology
(Valsiner, 1989), transcultural child psychiatry (DiNicola, 1992), and
cultural family therapy can provide us with powerful tools for understanding and helping children in cultural flux, whose identities
can be complex, confusing and transitory. Applied in these contexts
of cultural change, cultural family therapy may be thought of as
"threshold therapy." The defining image for the twentieth century
may come to be the endless exiles created by countless revolutions
and wars. The worldwide conditions of migration and exile in this
century have created untold problems and also a heretofore un-
imagined degree of cultural interpenetration. In future decades,
children and their families may feel more enriched than isolated by
such intercultural encounters. Our cultural future may be in the
hands of the creative individual adaptations of "third culture kids"

and their family and communal evolutions into "créole cultures." If we help children in cultural transition feel at home with their families in their new worlds, they may develop the mental health that Erikson envisioned to enjoy a future that is culturally enriched (rather than merely complex), offering many choices (not just confusion), and syncretic, plural (rather than transitory) identities, with each cultural encounter building upon the last.

Chapter 7

STONES AND BRIDGES

The Myth of Independence

Marco Polo describes a bridge, stone by stone.

"But which is the stone that supports the bridge?" Kublai Khan asks.

"The bridge is not supported by one stone or another," Marco answers, "but by the line of the arch they form."

Kublai Khan remains silent, reflecting. Then he adds: "Why do you speak to me of the stones? It is only the arch that matters to me."

Polo answers: "Without stones there is no arch."

—Italo Calvino,
Invisible Cities
(1978, p. 82)

In the search for interconnections between individuals, families, and culture, metaphor is one of our best tools. An evocative metaphor comes from the Italian writer Italo Calvino, who in a few words offers us a rich dialogue on stones and bridges, parts and wholes. This chapter examines "The Myth of Independence" as a connecting theme in Western psychological theories and therapies. Six aspects of the myth of independence are outlined to show the pervasive implications of this concept: development, gender, family functioning, pathology, culture, *and* therapy. *Two aspects are explored in depth: (1) how independence has become enshrined as an ideal goal in family therapy in the guise of descriptions of family functioning, and (2) how, from a cross-cultural view of attachment, import/export of psychological theories and therapies between the West and other societies can be problematic.*

THE MYTH OF INDEPENDENCE

Independence? That's middle class blasphemy. We are all dependent on one another, every soul of us on earth.

—George Bernard Shaw, *Pygmalion* (1916/1940, Act V, p. 89)

In this chapter, I want to explore a notion that has become a powerful myth in Western societies. That notion is *independence* and its many permutations in Western therapies and social sciences. It shows up in family therapy in three key ways: (1) in the uncritical acceptance of the idea that a key goal of adolescent development is independence from parental support, (2) in the way family functioning is described—and prescribed as a normative goal—chiefly in Salvador Minuchin's (1974) notion of "enmeshment" as a failure of differentiation (and therefore a kind of pathological dependence), and (3) in the indiscriminate use of the term "enmeshment" as a cultural misperception, whereby many, if not all, members of some cultural communities are labeled as enmeshed.

My argument is that in each case a kind of cultural stereotype is in place, which members of the dominant majority do not see and cannot sidestep. Regarding the first point, adolescence as a time of "independence" is a cultural and historical construction and not the given that most North Americans assume. As to the second two points about Minuchin's term "enmeshment," I have frequently and pervasively observed that mainstream therapists have systematic misperceptions about "ethnic" families in North America. Here is a clear example from the chapter on Italian families in *Ethnicity and Family Therapy*, where the authors caution that:

> The therapist must learn to differentiate between intense closeness and *pathological enmeshment* in Italian American families. . . . In the final phase of treatment, the therapist will be presented with the therapeutic issue of how to *extricate him- or herself from the system.* Families may attempt to "*absorb*" therapists and make them *auxiliary family members.* (Giordano & McGoldrick, 1996, p. 579, emphasis added)

This is a two-stage cultural misperception: (1) the creation of an outsider group, and (2) the imposition of a cultural stereotype.

1. *Creating outsiders*. This starts by seeing the family as an "ethnic" group ("outsiders"), rather than understanding its "presenting culture" as part of a unique family worldview. The reason why "ethnic" implies "outsider" in the above case is that, despite the fact that the majority of Italian American families have been in the United States for several generations, the authors highlight the vestiges of their Italian ancestry and the continuing differences, rigidly portraying Italians as "unmeltable ethnics" (see Novak, 1971). What is not addressed are such questions as: How does living in the United States shape the acculturation of immigrants and the enculturation of their children? Would Italian families in Brazil or Australia retain the same presenting culture that Giordano and McGoldrick (1996) describe among Italian Americans? After decades of living in the United States, the children of these families have been enculturated as "Americans." There are many possibilities for how American immigrants and their children might define themselves and how they might bring the two cultures together—from assimilation as "Americans" and the exciting prospects of cultural hybrids as "Mexican-Americans" or "Chinese-Americans," to the persistence of their cultures of origin as a barrier to the American ideal of integration into the "melting pot" (which Giordano and McGoldrick imply for Italian families)—a phenomenon described as "the unmeltable ethnics" (Novak, 1971) and estrangement as "outsiders" (the Amish and Hassidic Jews among religious groups).

2. *Imposing stereotypes*. Once we have created a category of "outsiders" by the use of the term "ethnic," the family can be shoe-horned into a cultural stereotype. The stereotype here is of Italian Americans as "enmeshed," which, even if true, has the potential to ignore the value of a family-oriented way of being and to misconstrue the experience of not fitting in with such an orientation. This misperception is not an isolated case; it is, in fact, a rather common one. My argument about the myth of independence in our culture predicts that the flip side of this stereotype will be problems with separation-individuation in children, resulting in a lack of differentiation. Another recent cultural perspective on family therapy states flatly that, "Italian Americans traditionally consider the family of prime importance and are reluctant to support members' differenti-

ation'' (Kaslow et al., 1995, p. 630). Differentiation is also addressed as a problem in the chapter by Giordano and McGoldrick (1996). Further on in this chapter, I will suggest alternative models for ''enmeshment'' (familism) and ''differentiation'' (interdependence).

For stereotypes to work, one has to be willing to see others in categorical terms. When this is done repeatedly and without reflection, a strange mindset occurs called ''hardening of the categories.'' Why does this occur? It is most likely to occur when a theory or an approach is developed within one society (or cultural community) and uncritically applied to another.

While alternative and competing ideas are emerging in family therapy and cultural psychology, we need to explore the myth of independence carefully in order to divest ourselves of this myth. Independence is a powerful and persistent underlying assumption in social science (Waterman, 1981), appearing as an ideal goal in theories as diverse as those of psychoanalyst Margaret Mahler (1963) and family therapist Salvador Minuchin (1974). The words associated with psychological theories that invoke states of dependence betray their status as conditions to be avoided, grown out of, and treated: *dependency, enmeshment, fusion,* and *symbiosis.* Conversely, *autonomy, independence, individuation,* and *self-control* are set as normative goals for development and prescriptions for therapy.

INDEPENDENCE: A PERVASIVE MYTH

Various aspects of the myth of independence burden psychological theories with their covert assumptions (see Table 7.1). The first aspect concerns *development.* Here the myth of independence is seen in the common assumption that separation-individuation is the major goal of adolescence. The second aspect relates to *gender;* in the myth, females and males are seen as having the same developmental paths, behavioral styles, and family interactional patterns with regard to attachment. In the third aspect, normative judgments related to independence are made about *family functioning;* for instance, consider the construct of enmeshment/disengagement developed by Minuchin and associates (1967). The fourth aspect

Table 7.1. Six Aspects of the Myth of Independence and Their Corollary Assumptions

ASPECT	COROLLARY ASSUMPTION
1. Development	Separation-individuation is the major goal of adolescence.
2. Gender	Attachment behavior is the same in both sexes.
3. Family Functioning	Normative judgments are made about family life (e.g., about ''boundaries'').
4. Pathology	Attachment styles predispose to, precipitate, and prolong mental illness.
5. Culture	There is little cultural variation of attachment behavior, considered universal.
6. Therapy	These assumptions form the framework and shape the goals of psychotherapy.

reveals a bias toward *pathology,* as certain family interactional styles are assumed to be enduring and inherently pathogenic, predisposing to, precipitating, and prolonging serious mental illness such as anorexia nervosa and schizophrenia. The fifth aspect is a *cultural blind spot,* that is, the assumption that these concepts are human behavioral universals, applying across classes and cultures. The sixth aspect has the greatest impact: when autonomy and independence are assumed to be normative ideals, they form part of the accepted framework and implicit goals of *therapy.*

This chapter addresses two aspects of the myth. The ''Familism'' section questions the normative judgments of family functioning represented by Minuchin's structural theory of family therapy and offers alternative approaches. ''Conviviality'' takes a cross-cultural view of attachment, looking at import/export problems with psychological theories and therapies between the West and other societies.

"NO MAN IS AN ISLAND"

Before moving on to the main argument, another conceptual point needs underlining. Since independence and its corollaries are construed positively, dependency and its associated qualities are construed as pathological. This blinds theorists and therapists to the implications of extremes of independence—isolation and abandonment. Why do we focus on the negative features of dependency, but not on the costs of independence?

Leading scholars in many fields, from Jerome Bruner (1990) and Richard Shweder (1991) in psychology to Charles Taylor (1989) in philosophy, have demonstrated that this is due to the Western focus on the atomistic individual as the starting point for psychological inquiry. "[By] habit and tradition," as Bruner (1990) puts it, Western psychologists "think in rather individualistic terms" (p. 11). And instead of imagining this as simply our folk psychology, what comes natural to us given our history, Westerners want our view of the world to be the human view through the ethnocentric assumption of *universalism*. Shweder (1991) writes that this "concept of the autonomous distinctive individual living in society" (p. 150) is precisely what makes Western culture unique among world cultures. Philosopher Charles Taylor examines and rejects this "disengaged image of the self." Although "we cannot but reach for this language," which is embedded in modern life, Taylor (1989, p. 177) convincingly demonstrates that "it was not always so."

Taking a long-range view, we may trace the origin of this emphasis through the cultural shift from the Elizabethan metaphors of relatedness, as expressed in the work of English poet John Donne, to the Romantic Movement of the latter eighteenth century, marked by an extreme assertion of the self and the value of individual experience. This was a shift from others to the self. "No man is an island," wrote Donne, all individuals are connected to the mainland and through this connection the "defects of loneliness" are controlled (1962, p. 61). In contrast, Western psychology is a descent down the "spiral staircase of the self," in Michel de Montaigne's memorable phrase (cited by Steiner, 1975, p. 120). Psychology and the human sciences, deeply influenced by Freud, have been preoccupied with the individual in society. Minuchin characterized this approach as "a product of the romantic idea of the hero and his struggle against society; it is about man out of context'' (cited in Malcolm, 1978, p. 73).

William James observed that "we are gregarious animals" with "an innate propensity to get ourselves noticed . . . favorably by our own kind" (1890, p. 293). He imagined that:

> No more fiendish punishment could be devised . . . than that one should be turned loose in society and remain absolutely unnoticed by all the members thereof. (James, 1890, p. 292)

Frieda Fromm-Reichmann, in her fine paper on loneliness, agreed with novelist Thomas Wolfe that "the essence of human tragedy [lies] in loneliness, not in conflict" (1959a, p. 8). Remarking on the perceived emotional coldness of mothers of schizophrenics, Fromm-Reichmann coined the now disparaged term "schizophrenogenic" parents (1959b). A similar notion became popularized as the "refrigerator" parents in Leo Kanner's (1948) description of the parents of autistic children. Reflecting on her life's work, Margaret Mahler stated:

> I have maintained a rather personal interest in . . . the fact that lifelong . . . emotional dependence on the mother is a universal truth. (1963, p. 307)

Between them, these two pioneers in relational psychology, Frieda Fromm-Reichmann and Margaret Mahler, framed the issues of this chapter poignantly: the tragedy of loneliness and the inevitability of dependency.

FAMILISM: CHALLENGING ENMESHMENT

> The more a system develops in complexity, the more it can develop its autonomy and multiply its dependencies. We construct our psychological, individual and personal autonomy through the dependencies we undergo, which are those of the family and of school.
>
> —Edgar Morin (1982, pp. 194–195, my translation)

Despite the conceptual sophistication of family theory and the advances it represents in the understanding and treatment of human problems, many family therapists have incorporated, almost whole, some major untested assumptions of psychodynamic psychotherapy. Among these are the developmental model of object-relations theory (Stewart et al., 1975) and the myth of independence. Furthermore, the work of two influential groups—Bateson's Palo Alto project represented by Jay Haley (1976a) and the Philadelphia Child Guidance Clinic represented by Salvador Minuchin (1974)—have added a new dimension to the myth of independence: normative judgments of family functioning.

Haley (1963, 1976b) stressed power and authority, arguing that its diffusion between generations produces family problems. Gregory Bateson, the founder of the Palo Alto group, did not concur with this approach. Bateson argued that power, as a mechanistic metaphor from nineteenth-century physics, was unsuited to modern cybernetics and systems theory. With this conceptual confusion, Bateson warned that we should not rush to ''take it on the wards and try it'' (1978, p. 41). Minuchin (1974) elaborated a structural theory that analyzes family hierarchies, subsystems, boundaries and certain aspects of family relating styles, the chief of which is his bipolar construct *enmeshment/disengagement*. This reflects an emphasis on independence, touching on three aspects of the myth (see Table 7.1): separation-individuation as the goal of development, normative judgments of family functioning, and a pathological bias in assuming that an enmeshed family predisposes its members to psychosomatic illness. At first, it would appear that enmeshment is a metaphorical, descriptive term used loosely in clinical work, but a close reading of Minuchin's work allows no ambiguity:

> A pathologically enmeshed family system is characterized by a high degree of responsiveness and involvement. (Minuchin et al., 1975, p. 1033)

Enmeshment is reflected in:

1. interdependence of relationships,
2. intrusion on personal boundaries,
3. poorly differentiated perceptions of self and of other family members,

4. weak family subsystem boundaries (Minuchin et al., 1975, p. 1033).

Capturing the essence of this description, Nathan Epstein called such families "huddlers" (Epstein et al., 1964). David Reiss (1971) has studied the problem-solving styles of families, using a similar continuum whose poles are "consensus sensitivity" (seen in families with a schizophrenic member) and "interpersonal distance sensitivity" (seen in families with a delinquent member). Significantly, Reiss recognized the contribution of "ethnicity" to these family interactional styles in a more positive way that does not equate family problem-solving styles with specific groups (Sugarman, 1983).

In the 1970s, Selvini Palazzoli and the Milan group, employing a systems theory approach to family therapy, avoided labeling family interactional styles. In reading their cases, one is not tempted to call the families "enmeshed" (see DiNicola, 1984). Instead, one discovers the misery that ensues when individuals are excluded rather than integrated into the family system. The story of little Marella, treated by the Milan group, illustrates this poignantly.

Marella: "Conspiracy of Silence"

Marella, a child of two years and two months, was presented by her parents with anorexia (loss of appetite) of six months' duration, coincident with the birth of her baby brother, whom Marella had not yet seen (Selvini Palazzoli et al., 1974). This case has four elements:

1. the exclusion of the mother from her husband's family;
2. the unavailability and condescension of the husband to his wife and child;
3. the birth of the new baby as a non-event; severely damaged and hospitalized, "For Marella he is only a sort of phantom" (Selvini Palazzoli et al., 1974, p. 435);
4. finally, the death of the baby, which was kept a secret from Marella.

To dramatize breaking this wall of silence, a funeral ritual was prescribed, which involved all family members burying the baby's clothes. Included in the family in this way, the child responded with a dramatic resumption of eating and talking.

In my reading, the interventions of the Milan group typically address such exclusions. For example, the "odd days/even days" prescription in which parents alternate being in charge of the identified problem serves to unite parents by showing them that their behavior is working at odds in the family (Selvini Palazzoli et al., 1978a). Another approach, Selvini Palazzoli's "invariant prescription" (1986b; Selvini Palazzoli & Prata, 1982a; Selvini Palazzoli et al., 1989) is a series of staged interventions in which the parental couple meets alone with the therapist and is given the prescription to spend increasing amounts of time together away from their children. This method of therapy is aimed at bringing the parents together.

Minuchin (cited by Goldner, 1982) saw this as Selvini Palazzoli's move in a structural direction (working on family structure by addressing the parental functions and the sibling interactions as subsystems) and an acknowledgment of his notion of family boundaries. Another interpretation is that this prescription allows all the children (including the symptomatic one) to be on an equal footing (DiNicola, 1984). With the parents keeping a secret from all the children, the symptomatic child becomes part of the sibling group in sharing a common problem—what to make of the parents' behavior. This short-circuits favoritism and scapegoating alike.

Based on observations from their method, Selvini Palazzoli and Prata argued that psychotic symptoms arise when "the patient becomes the one who does not know while the others know. Somehow, feeling cheated, he reacts accordingly" (1982a, p. 242). This hypothesis "could explain the first explosion of psychotic behavior as a dramatic protest" (Selvini Palazzoli & Prata, 1982a, p. 243) against exclusion. The Milan group emphasized secrets and their functions in family life (Selvini Palazzoli & Prata, 1982b). Their refusal of secret knowledge from individual family members is an insistence on the therapist's neutrality, blocking private coalitions (among family members or with the therapist). This highlights the exclusionary power of such information and relations.

Addressing private coalitions and secrets as exclusions is not the same as invoking boundaries in the normative way of structural theory. The systemic approach of the Milan group (in the 1970s and 1980s) did not assume where such boundaries should be. They took a neutral, meta-view of the family, asking what functions such information and relations (such as accusations, coalitions, identifications, revelations or secrets) might serve. In comparison, enmeshment is a generic concept that does not lead to specific hypotheses or interventions. "What we *must* understand," Selvini Palazzoli commented, "are the specific games in the families, and the position of the members in the game."[1]

The concept of enmeshment may be construed as a problem in cross-cultural perception. Enmeshment, so often diagnosed in ethnic families in North America, is perceived when people are seen *out of cultural context*. If the behaviors that enmeshment labels do occur, what function do they serve in the family? Can we reframe the concept in a nonpathological way? Frank Pittman's (1984) review of an American film criticizes the pathology implicit in family therapists' use of enmeshment and its implication that leaving home is an all-or-nothing affair: *"Terms of Endearment* has made enmeshment seem secure, reciprocal, and liberating. It makes it respectable not to totally leave home" (p. 61).[2] If North American family therapists step outside their narrow and often ethnocentric framework, they could see how constraining such notions are.

The concept of *familism* offers an alternative to enmeshment by taking culture into account. The term has a long history and is not always neutral. Anthropologist Edward Banfield (1958) coined the term "amoral familism," which has a very negative connotation, while family therapists Fredda Herz and Elliott Rosen (1982) apply it more positively to describe the centrality of the family in Jewish life as deriving from the Bible. One of the commonalities in the use of the concept of familism is that the family as a natural group coheres to form a whole, with a united front to others. Familism is family centeredness and nurturance. Rather than diagnosing enmeshment in ethnic groups that stand apart from the cultural mainstream, familism helps us to understand how cultural conditions can shape the family's attachment style. This knowledge can be used clinically when conducting cultural family therapy.

French social historian Philippe Ariès (1977) places the development of familism in historical context. Two centuries ago, he argues, an emotional revolution took place. Feelings that had been diffuse, "spread out over numerous natural and supernatural objects," became "focused entirely within the family" (Ariès, 1977, p. 229). Consequently, "the individual must recede into the background for the sake of the family unit" (Ariès, 1977, p. 230). For Ariès, familism created a sanctuary, "The only place where a person could . . . escape the inquisitive stare of industrial society" (Ariès, 1977, p. 230).

While familism may be the product of certain economic and social conditions, examining the family life cycle (Carter & McGoldrick, 1989) helps us understand that any attachment style has relative merits. Different family attachment styles are more or less adaptive for individuals at various phases of their development. Placing the family life cycle into the context of time and place—what I call the "cultural family life cycle"—allows us to perceive more adaptive possibilities in different ways that families negotiate life cycle issues.

Familism, for example, can be quite adaptive at extremes of the life cycle. The very young and the very old and those with developmental disorders who cannot totally separate are well served by familism. Adolescents and young adults, conversely, require relatively less investment in family relations. Turmoil and the rupture of relations as outlined by Anna Freud (1958), however, are not inevitable.

The "turbulence model" of adolescence has been challenged (Slaff, 1981) by both clinicians and researchers. First, not all adolescents rebel and move away from the family (Masterson, 1968; Offer, 1969). Second, gender differences are becoming evident in the adolescent's handling of maturation. Carol Gilligan's (1981) notion is that the two genders speak in different voices. McDermott and associates (1983) portray the adolescent girl as "a connected person," struggling for individuality within the family and using the family as an emotional vehicle for defining herself. This is in contrast to the adolescent boy, "a separate person" who seeks his own space on his own terms. The French systems theorist Edgar Morin describes the connected person well in his theory of the open system—"a system that can nourish its autonomy, but through its dependence on its external milieu" (Morin, 1982, p. 194, my translation).

The conclusions of the McDermott study speak to the heart of the myth of independence:

> We need not consider the complete differentiation of the self from the family to be the ideal goal. Individuals who retain strong ties and an orientation to relationships may be more, rather than less, mature . . . maturity follows a spectrum from dependence to independence. Yet various points . . . such as interdependence, may be more functional than an end point of independence. (McDermott et al., 1983, p. 1321)

CONVIVIALITY: INTERDEPENDENCE IN CROSS-CULTURAL PERSPECTIVE

The question of psychotherapy in different cultures can be imagined as an "import/export" problem (DiNicola, 1985b). The West has exported a model of dynamic psychotherapy based on three ethnocentric assumptions—the *individual* as the focus of therapy, personal *independence* as a therapeutic goal, and *introspection and insight* as a therapeutic method (based on Prince's review; see DiNicola, 1985c). As Clifford Geertz makes clear, among world cultures, Westerners have a peculiar view of

> the person as a bounded, unique, more or less integrated motivational and cognitive universe . . . organized into a distinctive whole and set contrastively both against other such wholes and against its social and natural background. (1983b, p. 59)

Because such assumptions rarely resonate with other cultural traditions, Western psychotherapy has met with little acceptance in other societies. Nevertheless, the development of mental health services has meant that Westerners or Western-trained native practitioners carry these assumptions with them, applying them to elite, educated, and urbanized groups (Prince, 1972).

Pande, an East Indian psychiatrist working in the United States, interpreted Western psychotherapy as a disguised dependency, invented by a society which prizes "self-direction and independence in life" above all (1968, p. 426). Pande argues that psychotherapy, as a "magnificent ruse for fostering a long-term and intimate relationship," copes with needs that are met more directly in "other societies that are oriented toward interdependence" (1968, p. 426). Seen in cross-cultural perspective, psychotherapy is an "undertaking to meet the deficits in the Western way of life and to cope with the negative psychological implications of its premises" (Pande, 1968, p. 432).

Examining indigenous healing beliefs and practices and models of psychotherapy in societies that do not subscribe to the myth of independence may lead to valuable imports for Western therapists. Given the problems that are generated by therapy models that subscribe to the myth of independence, such imports are potentially helpful to specific groups in our own societies. Problems exist in the delivery of services to the chronically poor (Prince, 1969), disadvantaged minorities (Hines & Boyd-Franklin, 1982), and cultural and immigrant groups in our own society (Vargas & Koss-Chioino, 1992)—groups that I have characterized as "the Third World in our own backyard" (DiNicola, 1985d).

Of course, the Western emphasis on individualism and independence is not universal. Many other cultures are more "sociocentric" in their conception of the individual-society relationship. Indeed, cultural psychologist Richard Shweder notes that "members of sociocentric organic cultures," like India and Japan, must find independence "alien"—"a bizarre idea cutting the self off from the interdependent whole, dooming it to a life of isolation and loneliness" (Shweder, 1991, p. 154, citing the work of Indian psychoanalyst Kakar). Cultural alternatives to the myth of independence from two non-western societies, India and Japan, are examined below.

INDIA: THE *GURU-CHELA*
(MASTER-DISCIPLE) RELATIONSHIP

Jaswant Singh Neki (1976a, 1976b) explores dependence as the dynamic of therapeutic relationships in India and in the West. Analyzing therapist-patient relationships in psychotherapy, Neki (1973, 1974) argues that, since dependency longings are considered a sign of morbidity, Western therapists minimize their own influence. In contrast, the Hindu ideal of maturity is a "satisfying and continuous dependency relationship" (Neki, 1973, p. 756). Accordingly, Neki suggests that the *guru-chela* relationship may serve as a therapeutic paradigm with Indian patients. In the *guru* (or master) role, the therapist will be more active, directive, instructive, and available, while as a *chela* (or disciple), the patient will be accepting and obedient, entering a lifelong friendship. Congruent with the insights of cultural psychology and cultural family therapy, Neki (1973) asserts that a therapeutic paradigm must resonate with the total cultural pattern and that the *guru-chela* relationship suits Indians well.

Bhatti and associates (1980) trace the development of family psychiatric ward treatment in India from the 1950s, independent of Western developments at the same time. They credit Indian psychiatrist Vidyasagar with discovering that family admission is a powerful therapeutic act. What began as makeshift accommodations for out-of-town family members became so popular that there were eventually 20 family units at the National Institute of Mental Health and Neurosciences at Bangalore. This speaks for the Indian emphasis on family relationships and interdependence.[3]

Citing the advantages of family ward treatment, Bhatti and associates emphasize "faster and more extensive recovery," with shorter hospital stays (1980, p. 197). Echoing the goals of community psychiatry, they note that, since patients are not separated from their families, they are "spared feelings of isolation, rejection and hostility" (1980, p. 197). Moreover, family members can learn to modify their behavior in relation to the patient. An important feature is the patient's choice of a preferred relative. Hospital stays with a preferred relative are significantly shorter. This has remarkable congruence with sociologist George Brown's (1959) finding at the Maudsley Hospital in London that schizophrenics discharged to live with siblings or in "lodgings" had lower relapse rates than when sent to spouses and parents. While some family relationships may precipitate or prolong mental illness, the Indian orientation to familism demonstrates that there are clearly ways to structure the family's contacts to promote well-being.

Brown's study gave rise to a generation of research on "expressed emotion" (EE), a complex measure of family interactions in families of schizophrenics. Researchers have made transcultural comparisons of EE, including several studies in North India (Leff et al., 1987; Wig et al., 1987a, 1987b). Transcultural work is needed and welcome, but the North India studies have serious limitations. Basically, the researchers opted to test the cross-cultural reliability of British ideas of family interaction rather than to explore cultural differences (see my critical review, DiNicola, 1988a, and my discussion of EE in Chapter 4).

JAPAN: SURROUNDED BY *AMAE* (INDULGENT LOVE)

In Japan, where dependency is a key social dynamic, Takeo Doi (1973), a Western-trained Japanese psychiatrist, explores an emotion that is central to Japanese experience. *Amae* refers to the indulgent, passive love that surrounds the individual in the family. Noting the lack of this word in Western languages, Doi contrasts the ideal of self-reliance in the West with that of interdependence and the indulgence of weakness (*amae*) in Japan. When a dependent, indulged child is called *amaekko* in Japan, it is a term of endearment. In contrast, listen to the words that Western society and therapists have developed for dependent relationships: enmeshment, fusion, symbiosis, and *folie à deux*. Using this contrast, Doi examines psychological problems such as fears, dystonic homosexual feelings, and disorders of the self (alienation, guilt, and the feeling of being victimized). He posits that different social relations in Japan have implications for therapy. These implications have been taken up by a number of Western visitors to Japan.

An illustrative case was related by a Japanese school counselor at an American school in Tokyo. Taro is a seven-year-old Japanese boy who had studied at the school for two years when he suddenly refused to attend school for several months. When he started to attend sporadically again, the school implemented a plan for his reintegration. Regular daily attendance for a shortened day at fixed times was prescribed, as the "American" context demanded. On the other hand, a mother and child clinic in Tokyo recommended the Japanese approach, which is to simply let the child attend at will, getting his education "on demand." This story contrasts the regulator approach of the American school with the more facilitating attitude of the Japanese clinic (cf. Raphael-Leff, 1983).[4]

In a review of psychoanalytic therapy in Japan, Alan Roland

(1983) analyzes how social patterns affect the therapist-patient exchange. Supervising a group of Western-trained Japanese psychotherapists, Roland was struck by the therapeutic progress made despite "an extraordinary minimum of interpretation and investigation" (Roland, 1983, p. 500). This is a puzzling finding, since a cardinal tenet of psychoanalysis is that interpretation is the major curative factor. Roland reviews the hierarchical nature of Japanese social relationships and claims that in Japan the patient and therapist enter a qualitative mode of hierarchical relationship (as opposed to a structural one—see Hsu, 1971). Within such "emotionally connected" and "enmeshed hierarchical" relationships, Roland states, individuality can be kept by having a "highly private self" (1983, p. 501). This inner self is kept privately and communicated indirectly.

Western-trained therapists returning to Japan had to readjust "because they became far too direct" (1983, p. 502; see Prince, 1972). Japanese therapists have developed non-intrusive interventions, techniques that "minimize the patient's vulnerabilities" (Roland, 1983, p. 504) and use humor and subtle adjustments of the hierarchical positions between patient and therapist. In outlining the parameters that have been changed to make therapy workable in Japan, Roland uses language that is closer to structural family therapy (e.g., enmeshment). By underplaying two key aspects of analytic technique—interpretation and transference—the Japanese have developed a psychoanalytic approach that is attuned to Japanese social relationships, which stress nurturance and dependence.

Again, it is interesting to note the Western language Roland uses in describing Japanese relationships as "enmeshed hierarchical." The highly private Japanese self is addressed more directly by the Nobel Prize-winning novelist Kenzaburo Oe. Oe applies the image of Ralph Ellison's *Invisible Man* to the Japanese. "The majority of Japanese images are masks," says Oe, who laments that while Japanese technology and economic power are visible, "we are inscrutable in the eyes of Europeans and Americans" (Remnick, 1995, p. 42).

Although Minuchin's structural family therapy is known in Japan, a Western transcultural psychiatrist visiting Japan found that Japanese psychiatrists did not find it useful because of the different family patterns there.[5] Minuchin himself suggests that an intergenerational model (Boszormenyi-Nagy & Spark, 1973) may provide a better basis for the development of Japanese family therapy. Falicov (1986) notes that Carl Rogers' client-centered therapy has been well-received in Japan. This is because Rogers' therapeutic method has explicitly developed what Roland discovered serendipitously: a respect for the individual and, in Japan, a relational style that fits the culture.

Ivan Illich's term *conviviality* (1973) warmly conveys the interdependence of family and social relations in many cultural contexts. Illich defines conviviality as "individual freedom realized in personal interdependence" (1973, p. 24).[6] Conviviality is "relative and relational," like Edgar Morin's notion of autonomy (1982, p. 195). We struggle to capture experience in fresh words that will not shackle thought or impose out of habit notions that hold contradictions or force dichotomies on continuous experience. Such language changes are not merely cosmetic; rather, they are the logical consequence of divesting therapy of the myth of independence. That is a first step toward a new language of therapy. To return to the opening theme of the tragedy of loneliness and the inevitability of dependency, Morin (1982) implies that as we steer away from either/or dichotomies toward joining constructions, what counts is not the quantity of each thing joined, but the shape and mold of their combination:

> this is not to say that the more one is dependent, the more one is autonomous—there is no reciprocity between these terms—but that one cannot imagine autonomy without dependency. (Morin, 1982, p. 195, my translation)

Chapter 8

STONES WITHOUT BRIDGES

Four Orphan Cases

The center of gravity no longer lies in the individual but in
the relations between things.

—Robert Musil,
The Man Without Characteristics
(cited in Baumeister, 1986, p. 86)

*I*n this chapter, I present four women who are among the "orphan cases"
of my therapeutic work. In each case, the impediments to working more
fully with their families limited the elucidation of their predicaments. Cut
off from a more complete relationship to her family and society, each of
these individuals suffered in a unique way. They illustrate the psychological, social, and cultural implications of the myth of independence, which
brings us to my sixth conceptual tool, bridges—understanding cultural
aspects of the family life cycle.

"THE SPIRAL STAIRCASE OF THE SELF"

The community stagnates without the impulse of the individual. The impulse dies away without the sympathy of the
community.

—William James[1]

These four individuals are among the "orphan cases" of my therapeutic work. They illustrate the psychological, social, and cultural

implications of the myth of independence. Although individual psychotherapy represents a major or minor aspect of their treatment—from Erica (who was seen exclusively in individual psychotherapy) to Hannah (who was seen individually by several members of our Eating Disorder Program, but whose major psychological treatment was in family therapy)—their personal stories demand to be understood in their family and cultural contexts. These contexts can be created by placing the stories of these individuals in their "cultural family life cycle." By *cultural* family life cycle, I mean each family's growth and change understood in its given time and place. I call this narrative process of recreating the cultural context for the family life cycle in therapy "bridges," my sixth conceptual tool of CFT. Denied a history (as were Erica and Antonella) or a voice (as was Ismet), experiencing conflict between their inner worlds and their outer worlds (Hannah, Ismet), these women had no recourse but to descend down "the spiral staircase of the self" described by Montaigne. In each case, there were impediments to working more fully with their families.

In some cases, I knew the family members well and worked with them (Hannah, some consultations with Antonella's family). In Ismet's case, I met some of the family members who were valuable as informants, but I did not have permission to discuss her dilemma with them. In Erica's case, while she attended sessions on her own, her mother was always a looming presence in our sessions.

Only one of these woman, Erica, participates in a culture that overtly endorses the myth of independence. The others do not, for religious or cultural reasons. Hannah's religion, Jehovah's Witnesses, requires strict adherence to the faith and a comparatively clear set of boundaries between adherents and nonadherents to the faith. This is doubly true for Ismet, a Pakistani Muslim, whose country of origin is ruled by *sharia*, Islamic law, and whose family lives by a code of honor and propriety. Antonella is somewhere in between: in practice, Italians have become quite independent-minded in their socialization, but they tend to maintain family ties for support throughout the life cycle.

Cut off from a more complete relationship to her family, each of these women suffered in a unique way. Erica, denied access to her parents' experience as Holocaust survivors, lived her life as a series of discrete episodes and events, which she struggled to connect meaningfully. Hannah's life only made sense inside the sacred circle of her family and her congregation; when her older sister left the religious fellowship, another tempting but forbidden world opened up to Hannah. For Ismet, it was not the outside world that held temptation and danger, but events within her own Muslim family, which, if revealed, would bring dishonor and shame. Both Hannah and Ismet had a world of meaningful ties given to them, but the cost of membership was expressed through their bodies. And finally, Antonella is the ultimate stranger. In a world of migrants, in a book of stories about people estranged from their families and their cultures, Antonella made the most radical migration. When her sojourns with extended family members—migrations across cultures, across age barriers, and even within herself, did not sustain her—she looked to the nonhuman world for companionship.

Antonella: "A Stranger in the Family"

[T]he smallest divisible human unit is two people, not one; one is a fiction.

—Tony Kushner (1994, p. 25)

Ottawa in the early 1990s. Antonella Trevisan, a 24-year-old woman, was referred to me by an Italian colleague, Dr. Claudio Angelo, who had treated her when she returned to Italy. When Antonella came to Canada to live with a man she had met through her work, Dr. Angelo referred her to me. Antonella's presenting problems concerned two areas of her life: her eating problems, which emerged after her emigration from Italy, and her relationship with her partner in Canada.

Antonella's predicament. My initial psychiatric consultation (conducted in Italian) revealed the complexities of Antonella's life. This was reflected in the difficulty of making an accurate diagnosis. Her food-related problems had some features of eating disorders, such as restriction of intake, the resulting weight loss, and a history of weight gain and being teased for it. What was missing was the "psychological engine" of an eating disorder: a drive for thinness or a morbid fear of fatness. Her problem was perhaps better understood as a food-related anxiety arising from a ''globus'' sensation (lump in the throat) and a learned avoidance response that generalized from one specific situation to eating in any context.

Although it was clear that her weight gain in late adolescence and the teasing and insults from her mother had sensitized her, other factors had to be considered. Antonella showed an exquisite rejection sensitivity that both arose from and was a metaphor for the circumstances of her birth and adoption. Her migration to Canada also seemed to generate anxieties and uncertainties, and there were hints of conflicts with her partner. Was she also reenacting another, earlier trauma? In the first journey of her life, she was given up by her birth mother (or taken away?) and left on the steps of a foundry. In the first year of her life, Antonella had shown failure to thrive and developmental delays. And she had, at best, an insecure attachment to her adoptive family, predisposing her to lifelong insecurities.

A therapeutic buffet. After my assessment, we faced a choice: whether to treat the eating problem concretely, in purely behavioral terms, or more metaphorically, with some form of psychotherapy. Given the stabilization of her eating pattern and her weight and the larger context of her predicament, we negotiated to do psychotherapy. There were several components to her therapy. Starting with a psychiatric consultation, three types of therapy were negotiated, with Antonella sampling a kind of ''therapeutic buffet'' over a period of some two years: individual therapy for Antonella, couple therapy for Antonella and Rick, and brief family therapy with Antonella's adoptive family visiting from Italy.

The individual work with Antonella was at first exploratory, getting to know the complex bicultural world of the Italian Alps, how she experienced the move to Canada, examining her choices to move here and to live with Rick. Sessions were conducted in a mix of Italian and English. At first, the Italian language was like a ''transitional object'' in her acculturation process; slowly, as she gained confidence in her daily life, English began to dominate her sessions. Under stress, however, she would revert to Italian. I could follow her progress just by noting the balance of Italian and English in each session. (This does not imply any superiority of English or language preferences; rather, it acknowledges the social realities of the culture making its demands felt even in private en-counters. This is the territory of sociolinguistics; see Douglas, 1975a, 1978; Crystal, 1987.) Like Italian, these individual sessions were a secure home base to which Antonella returned during times of stress or between other attempts to find solutions.

After some months in Canada and the stabilization of her eating problems, Antonella became more invested in examining her rela-tionship to Rick. They had met through work while she was still in Italy. After communicating on the telephone, she daringly took him up on an offer to visit. During her holiday in Canada, a romance developed. After her return to Italy, Antonella made the extraordi-nary decision to emigrate, giving up an excellent position in indus-try, leaving her family for a country she did not know well. Rick is 22 years her senior and was only recently separated from his first wife.

In therapy she not only expressed ambivalence about her situa-tion with Rick but enacted it. She asked for couple sessions to discuss some difficulties in their relationship. Beyond collecting basic information, couple sessions were unproductive. While Rick was frank about his physical attraction to her and his desire to have children, Antonella talked about their relationship in an oddly detached way. She could not quite articulate her concerns. As we got closer to examining the problems of their relationship, Anto-nella abruptly announced that they were planning their wedding. The conjoint sessions were put on hold as they dealt with the wed-ding arrangements.

Her parents did not approve of the marriage and boycotted the wedding. Her paternal aunt, however, agreed to come to Canada for the wedding. Since I was regarded by Antonella as part of her extended family support system, she brought her aunt to meet me. It gave me another view of Antonella's family. Her aunt was warm and supportive of Antonella, trying to smooth over the family dif-ferences. A few months later, at Christmas time, her parents and sister visited, and Antonella brought them to meet me. To under-stand these family meetings, however, it is necessary to know An-tonella's early history.

A foundling child. Antonella was a foundling child. Abandoned on the steps of a foundry in Milan as a newborn, she was the subject of an investigation into the private medical clinics of Milan. This revealed that the staff of the clinic where she was born was "paid off to hide the circumstances of my birth." As a result, her date of birth could only be presumed because the clinic staff destroyed her birth records. She was taken into care by the state and, as her origins could not be established, she was put up for adoption.

Antonella has always tried to fill in this void of information with meaning that she draws from her own body. She questions me closely: "Just look at me. Don't you think I look like a Japanese?" She feels that her skin tone is different from other Italians, that her facial features and eyes have an "Asian" cast. With a few, limited facts, and some speculation, she has constructed a personal myth: that she is the daughter of an Italian mother from a wealthy family (hence her hidden birth in a private clinic) and a Japanese father (hence her "Asian" features). It is oddly reassuring to her, but also perhaps a source of her aloofness from her family.

At about six months of age, Antonella was adopted into a family in Merano, in the Italian Alps, near the border with Austria. This is a bicultural region where both Italian and German are spoken and services are available in both languages (much like Ottawa, which is bilingually English and French). Her father, Aldo, who is Italian, is a retired FIAT factory worker. Annalise, her mother, who is a homemaker, had an Italian father and an Austrian mother. About her family she said, "I had a wonderful childhood compared to what came afterwards." Years after her adoption, her parents had a natural child, Oriana, who is 15.

She describes her mother as the disciplinarian at home. Her mother, she said, was "tough, German." When she visited her Austrian grandmother, no playing was allowed in that strict home. Her own mother allowed her "no friends in the house," but her father "was my pal when I was a kid." Although she had a good relationship with her father, he became "colder" when she turned 13. Her parents' relationship is remembered as cordial, but she later learned that they had many marital problems. Mother told her that she married to get away from home, but in fact she was in love with someone else. Overall, the feeling is of a rigid family organization. Her father is clearly presented by Antonella as warmer and more sociable. Mother is experienced by the patient as "tough" but crying all the time, feeling betrayed by everybody.

"A family visit from the Italian Alps." When her family finally came to visit, Antonella brought them to see me. At first, the session had the quality of a student introducing out-of-town parents to her college teacher. They were pleased that I spoke Italian and knew Dr. Angelo, whom they trusted. I soon found, however, that the Trevisans were hungry to tell their story. Instead of a social exchange of pleasantries, this meeting turned into the first session of an impromptu course of brief family therapy.

Present were Antonella's parents, Aldo and Annalise, and her sister, Oriana. Annalise led the conversation, relegating Aldo to a support role. Oriana alternated between disdain and agitation, punctuated by bored indifference. Annalise had much to complain about: her own troubled childhood, her sense of betrayal and abandonment, heightened by Antonella's departure from the family and from Italy. I was struck by the parallel themes of abandonment in mother and daughter. Mother clearly needed to tell this story, so I tried to set the stage for the family to hear her, what Parry and Doan (1994) call "recruiting an audience." I used Antonella, whom I knew best, as a barometer of the progress of the session, and by that indicator, believed it had gone well.

When I saw them again some ten days later, I was stunned by the turn of events. Oriana had assaulted her parents. The father had bandages over his face and the mother had covered her bruises with heavy make-up and dark glasses. Annalise was very upset about Oriana, who was defiant and aggressive at home. For her part, Oriana defended herself by saying she had been provoked and hit by her mother. Worried by this dangerous escalation, I tried to open some space for a healthy standoff and renegotiation.

Somehow, the concern had shifted away from Antonella to Oriana. Antonella was off the hook, but I waited for an opening to deal with this. I first tried to explore the cultural attitudes to adolescence in Italy by asking how the Italian and the German subcultures in their area understood teenagers differently. What were Oriana's concerns? Had they seen this outburst coming? The whole family participated in a kind of sociological overview of Italian adolescence, with me as their grateful audience. The parents demonstrated keen insight and empathy. Concerned about Oriana's experience of the session, I made a concerted effort to draw her into it. Eventually, the tone of the session lightened. Knowing they would return to Italy soon, I explored whether they had considered family work. Since they had met a few times with Dr. Angelo over Antonella's eating problems, they were comfortable with the notion of family therapy. They all agreed to consider seeing Dr. Angelo as a family to find ways to understand Oriana and her concerns and for Oriana to explore other, nonviolent ways to be heard in the family. I agreed to meet them again before their departure and to communicate with Dr. Angelo about their wishes. On their way out, I wondered aloud about the apparent switch in their focus from Antonella to Oriana. The parents reassured me that they were ready to let Antonella live her own life now.

When they returned to say goodbye, we had a brief session. Oriana and Antonella were oddly buoyant and at ease. The parents were relieved. Antonella had offered the possibility of Oriana returning to spend the summer in Canada with her. I tried to connect this back to the previous session, wondering how much the two sisters supported each other. I was delighted, I said emphatically, by the family's apparent approval of Antonella's marriage to Rick. It was striking that, even from a distance of thousands of miles away, Antonella was still a part of the Trevisan family. And Rick was still not in the room.

"Life Before Man."[2] To understand Antonella's attachments more fully, it is important to explore her passion for her Siberian huskies. From the beginning of her relationship with Rick she used her interest in dogs as a way for them to be more socially active as a couple, getting them out of the house to go to dog shows, for example. As her interests expanded, she wanted to buy bitches for breeding and to set up a kennel. Rick was only reluctantly supportive in this. Nonetheless, they ended up buying a home in the country where she could establish a kennel. Her haggling with Rick over the dogs was quite instrumental on her part, representing her own choices and interests and a test of the extent to which Rick would support her.

But I think there is something deeper, too. From the first days of her life, Antonella was rejected by her birth parents, literally abandoned and exposed, and later adopted by what she experienced as a non-nurturing family. Having thrown her net wider afield, she looked to Canada, and to Rick, for nurturance and for identity; but it was only partly there. She turned to the nonhuman world for the constancy of affection she could not find with people. Her huskies gave her pleasure, a task, an identity. She spent many sessions discussing their progress, showing me pictures of her dogs and their awards. As it happened, my secretary at the time was also a dog lover who raised Samoyed dogs (related to huskies) and the two of them exchanged stories of dog lore.

Is there something, too, in the mythology of Canada that helps us understand Antonella? Does Canada, the New World, still hold a place in the European imagination for radical departures, identity makeovers? Or does Canada specifically represent the "malevolent North," as Margaret Atwood (1995) calls it in her exploration of Canadian fiction? Huskies are a Northern animal, close to the wolf in their origins and habits. In Chapter 5, we met River Running, a white boy with the "Grey Owl Syndrome," wishing to be Native. Are we seeing with Antonella something akin to that? Bypassing the human world, she makes her identification with a new world through its animals. If people have failed her, then she will leave not only her own tribe (Italy), but skip the identification with Canada's Native peoples, responding to the "call of the wild" to identify with a "life before man" (to use another of Atwood's evocative phrases), finding companionship and solace with her dogs.

In *Bear*, Canadian novelist Marion Engel (1976) portrays Lou, a woman who lives in the wilderness and befriends a bear. Lou seeks her identity from him: "Bear, make me comfortable in the world at last. Give me your skin" (Engel, 1976, p. 106). After some time with the bear, the woman changes: "What had passed to her from him she did not know. . . . She felt not that she was at last human, but that she was at last clean" (Engel, 1976, p. 137). And Antonella? I met her again in a gallery in Ottawa, rummaging through old prints. She was asking about prints of dogs; I was looking for old prints of Brazil. How was she, I asked? "Well . . . ," she said. Was that a healthy "well" or the start of an explanation? "Me and Rick are splitting up," she said without ceremony, "but I still have the huskies." For each of us, the prints represented another world of connections.

Erica: "The Past Is a Foreign Country"

The past is a foreign country: they do things differently there.

—L.P. Hartley (1953, p. 1)

Montreal, early 1980s. Erica Gershon was a successful single woman in her mid-thirties, a child of Polish Jewish Holocaust survivors who was born and raised in Montreal. Erica was referred for individual psychotherapy to my psychotherapy supervisor, who conducted research on Holocaust survivors and their families in Montreal (see Sigal, 1986; Sigal, DiNicola, & Buonvino, 1988; Sigal & Weinfeld, 1989). She became the formal long-term psychotherapy case required for my residency in psychiatry at McGill University. The psychiatry resident who had seen her in the assessment clinic suggested that a geographic relocation might be as beneficial as psychotherapy. This turned out to be prophetic, as Erica eventually moved as a way to deal with the difficult issues with her mother.

Although Erica was seen in individual psychotherapy, her parents had a palpable presence in our sessions. Her memories of her deceased father were warm ones, interrupted by intrusions of her mother's firm resolve to leave the past behind. But her mother is someone Erica never left behind. She had a profound reach into Erica's life, expressed in her hypochondriacal concerns and her staging of medical emergencies that required Erica's immediate response from her apartment across the city. For Erica, it was not a question of going back home or not going back home; rather, she had never found her place at home and as a consequence there was no way out. "To get out of it, you have to get into it": to leave home, to be an adult, Erica first had to make her peace with her mother.

"Off the dial." Raised in a family environment of secrets and guilt that were never named, Erica reenacted the vicarious trauma that her parents transmitted in spite of themselves. At the beginning of our sessions, she had an out-of-town lover who was kept a secret from her family. Dietrich was a German immigrant living in Can-

ada. Although she felt she could not tell her mother about him, Erica did not understand her ironic attraction to him. For her, seeing Dietrich was a series of encounters, the pattern of which was beyond her grasp. Each weekend with him was its own experience, untethered to the last one or to any thought of another.

In *Immortality*, novelist Milan Kundera (1991) pursues the meaning of a central metaphor, the dial, through the erotic life of a character called Rubens. When his marriage (''a mere parenthesis in his life,'' p. 288) ends, Rubens lands *''beyond the border of love''* (italics in original, p. 288). Rubens discovers that he is off the dial of progress, not only in his love life but in his painting as well. He later discovers a different kind of love ''beyond the border of love,'' an episodic love without continuity, restricted to the ''erotic sphere,'' unrelated to the course of his life. Like Rubens, Erica had an affair with Dietrich that had no influence on the rest of her life. The restrictions that Erica imposed on it created the erotic charge for her, a charge she had no desire to dissipate by making it public. The internal evidence of our sessions suggests, in fact, that even sharing it in therapy may have dulled its emotional impact for her.

In her next affair, she went out with a man ten years her junior. He, too, was kept a secret from her mother. When the young man told his father about Erica, the father approved, ''After all, you don't learn to ride on a new bicycle.'' Erica registered no emotion in retelling this story in therapy. She had a vague idea that it was meant to be funny, but expressed neither anger nor shame. Off the dial, beyond the reach of metaphor, the whole relationship, not to mention any degrading comments, had no impact on her life.

''A disguised dependency relationship.'' In my view, Erica's psychotherapy was ''one-person'' family therapy. The sessions offered her what she could not ask for and did not get from her mother or from her lovers: dependence upon a nurturing parental figure, reflecting back to her a sense of who she was. As such, it was what Indian psychiatrist Pande calls a ''disguised dependency relationship'' in a culture that pathologizes such needs in adults. Erica's presenting problem was a stark and moving plaint: ''I have no memories, I have no childhood, and no past.'' For Erica, the past is a foreign country—something that happened to other people, in another place. In spite of her intelligence and professional success,

there was a concreteness to her emotional world. She was in psychotherapy for three years. I did not invoke the concept of alexithymia to describe her concreteness, though something like that is described in the language of survivors. My objection to the concept of alexithymia is that it is a temptation to teach people the meaning of their experience and "the words to say it" (to use a phrase by novelist Marie Cardinal, 1983). Rather than invoking psychopathology, I was more willing to accept her life as she lived it—holes, gaps, and all. Therapy was aimed at learning to sit with those gaps and to stitch a life out of what was accessible to her.

"Knowing and enduring." Hannah Arendt (1968) claimed in her brilliant essay, "On humanity in dark times," that we cannot master a past like Nazism: "The best that can be achieved is to know precisely what it was, and to endure this knowledge, and then to wait and see what comes from knowing and enduring" (p. 20). One cannot easily appropriate for oneself what one's parents have declared off limits. In therapy, Erica had been able to recount many details from her parents' lives and from her own childhood. She had provided many still shots, sometimes vivid and informative, but often disembodied fragments of a life. After three years of therapy, it was like a David Hockney photo collage, with individual still shots coalescing into a recognizable portrait. But no matter how detailed, that portrait is not a movie, there is no narrative flow. What Erica still lacked was the ability to put it all together into a coherent story.

Erica could not recapture the memory of a childhood that was denied and forbidden. It was as if, in trying to suppress the pain, her parents suppressed too much. But something leaked through anyway: you cannot keep everything to yourself. Erica's mother did pass something on, coded not only in Polish and Yiddish, but in a complex series of injunctions about what can be said and felt and remembered.

In an essay about "knowing what you are not supposed to know and feeling what you are not supposed to feel," John Bowlby (1979) described this forbidden territory of feelings, knowledge, and memories in families. Perhaps the playwright Eugene Ionesco put it best: "There are no words for the deepest experience. The more I try to explain myself, the less I understand myself. Of course, not everything is unsayable in words, only the living truth'' (cited in Steiner, 1975, p. 185). Philosophers gave up—''Poetry after Auschwitz is barbaric'' (Theodor Adorno); playwrights gave up—''no words for the deepest experience'' (Eugene Ionesco), *Act Without Words* (Samuel Beckett); theologians gave up—''God was silent'' (Jonas, 1987, p. 10). Who talked? Patients talked to their psychiatrists. Leo Eitinger (1980) noted that, ''It was only—or rather *mainly*—psychiatrists who were able to find 'any bad results' in the Jewish survivors from their sojourn in the concentration camps'' (p. 234).

What did they find? A major theme in all the literature on Holocaust survivors and their families concerns memory and silence. Saul Friedlander (1980), who is a historian and a child survivor, entitled his personal account, *When Memory Comes*. Nadine Fresco's (1984) evocative conversations with fellow survivors is called, ''Remembering the unknown.'' Grubrich-Simitis (1984) offers a model for understanding and working with the lost memories of survivors. Survivors not only lose their memories, she observes, but they become concrete. Survivors inhabit ''a world beyond metaphor'' (coined by Herzog, cited by Grubrich-Simitis, 1984). The aim in their therapy ''is to overcome concretism and to restore metaphoric function'' (Grubrich-Simitis, 1984, p. 303). Like Erica, the people that Grubrich-Simitis saw in therapy came from families that developed a ''pact of silence''—their parents' traumatic memories were never talked about. John Sigal describes ''a special, psychologically unhealthy quality of the relationship between survivors and their children, which resulted in difficulties for the children'' (Sigal, 1986, p. 364). He reported ''an unusual degree of mutual involvement, an enmeshment between parent and child'' (p. 364). ''Enmeshment'' here has a specific meaning. The parents had expectations that became burdens for their children: to share the intensity of mourning and to replace the dead relatives and become idealized, perfect versions of them.

This did not happen only to survivors. The enormity of the experience was so great that even courageous witnesses were cowed into silence. German philosopher Theodor Adorno said in an often-quoted phrase, ''Writing poetry after Auschwitz is barbaric.'' Author-survivor Elie Wiesel wrote, ''Auschwitz means death . . . of language and . . . of time'' (cited by Grubrich-Simitis, 1984, p.

309). There has also been discussion of the "hollowness," the fail-ure of language, particularly German,[3] at the cultural level.

All of the foregoing is a series of metaphors—"remembering the unknown," "pact of silence," "hollowness," "death of lan-guage." These are ways of saying *in words* that some events are so far outside our previous experience that the words we have seem inadequate. What I object to—and resist—is the idea that the diffi-culty in finding the words for this is some kind of basic cognitive or expressive deficit called "alexithymia" and *pensée opératoire* in psychosomatic patients or "concretism" in Holocaust survivors.[4] When the conditions are right, if they are safe and other people listen, survivors can and do remember their experiences; they can and do find the words to convey horror. Somehow, we have to overcome this temporary impotence of words. Some survivors have done it; the very writers who despaired of finding the words have done it (e.g., Elie Wiesel). We have to reach beyond the numbing facts that render us literal and concrete, even if we have to invent a new language to do it.

In the kind of synchrony of events that I no longer find unusual, Erica ended her dependencies on her mother and on therapy by moving to Toronto. I was ending my training and was to leave myself a few months later. This was the "geographic cure" that had been suggested several years earlier. Erica had changed in subtle ways: she made choices that were more personally meaning-ful to her. She had found an excellent position in Toronto and was reconnecting with other friends who had moved there. She had slowly weaned her mother from a dependence on Erica's involve-ment in every aspect of her life. In any case, she was prepared to leave. In a book so taken with words and narrative in therapy, this case is about the failure of words and memory. Within the limited scope of my knowledge about her in therapy, Erica remained be-yond the reach of metaphor.

If I had to do it again, would I change anything? Yes. Early on in therapy, I would suggest that Erica bring her mother into the ses-sions more directly, by doing family-of-origin work (Framo, 1976) or even by inviting her mother to participate. I would have worked on what was already shared between them, opening space for the creation of further memories, new stories about the past. New re-search on memory suggests that when new stories are told about ourselves, they eventually become memories of our own. In his fascinating study of autobiographical memory, psychologist John Kotre (1995) concludes:

> Are these memories false? Not necessarily. Whatever their mix of fact and fantasy, they are the means by which an individual's identity is grafted on to a group's. They are the glue that binds a child to a family, a player to a team, a patient to a school of therapy, a devotee to a religion, a citizen to a nation. It makes *me* one of *them*. (p. 229)

If Erica's mother could have done this, she would have passed on her history to the person for whom it mattered most. With this transmission, perhaps the mother would not have needed medical crises to bring her daughter to her side.

Hannah: "From the Cradle"

Only in an enlarged research context that considers meaning as well as behavior will we be able to understand how anorexia nervosa is experienced and why it has become the characteristic disorder of the female adolescent in our day.

—Joan Jacobs Brumberg
(1985, p. 104)

Hannah Davies was a 16-year-old adolescent admitted to hospital in the early 1990s. Her parents are British immigrants from Northern England. They live in a small town near Kingston, Ontario where their family and social life revolves around being Jehovah's Witnesses. The faith gave the immigrant parents a community to participate in and a meaningful direction for their family. Hannah, they stated with quiet pride, was raised in the faith "from the cradle." Hannah was admitted for further investigation of a number of different problems:

1. eating disorder: anorexia nervosa, restrictive subtype (APA, 1994);
2. thoughts of harming herself;
3. mood disturbance;

4. various somatic complaints: dizziness, occasional fainting episodes, symptoms of "mono" including fatigue;
5. family issues.

Except for her weight loss, most of her problems, for which she already had many consultations, were only vaguely defined. Hannah lived with her parents and her two younger siblings. Her older sister, Esther, who was 19, had left home and the faith.

A meeting with the elders of Kingdom Hall. After her admission, members of the child psychiatry inpatient treatment team expressed concerns about whether her religious beliefs would interfere with her treatment. I suggested that we ask the family directly if they had any concerns or reservations about our treatment approach and to learn more about their faith. Mr. Davies, we discovered, was one of the elders of their congregation or Kingdom Hall. I asked to meet with the family to discuss their faith and our treatment plan for Hannah. The response was gratifying: they convened a group of elders of the congregation along with the Davies family.

They were very informative about their faith, answering all our questions. We in turn described our treatment plan. Nothing in their faith, they reassured us, stood in the way of our plan. In fact, they wanted to reassure us of their complete support. Hannah was a highly valued member of the congregation, raised in their faith "from the cradle." She had taken her "fellowship" in the faith at the unusually young age of twelve. Her family was clearly held in high esteem by the elders, as was Hannah herself. The meeting was quite a long one. The treatment team learned a great deal about Jehovah's Witnesses and the elders were assured that we were committed to working with them collaboratively. Throughout the meeting, I had expressed great curiosity about their faith. At the end, the leader of the elders turned to me and thanked me for my interest and extended a very sincere invitation for me to visit their Kingdom Hall.

The price of fellowship. What we learned from Hannah herself, however, was that her older sister, Esther, had left home and the faith. Esther wrote the elders a "letter of disassociation." The congregation responded by cutting her off—she was "disfellowshipped."

This put a fence between her and the congregation, including her family. Although Hannah could speak to her, the family was vigilant over the older sister's influence on Hannah and the other siblings.

Publicly, Hannah acquiesced. Privately, however, she was distressed. Although she expressed no personal qualms about the faith, she was upset by her sister's predicament. As outside observers on the treatment team, we saw disfellowship as "a fiendish punishment," as William James put it: Hannah's sister had been "turned loose in society" and cut off from her own kind. To us (and we sensed it was Hannah's feeling as well), it appeared to be a religious version of *Invisible Man*, Ralph Ellison's (1952) story of a nameless young black man's search for his own identity. He is "invisible" because the people he encounters "see only my surroundings, themselves, or figments of their imagination" (Ellison, 1952, p. 3).

My construction of anorexia nervosa (DiNicola, 1990b, 1990c) is of a complex chameleon-like illness that takes its form from prevailing social views of the body. At first, this seemed paradoxical: Hannah lived in a relatively enclosed social circle. Where had she picked up such ideas? Most likely at school and from her social contacts. Indeed, it is reasonable to suggest that, given the distress that she felt within herself and her family, the larger society provided a model for the expression of her distress in the one arena within her absolute control: her body. Anthropologist Margaret Mead suggested this possibility during times of cultural change:

> periods will be found in which adequate social forms for the expression of points of strain and tension in the personality will be forced back upon [her] own body for symbolic expression. (1947, p. 72)

This is how a young woman who is not part of the cultural mainstream developed what social historian Joan Jacobs Brumberg calls "the characteristic disorder of the female adolescent in our day" (1985, p. 104).

Therapy: Opening space for health. Hannah's treatment had several components:

1. Admission to an adolescent inpatient unit for the treatment of her eating disorder.
2. Hospitalization was a powerful act, creating a temporary home for her and a space between Hannah and her family. In an earlier era of the treatment of eating disorders, this was called a "parentectomy." It created space for her: time for reflection, an opportunity to work on her eating in a different context.
3. In family sessions, we asked the questions she could not, thereby opening up a dialogue with her parents. Hannah, for example, would not openly express her distress about her sister. It happened more subtly, indirectly. A dialogue took place about Hannah, about the family in their presence: a reflection on themselves in which they took part. The parents made some accommodations to her; she made some adjustments in her attitudes and her behavior.
4. Finally, we were "witnesses" to her predicament. In a context of change, we could be an audience for her story. Hannah did the rest.

Her course in hospital included numerous episodes of unresponsiveness, one serious enough to trigger an admission to the intensive care unit. However, no cause was found for her episodes of unresponsiveness (everything from conversion disorder to a sleep disorder was considered). Her suicidal ideation improved rapidly and there was good steady, symptomatic progress of her anorexia nervosa.

What I suspect really happened is this. Hannah thought through her commitment to her family and her faith: the benefits of their support and the comforting teachings of Jehovah's Witnesses weighed against the price of being shunned, of disfellowship, and the impact of being ill. I think that in the end, she got better through an effort of will, a decision to be healthy in her predicament. Several follow-up sessions confirmed that things were going rather well, although her somatic symptoms were still mildly present. Her mood and weight were stable. My impression was that her eating disorder was stable but not cured. She joined the psycho-education groups offered to adolescents and their families with eating disorders.

Therapy as a silent witness. When I did research on Jehovah's Witnesses, I discovered that a lot of people think of this religion as a sect or a cult, with all that those words conjure up.[5] I am not very impressed with these arguments: religion is not something that stands up to the demands of logic. I would hate to appear before a committee to explain my love for my family, my commitment to an open society, and other irrational enthusiasms. Religion is a meaning system: it thrives on belief, on shared symbols, transcending what can be shown, going "beyond the information given" in Jerome Bruner's phrase, reaching for something outside of direct human experience, something numinous. In a celebrated essay, Rabbi Joseph Soloveitchik put it this way:

> Reason does not lay down the path along which the man of faith walks. Only after the fact, can reason describe it. The latter walks behind, not in front of the man of faith. (Resdin, 1979, p. 219)

Sigmund Freud's (1927) essay on the subject of religion was called *The Future of an Illusion*, as if religion were something neurotic, something primitive, to be grown out of. Perhaps in the hands of someone else, Hannah's faith would have been put on the table of therapy like food restriction or another symptom of illness: I refused to do this. We must not confuse disease, illness, suffering, and predicaments: we must resist the reduction of predicaments to diseases, but also the conflation of disorders and predicaments. They are different, if connected, realms. What made Hannah's problem a predicament, something with a moral charge to it, was the fact that it was a lonely, personal dilemma requiring her own choices. Her faith could not be argued out, only animated by her own belief, her own convictions of what made life sensible to her.

I am very clear about what I did for her as a physician, as a psychiatrist, and as a therapist (these are all different roles). As a physician, I investigated her physical complaints, as a psychiatrist I offered her a path away from self-starvation, as a family therapist, I opened space for a family dialogue. She was healthy enough to face the irreducible human dilemmas of her family and her faith (this is not a space for psychiatry or for therapy to do its work, but to get out of the way). In our culture, unlike Neki's model for working in

India, therapy cannot give people the meaningful connections they lack in their lives. In our culture, therapy is a path, not a destination. After I did my practical work as a physician, and a little work with Hannah and her family as a therapist, I did what physicians, healers, and shamans have done for millennia in all the world's cultures: I set up a quiet watch on the sidelines, bearing silent witness to her suffering.

Ismet: "A Pain With No Name"

At times the body speaks what the tongue cannot utter.

—David Taylor (1985, p. 134)

Ismet Farida Aziz was admitted to the Montreal Children's Hospital in the early 1980s for investigation of abdominal pain of unknown origin. When medical investigations could not resolve the problem, a psychiatric consultation was sought. I started by asking Ismet about herself and learned that she was a 17-year-old Pakistani Muslim, born in Mirpur in Northern Pakistan. Always curious about the meaning of names, I learned that Ismet means "demure" and that Farida means "blessing." Her family had moved to Montreal when she was a child. She appeared to answer these questions truthfully but with a modest reserve. Although she was willing to let me talk to her, I soon found her reluctant to share much about her pain or her ideas about it.

After a while, I stumbled onto a way to communicate with her. I discovered that she was unwilling to actively inform me, but somewhat willing to passively answer some of my questions. At first, it was a version of the guessing game "hot and cold"—she would let me know if I was getting closer to her concerns or farther away. As I built trust with her, it became more like "twenty questions"—she actually answered some questions, up to a point. In this first session, I did not get very far, but I started to build rapport with her. The session ended when her family appeared at the door and Ismet had a startle reaction. I sensed it was time to end the interview. Looking back at her as I left, I noticed a deep blush covered her face and was spreading down her neck. The abrupt change in her demeanor puzzled me.

When I returned later, I found her more willing to talk. Her description of her pain was vague and somewhat inconsistent. I remembered what my mentor in medical school had taught me: "Treat your patient as if you are the only physician she will see." Given Ismet's reserve, I questioned how much the medical service had been able to accomplish with her. So I methodically started going through body systems. When I started asking her questions about her reproductive system, she had the same reaction I had noticed when her family visited earlier. She became hypervigilant, looking around excitedly and nervously, as if she expected someone to be listening to us.

We now have a way to understand such reactions as part of posttraumatic stress disorder (PTSD; see *DSM-IV*, APA, 1994; DiNicola, 1996b). They are exaggerated startle reactions that become conditioned responses in traumatic contexts. Her responses were doubly worrisome: there was clearly some troubled area of her life that she could not or would not discuss. A psychiatric colleague, Pierre Leichner,[6] has a model of the sometimes contradictory and puzzling responses to sexual abuse. He notes two overall patterns: "repressed-denied" vs. "expressed-amplified" reactions. Ismet was clearly repressing and denying the origin of her distress. At that time, however, in the early 1980s, when I was just out of medical school, I did not have this expanded vocabulary to understand Ismet's predicament.

Transcultural reconstruction. For a therapeutic translation of her predicament, I first had to try to understand her culture and religion, the possible meanings of her pain for her, and what implicit rules she was observing in her medical presentation. The question was: what in her presenting culture could help me understand her presenting complaint?

Her culture, her family, her religion made it enormously difficult for Ismet to give words to her predicament in a Western context. In fact, these did not appear to be merely impositions from the outside, but a core part of her own make-up, the stuff of her identity. What she herself felt, what generated sense-making in her life, militated against even looking for a way to say it.

In spite of these injunctions against expressing herself, I was able to put this picture together through a kind of transcultural reconstruction of her experience. After her older sister's arranged marriage with a man from Mirpur, their native city in Pakistan, the newly-wed couple moved in with the Aziz family in Montreal. With both parents and her older siblings at work, Ismet sometimes found herself at home alone with her brother-in-law. This situation eventually led to sexual contact between the two of them. Of course, because of her age and status, this can only be construed as sexual abuse from a Western psychiatric perspective. What I did not know was whether Ismet experienced it as abusive. I believed she did because of her indefinable pain and distress. On the other hand, the medical team, including the social worker, pointed out that she might have other reasons for her concerns: perhaps she was worried about getting caught or being pregnant. When I negotiated with her to do a pregnancy test, she was both concerned and relieved. Relieved to have the issue addressed; concerned as to whether her family could find out. I assured her that I could not do the tests without her permission, nor would I share the results with anyone else. I took this opportunity to reassure her that due to her age, she could control the flow of information. I would not reveal anything to her family (or to the child protection team of the hospital) without her permission. With this reassurance, more of the story emerged.

She told me that she, too, was engaged to be married. Her intended was Mughram, a young man in Pakistan, chosen by her family. Mughram was to visit in the next few months. If all went well, their wedding would take place in the next year or two. I surmised that Ismet was worried about the loss of her virginity, which her future husband would discover, bringing shame and ruin on herself and her family. In the end, she was not pregnant. Her abdominal distress resolved. She returned to her family and to her predicament.

When I read Salman Rushdie's novel *Shame* (1983), I felt a shock of recognition. Rushdie's novel has its origins in a newspaper report of a Pakistani father in London who murdered his daughter ''because by making love to a white boy she had brought such dishonour upon her family that only blood could wash away the stain'' (1983, p. 123). It brought home to me how much had been at stake for Ismet. This is not to say that I suspected her family would be violent, but that Ismet's family surely shared the same sources of meaning, the same ''social and sexual codes'' imposing on women "the intolerable burdens of honour and propriety" (Rushdie, 1983, p. 189). Writing as an Asian, Rushdie (1983) laments:

> We who have grown up on a diet of honour and shame can still grasp what must seem unthinkable to peoples living in the aftermath of the death of God and of tragedy: that men will sacrifice their dearest love on the implacable altars of their pride. . . . Between shame and shamelessness lies the axis upon which we turn; meteorological conditions at both these poles are of the most extreme, ferocious type. Shamelessness, shame: the roots of violence. (p. 124)

Rushdie and his novel are haunted by that story, and my account of Ismet, too, is haunted by this sickening possibility. Ismet's story is another of those incomplete, impossible stories of my practice. Without an end, without resolution, they haunt my therapeutic work. And Ismet sometimes joins Nikolai, the Russian/Jewish boy of Chapter 1, in a kind of Greek chorus in the room when I am helping families to imagine livable solutions to impossible predicaments. "All stories are haunted by the ghosts of the stories they might have been," Rushdie wrote (1983, p. 125). Like stories, therapy, too, is haunted by other possibilities, other rationalities.

And in the end, what could I call Ismet's nameless pain? The name of an emotion that comes out of the interplay between the authoritarian repression of women in the name of "honour and propriety" and the pride some men take in defending such values. Shame. Expressed through her body, speaking what her tongue could not utter.

Part III

FAMILIES AS
STORYING CULTURES

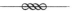

When families are viewed as interpretive communities or storying cultures, family narratives are rich with meaning. Like all cultures, families tell stories of themselves—stories about who they are, about where they have been, and where they are going. . . . To tell one's story is to construct one's life.

—David Paré,
"Of Families and Other Cultures"
(1995, p. 13)

Chapter 9

A GARDEN OF FORKING PATHS

Exploring a Family's Alternities of Being

All stories are haunted by the ghosts of the stories they
might have been.

—Salman Rushdie,
Shame (1983, p. 125)

*T*his chapter illustrates the use of family narrative as a conceptual tool
for CFT. Stories, my seventh conceptual tool, examines the evolving
narrative of family life and therapy as a garden of forking paths. I pick up
the story of the Shami family, introduced in Chapter 1, and follow their
therapeutic story over 12 sessions to its completion. It demonstrates all the
tools introduced so far—spirals of negotiation, cultural and therapeutic
translation, playing with insider and outsider roles, peering through the
masks of cultural costume and camouflage, examining cultural strategies,
and building bridges between individuals and families.

"ALTERNITIES OF BEING"

"Woods" is a metaphor for narratives that Umberto Eco (1994)
explores in his work on the construction of texts. Eco takes his root
metaphor from a story by Jorge Luis Borges, "The Garden of Forking Paths" (1964). In this chapter, I pick up the story of the Shami
family we met in Chapter 1. The story of their therapy is a walk
through the woods of the Shami family's predicament, each session
offering many forking paths. Each choice made, each turn to one
side or the other, led to another part of the woods. This was true

not only for the parts of their past that were explored, but also for the different possible futures that presented themselves for consideration, futures that we as therapists helped the family define, comprehend, and prepare to live in.

At times, these possibilities were so intense, so palpable, and we came so close to the edge, that there was a sense of vertigo from the heights we reached and the depths yawning below us. We felt haunted by the ghosts of other stories, not from far away or long ago, but right there in the session, as it unfolded. These possibilities are what George Steiner (1975) describes as "alternities of being." My seventh conceptual tool for CFT is the *stories* that metaphorically express the evolving narrative of family life as "alternities of being" and therapy as "a garden of forking paths."

Contrasted against the "alternities of being" were the many possible sets of lenses offered to and, at times, forced onto this family's experience. The challenge is not simply represented by the "Rashomon effect"—seeing the story from each person's point of view (see Elizur & Minuchin, 1989). It is not just about different persons with different and incompatible stories; rather, it concerns "different cultures, different rationalities" (Marshall Sahlins, cited by Geertz, 1995), even within Canadian society. Here are some of the multiple lenses we will encounter in my construal of their story:

Cultural lenses. The Shami family brought not one, but several cultures to therapy: the cultures of Islam and Christianity in the Middle East; the cultures of Lebanon and the culture of a place with no exact boundaries, Palestine; and, of course, their construal of Western culture, living in Canada.

"Orientalism." This is the term that Edward Said (1979) uses to describe the West looking at the East, a filter through which Westerners have sifted, selected, and shaped the experience of diverse peoples of the East into Others. I believe that this lens is one of the two key reasons behind their predicament; it was actively at work at Samya's school and in the children's agency.

The Western philosophy of childhood. This has led, inevitably, to the construction of "childhood" in individualistic terms, set in opposition to family, institutions, even the state, in the assertion of "children's rights" (Archard, 1993; Matthews, 1994; cf. DiNicola, 1995). The construal of Samya's "rights," asserted aggressively, in isolation from her family and in ignorance of the cultures that infuse meaning into her life, is the second key reason why the Shami family found itself in a battle with Canadian society and why Samya was caught as a pawn in the middle.

Three more lenses were brought to bear for the cultural and therapeutic translations of the Shami family's experience:

Transcultural child psychiatry. The knowledge of this field, which poses "developmental questions about children's mental disorders in the context of culture" (DiNicola, 1992, p. 26; presented in Chapter 4) can help us understand two aspects of Samya's predicament—the cultural and the developmental. The "royal road" for this task is the redescription of children's predicaments—drawing new maps, forging new tools, inspiring fresh metaphors, and coining alternative vocabularies for children's experience.

A critique of paternalism. While attempting to harness the authority that their culture of origin invested in the elderly as a working method, we were also richly aware of the domineering presence of Khaled, Samya's father. What we offered was a gentle, workable alternative that they could integrate into their family in their effort to live more comfortably in Canadian society.

Cultural family therapy. Finally, by adopting multiple lenses to create multiple descriptions, by trying to step outside of the dominating ideology of "Orientalism" as we worked with this family, and by being aware of the roots of the Western construction of childhood, we used the knowledge of transcultural child psychiatry and a critical perspective of paternalism to conduct cultural family therapy with the Shamis.

SAMYA: "ABOVE MY HEART, ABOVE MY GOD"

Presenting problem. Ottawa in the summer of 1990. Samya is a 13-year-old adolescent who accused her father, Khaled, of physical and sexual abuse. In the course of an investigation of physical abuse discovered at her French Catholic school, Samya made an allegation of sexual abuse by her father when she was 12 years old. When her sister, Soha, who is a year younger, was questioned by the school and the agency, she claimed that she had also been molested. Both Samya and her sister Soha were removed from her home by the French children's protection agency. During her stay at a group home, Samya was raped. Her parents were angry, accusing the agency and the group home of unreasonably removing Samya from the parental home and then failing to protect her. They blamed the agency for Samya's behavior and for the rape, angry that her social worker had supported "Samya's right to sexual expression."

When charges were laid against the father, the case went to court; the judge requested a child and family assessment through a special clinic that conducts court-mandated psychiatric evaluations. Soha recanted her allegations unequivocally, claiming that Samya had told her what to say, and returned home. Samya gave such vague and inconsistent testimony that the court was unable to render a clear judgment. Khaled, the father, frankly admitted that he had struck the children when disciplining them, in the manner of his culture of origin. He also stated that he hugged and kissed his children affectionately, but that he was never sexually inappropriate with them. Neither the agency nor the clinic was able to establish a working relationship with the family.

At this point, I was asked by the court to consult with the family as a transcultural psychiatrist and family therapist. I agreed to take on a clinical role with the child and her family if the court and the children's agency considered the investigation and legal issues resolved. In fact, they were stymied by the family but were happy to negotiate for a therapeutic rather than a legal solution. My own goal was clear: to pursue therapeutic change rather than to clarify the charges and countercharges. To that end, I gathered a therapeutic team. The heart of the team was a family therapy service consisting of social workers, psychologists, and psychiatrists, some of whom were in training. We also had available an Arabic-speaking staff psychiatrist from Egypt (whose culture the family pointedly identified as different from theirs) and their family physician, who was an Arab and their trusted ally. There were two other key resources. Dr. John Theis, a psychologist and family therapist, was on a year-long sabbatical with me to conduct and teach family therapy. Although he makes only one appearance in the text, Dr. Theis acted as a consultant throughout the Shami family's course of therapy. An East Indian woman who was a resident in child psychiatry and training in family therapy had two key roles: she was my co-therapist for the first six months of family therapy and she saw Samya and Rakia for alternating individual and mother-daughter sessions.

What follows is a psychological and therapeutic account of experiences (the "narrative truth"), rather than a journalistic rendering of actual events (the "historical truth"), which was outside of my agreement (cf. Spence, 1982). But there are rules, too. We cannot just fantasize any ending we want: writing imposes its own narrative truth. Narrative has to make sense, getting a story down on paper means putting things in order. To write this chapter, I transcribed every session verbatim, a tedious, time-consuming task. Watching a year's worth of session videotapes can be a numbing experience. It was only in the editing and shaping of the story that this family's experience emerged fully for me between the lines.

Presenting family culture. Samya and her family are from the Middle East. The family members variously identify themselves as "Arabic" (a racial, ethnic, and political affiliation), "Palestinian" (a historical, geographic, and political affiliation), "Lebanese" (where mother and father were raised), "Muslim" and "Catholic" (religious and political affiliations in the geopolitical context of Lebanon). Khaled, who was most vocal in his affiliations, ambiguously defined himself as Christian or Muslim due to his mixed parentage. After several childless marriages, Khaled had married a much younger Lebanese cousin, Rakia. The birth of Samya, their first child, inspired Khaled to leave the Middle East to live a new, more peaceful life. This man, who was passionately political and religious, declared that he held Samya "above my heart, above my God." Four more children followed: two girls—Soha and Salwa— and two young boys—Samuel and Salim. The older children attended French Catholic schools in Ottawa, an English-French bilingual Canadian city.

HEGIRA: FLIGHT AND RESETTLEMENT

In the Islamic tradition, a story is told about Muhammad, their prophet. When the leading families of Mecca were threatened by the changes he brought, Muhammad left for a place that later came to be known as Madina. Muhammad's move to Madina is called the *hegira*—

> the word has not simply the negative meaning of a flight from Mecca, but the positive one of seeking protection by settling in a place other than one's own. (Hourani, 1991, p. 17)

In order to understand Samya and her predicament, one has to understand the meaning of her family's move to Canada. For her father, Khaled, emigration was a kind of secular *hegira*—looking for a safe haven from the storms of his life in the Middle East. For Khaled and his family, Canada was a garden, a secular paradise. Unfortunately, it became a jungle, with unforeseen forks in the path. Playing with the alliteration of their children's names, Soha and Samya were nicknamed "Mecca and Madina" by their parents. This provides potent, culturally congruent metaphors for the family experience of the two sisters. If Mecca is home, the center of faith and meaning, then we can view Samya and Soha as having fled Mecca for protection elsewhere, in Madina. While Soha has returned to Mecca, Samya is still waiting in Madina—will it be a brief sojourn there, or a permanent settlement?

"CULTURAL QUESTIONS, HUMAN QUESTIONS"

Orientalism failed to identify with human experience, failed also to see it as human experience.

—Edward Said, *Orientalism*
(1979, p. 328)

What is the task of the first session in family therapy? A common answer is what Salvador Minuchin (Minuchin & Fishman, 1981) calls "joining" and what I call "meeting strangers"—entering the world of the family. But if we want to work in a collaborative context, a prior task is negotiation. In our very first session with the Shami family, we came to a definition of our work together. Our encounter could be described as "Arabian Nights" meets "Orientalism." After listening to different views of their problems, we spent much of the first session discussing their background, their presenting culture. In Chapter 1, I identified this negotiating process as "spiraling" or meeting strangers. Summarizing what I had understood, I tried to reframe their predicament not in psychiatric terms or as a protection issue:

Dr. DiNicola: These are important questions. Questions about your culture, your family . . .
Mr. Khaled Shami: Human questions, *human* questions!

I was trying to "read" them as part of a larger cultural story (what I mean by "Arabian Nights"), but Khaled, reaching across to me for recognition, reframed their predicament as a human story—and damn all else! He did not want to be understood as Other (represented by "Orientalism"). Of course, we needed to do both—they wanted to be understood in human terms, but there is no generic humanity standing outside of culture, so to know their humanity we had to know their culture. How could we accomplish both?

Cultural family therapy. A portal of entry into this family's culture opened for me at the outset. Having heard the father's complaints about the children's agency, the court, the lawyers, and Canadian society in general, I asked a few simple questions about the parents' view of the problem and what solutions would be acceptable to them. Pursuing questions about how such problems are experienced in Lebanon was unhelpful, as they denied that such things happen there (although this seemed unrealistic; see El-Islam, 1983; El-Islam et al., 1986). The question for me was: how could I enter a family culture marked by pride and mutual support (familism), whose solidarity was amplified through its involvement with the individualistic culture of North America, and whose wounded pride had made it rigid and defensive (through the protective functions of family myths)?

My approach to breaching this family's wall of solidarity was to join family members in their cultural style in order to understand their cultural assumptions. I should mention that I have a special interest in the Middle East, having briefly lived and studied in Israel. I could play with the options of adopting an insider role with this family or of taking an even stronger outsider role as an Italian student of Judaism working with Arabs.

Needless to say, one can only ''play'' with such options if these personal identifications are sincere and genuine. Furthermore, the beneficial use of one's personal, family, and cultural background as therapeutic resources requires both personal growth and clinical experience. Useful tips for this include: working with a co-therapist, collaborating with a cultural interpreter or culture broker, and attending experiential workshops on personal, family, and cultural issues.

So I posed this question: if a family problem occurs, to whom would you turn for help? The answer was unequivocal: to the elders of the family. Accordingly, they were invited to bring to a session one of the children's grandparents, whom I called the ''head of the family'' and their ''moral leader.'' It was a request they could not refuse because it was their suggestion, which was culturally sanctioned, as this quote from Arabic historian Albert Hourani (1991) suggests:

> such authority as existed lay with the elders, or heads of families, who preserved the collective memory of the group, regulated urgent common concerns and reconciled differences which threatened to tear the group apart. (p. 108)

Culture clash. As I read it, the stalemate between Samya's family and Canadian authorities was due to a cultural clash of values. In a bizarre irony, each party saw the other as having transgressed against Samya sexually. In their investigation of Samya's allegations, the agency perceived inappropriate sexual boundaries in her family interactions. As a result, the agency adopted a rigid stance toward her family, leaving no room for discussion of different cultural and family perspectives (the consequences of a deeply embedded Western assumption that our psychological theories are ''universal''). In a word, the agency saw Samya as sexualized by her family.

This feedback to the family about their child was not received as realistic or factual, but as a provocation. This was amplified by statements made to the family about Samya's right to express herself in a variety of ways, including dating and sexual activities. This was an image they could not support. The family felt that the agency gave Samya a license for sexual activity. When the family was forced to comply with the agency's plan of care for Samya, and she then made a further allegation of rape while in the society's care, Canadian society lost all credibility in their eyes.

The investigation was profoundly misguided: there was a confusion between the agency's definition of child abuse and the family's culturally sanctioned rules for individual behavior (Samya's, Khaled's) and family interactions (father-daughter). Since the parents felt that their entire family and cultural value system was under assault (the consequences of "Orientalism"), they avoided discussion of particular issues (Samya's allegations against her father). Samya and Soha first went outside the family with their complaints, but then retreated into the solidarity of the family, perjuring their own testimony. Confronted with legal sanctions, most of the family members (except Samya) preferred their own culturally sanctioned solutions to anything that an increasingly alien Western culture could offer. My therapeutic success with Samya's family was in positioning myself as someone who could resolve the differences between Canadian society and their own culture by negotiating goals that were acceptable in Canadian society achieved by means that were generated by their own culture.

Child abuse: "A generative metaphor." This family's predicament is very disturbing for me not only because of the distress expressed by all the members of the family, but because of the clear possibility that my society added significantly to their suffering. Power was used in a coercive way by almost all the actors in this family's drama—starting with the power of the accusations by Samya and Soha and the social power of the children's agency, triggering legal challenges and threats of abduction by the father.

In her thoughtful review of child sexual abuse, Claudia Konker (1992), a social worker and anthropologist, asserts that, "Each culture has a right to define appropriate social conduct on its own terms" (p. 150). Cultural beliefs generate norms for raising children and we use "parental, political, and professional power in support of those beliefs" (p. 150). In Samya's situation, each of these powers was pitted against the others. Samya's predicament supports Konker's conclusion that "child sexual abuse is, by definition, a cultural problem" (p. 151).

Cultural anthropologists can teach us much about the cultural contexts of the uses of power. In their critical review of how child abuse is imagined in our culture, two American anthropologists, Nancy Scheper-Hughes and Howard Stein (1987), argue that child abuse "functions as a generative metaphor." The identified individual child abusers serve as symptom-bearers for a social problem that is so broad they call it "normative." The child abuser as symptom-bearer distracts us from recognizing the extent to which we live in a society that fails to protect children.

BUILDING SOLIDARITY

Solidarity has to be constructed out of little pieces, rather than found already waiting . . .

—Richard Rorty (1989, p. 94)

In Chapter 1, I described the next session, when Samya's maternal grandfather, Mr. Massoud, who was visiting from Beirut, was brought in as a consultant. I called that session, "Two Old Men," referring to Mr. Massoud as head of the family and myself as head of the therapy team. By "going with their culture," we harnessed the authority that their family culture invests in the elderly to find new solutions. Was I, as a man, supporting a patriarchal family structure? Not quite. Meeting people on their own ground does not mean endorsing all their values. But there is an even more acute point to be made here: when people are in distress and at a loss, this is not necessarily the best time to ask them to defend or reject the ground on which they stand. Let me give an example from my work on eating disorders. Criticizing the family for participating in a patriarchal culture would be like asking young women who are starving themselves to reject the cultural sea of imagery that surrounds them, shaping their drive for thinness and their fear of being fat. While we do just that in our adolescent Eating Disorders

Program, where we offer critical media skills in psychoeducation groups, this is a long-term goal, which each young woman may choose for herself. With the Shami family, we have to balance our concerns about the domineering father against an all-too-common Western paternalism that arrogates a position of superior knowledge.

What made the encounter between "Two Old Men" possible is cultural translation as a therapeutic process. "Two Old Men" created a context for the whole therapy: it gave me an authority figure in the family to fall back on. Furthermore, the translation necessary to reach Mr. Massoud aligned me with their culture and served as a useful brake to slow things down when needed. Frequently, throughout the course of therapy, I turned to Mr. Massoud for support or clarification. But I also turned to him when something needed to be emphasized or to calm the family by slowing down the pace and flow of interactions. Their natural deference to him meant that when he talked, they listened.

By working patiently, slowly, with Mr. Massoud, we built trust between the family and the therapy team, first with him, then with Samya's parents and her siblings, and finally with Samya herself. Entering the world of the family, which I described as "spiraling" in Chapter 1, is not a "joining" technique, which, once accomplished, can be taken for granted as we move on to other therapeutic tasks. Always at the threshold of an ever-changing world, we cannot move on—we cross over and another threshold presents itself. Another name for cultural family therapy is *threshold therapy*. In cultural family therapy, this task never ends: our work is done at the borders of cultural communities and human interactions where the threshold therapist mingles with liminal people, moving between/among worlds. Solidarity, as Richard Rorty's quote suggests, is built moment by moment, session by session.

"THE PRINCESS AND THE ORPHANS"

In the third session, we continued to work with the family's culture, preparing the ground for our work with Samya by working with the other children in the family. I asked for someone in the family to act as translator for the sessions in order to continue to welcome Mr. Massoud in the family sessions. This was a choice; professional Arabic translators and colleagues were available. Although both Khaled and Rakia were reasonably fluent in English, I avoided using them as translators. The process of translation seemed to deepen their anxieties and frustrations, as they became more in touch with their pain and humiliation. For them, it was better to experience the session in English, as a way to distance themselves from their cultural and family myths, to open space for other ideas. This may seem either paradoxical or at odds with my notion of entering their culture. It is neither. I wanted to enter their culture in order to understand them and to stand apart from the cultural myths of my society. They needed to stand apart from their own myths in order to build a bridge toward my side of the river. I hoped our efforts would meet in the middle.

Later, I asked Samya to act as translator, as a way to reintegrate her into the family, but I wanted to prepare the ground through another child, who was reasonably fluent in Arabic and in a more secure position in the family. Soha, the next daughter, who was 12 years old, volunteered and did her best. What we discovered is that all the Shami children experienced difficulty speaking Arabic. Asking them to translate did more than create a special role for them; it enhanced the value of Arabic in this family. This was not lost on the parents, who were deeply touched by my asking the children to speak in Arabic with their grandfather. Over the course of therapy, we saw a clear improvement in the children's fluency and comfort in Arabic.

With all the shame that had visited this home, creating space for Arabic in our sessions gave them the message that they could be at home as Arabs in Canada. The Shami children lived in an Arabic Canadian home, where they spoke a mixture of Arabic, English and French. They attended French Catholic schools in a bilingual English-French city. They were learning to live in a complex, pluricultural world. The goal for them was to become comfortable in all these worlds, rejecting none of them, building bridges from home to the outside world. To sum up, we encouraged the parents to experience our sessions in English and the children to experience them in Arabic, each for different therapeutic reasons.

There was another reason for giving space to Samya's siblings in therapy. While the parents were always instrumentally adequate, due to their ordeal with Samya they had less time for the other children. In many ways, as we shall see, Samya was the highly valued ("above my heart"), first-born child who was made into a princess. Some of the other children complained about this. In team discussions, we began thinking of them as "orphans with parents."

"PLAYING WITH YES"

A gift from Mecca. When I greet the Shami family to usher them into the fourth session, Khaled introduces a guest, Jack Melville, an English-Canadian who is engaged to his niece. Everyone in the nuclear family is present, as well as Samya's grandfather. Still in the waiting room, Khaled shows me a beautiful string of green beads. "For you," he says, "a gift from Mecca." Placing them in my hands, he says the Arabic word for them—*sebha*. I recognize them: "Prayer beads! They're beautiful." They are a kind of rosary for Muslims, ever present in the hands of old men, invoking praise for Allah. I am very touched. Mr. Massoud catches my eye and raises folded hands to reveal his own string of beads with a muttered prayer on his lips—*sabeh'Allah.*

Dr. DiNicola: It's very nice to see that Samya is relating to her brothers and sisters. This is very important. So who's going to translate today? It was nice last time that the children tried. *(Soha is reluctant.)* Please ask Mr. Massoud: Is it time to start working?

    KHALED TRANSLATES.
    MR. MASSOUD NODS IN AGREEMENT.

Dr. DiNicola: Mr. Massoud says it's time to start working . . . Last week, Samya told me, "It's OK, you're part of the family." Did you mean that?
Khaled: Yes.
Dr. DiNicola: In my culture, if you're part of the family, you go home. . . . What about coming to your house?
Rakia and Khaled: No problem.
Dr. DiNicola (to Samya): What do *you* think?
Samya: I can't say anything, I don't live there.

Dr. DiNicola: That's an interesting point, because if I come to your house, I want you to be there.

Samya: You do? Why?

Dr. DiNicola: Because, if I'm part of the family, you, who was born into this family, should be part of the family too, right? Would you like to have meetings at your house? Instead of here? Sometimes we could meet here, sometimes we could meet there. (*to the whole family*) If we meet at your house, that's one way for Samya to visit home.

ALTHOUGH I ASK FIRST RAKIA THEN SOHA TO TRANSLATE, KHALED SPEAKS TO HIS FATHER-IN-LAW IN ARABIC.

———

Dr. DiNicola: So, Samya, you haven't been home in eight months?

Samya: Not at all, not even for a visit.

Dr. DiNicola: Would you like to have a session at home? We'll have you with us over there. First, I want to know: do you feel ready? (*to Soha*) Tell your grandfather, I'm asking Samya if she's ready to visit home.

Samya: Yes.

Dr. DiNicola: Samya, I'm not sure, I'm not sure that you're telling me yes.

Samya: I said yes.

Dr. DiNicola: When does yes mean *yes*?

Samya: When? Next week!

Dr. DiNicola: How can I be sure that you really want to do this?

Soha: How can you convince us?

Samya: How can I? I don't know!

Dr. DiNicola (to Soha): You want her to come home?

Soha: Yeah!

Dr. DiNicola: I'm not sure Samya. You know why I'm not sure?

Samya: Why?

Dr. DiNicola: Your father just told me that you say something on Friday [in family sessions] and then Monday, they get a different message from the agency. . . . Do you say one thing here and something different after?

Samya: No.

Dr. DiNicola: It's OK to be confused . . . but if you're confused, don't say "yes," say "maybe," or say "I'm not sure," or say "I have to think about it."

Samya: I said yes!

Dr. DiNicola: You're sure?

Samya: Yes!

FIRST KHALED TRANSLATES, THEN RAKIA TRANSLATES.

———

Khaled: My father-in-law says that when we meet here everything goes good, beautiful, but when we go home, we receive from the agency a different message *(a turning motion of his hand)*: "We are not happy because you convince Samya." Who's the boss? Agency say, "We are the boss. If we not agree, nobody can agree."

Dr. DiNicola: That's true, actually, but let's not make the agency more important than they are. They are important, but when we're *here*, let's not give them more importance than they have. *(to Rakia)* Please tell your father.

RAKIA TRANSLATES.

I said this many times: the people who are important are right here: first your father . . . the family. . . .

KHALED TALKING OVER ME, SIMULTANEOUSLY TRANSLATING.

My question is not: Is the agency ready for her to come and visit? My question is: Are *you* ready? *(looking at Samya)* Do you understand? I'm not asking the agency, I'm asking her. . . .

Samya: I said yes.

Dr. DiNicola: . . . because if she's clear—*(to Samya)* hear me, this is very important—*(to Mr. Massoud)* if she's clear, then the agency will not say what they said to you. I don't know if the agency is convincing her or she's confused. I'll take care of the agency. . . .

Khaled: I know . . .

Samya: I don't talk to the agency!

Dr. DiNicola (to Samya): . . . you have to be clear, I'm not asking you to make a decision today, but when you are ready. . . .

Samya (mounting impatience): . . . I said *yes!*

Dr. DiNicola: . . . when you are clear . . .

Samya (annoyed, bored): . . . I'm clear.

Dr. DiNicola: . . . then they [at the agency] will hear clearly, OK? This is a very important idea, because something very terrible has happened in this family.

Khaled: Yes *(bows his head).*

Dr. DiNicola: . . . and part of what's happened that's wrong—you see, it's not easy to see what's wrong with people, what hurt them, because what we see is their reaction. You know, if you cut yourself, you have a wound, you don't see the knife, you see the reaction, you see the scar.

Right now, I only see the scar, I can't see what happened. The terrible thing that happened in this family is: you let the agency become too important. Please tell your father: you let the agency become too important.

> RAKIA TRANSLATES.

Dr. DiNicola: Did he understand?

Rakia: Yes, but he doesn't agree, because we make fight with them.

————

Found in translation. We were very aware that in their Arabic conversations more than translation was going on. The team saw this as a kind of parallel process, two bridges across the same river. There was a therapy session conducted in English with Arabic translation for everyone's benefit. At the same time, a family reunion was taking place—the only time Samya and her family saw each other all week—experienced and communicated in Arabic. Both aspects of the sessions have therapeutic value. At times, I would connect the two parallel sessions by insisting on accurate translation.

Dr. DiNicola *(to Mr. Massoud):* They made the agency too important, by having arguments with them and giving them power. Tell your grandfather that this family made other people, outside [the family] too important.

Khaled: Not us—this *(pointing to Samya).*

Dr. DiNicola *(gently):* You mean "her." But as a family group, you let this become "crazy." Now, we have to work very hard to make it "uncrazy." I'll tell you what happened in my meeting with the agency.

You told me about your world. This is your gift to me *(holding up the prayer beads)*. I want to give you something back. I want to explain something about my world.

FIRST RAKIA TRANSLATES, THEN KHALED IS TRANSLATING INTO ARABIC. I TRY TO FOLLOW THE RHYTHM AND TONE, THEN I HEAR A WORD I RECOGNIZE IN ARABIC—SHARMUTA—AND STOP HIM.

Dr. DiNicola (concerned): I didn't say that! What did you say?
Khaled: I tell him this agency social worker like a prostitute . . .
Dr. DiNicola: I didn't say that!
Khaled: It's the same.
Dr. DiNicola: Please translate what I said.

I TURN TO THE CHILDREN TO HELP ME WITH THE TRANSLATION.

Samya: I can't remember what you said.
Dr. DiNicola: That's why translation is so useful, it makes you think—what did I really hear?

———

After this clarification, I explore several interconnected issues with the family. One is that Samya gives conflicting messages to different people. Another is the issue of power—how the parents gave Samya a sense of power by treating her like a princess, how Samya empowered the agency to act on her behalf by making her allegations, and how the parents entrenched the agency's power through their combative responses, confirming the agency's stereotypes of them as being "out of control." I performed a kind of shuttle diplomacy by going back and forth between the family and the agency. My goal is to open space for different mutual perceptions to break the rigid, black-and-white thinking.

Dr. DiNicola: I'm afraid that you blame the agency, that you blame other people—on that side *(indicating the parents)*. Or that you use the agency as an excuse not to come home—on this side *(indicating Soha and Samya)*. There are two sides.

I told the family that the agency was amazed when we met with them. "We didn't hear these things before," they said. "Their experience of your family and our experience of your family are two different stories," I told the Shamis. "How can people have two such strangely different stories?" By putting these two stories side by side, we opened space for the agency to see the family anew. In response, the agency acknowledged a difference. "No one had ever shown us these things," the agency said and acknowledged that, "We learned a lot from you." The agency asked for my recommendation. I described the sessions to them: "This is a good family, they're working hard, it's making a difference." After a long discussion, I said, "Just let me do my work."

After speaking with their lawyers, the agency phoned back. "We would like it if we stopped with the court right now, if it's all voluntary, but the lawyers told us it's not clear." Because Samya was still sending mixed signals to them, they felt an obligation to recommend continued guardianship over Samya for another three months. The judge would decide. "In my opinion," I reassured the family, "it's going to happen sooner, not later. At the end of three months, she's going to be home."

———

Dr. DiNicola: The agency is there to protect the children from their parents. I'm here to protect you from her. Because if she's not ready, she's more dangerous to you than you are to her. You gave her too much power when you put her "above my heart, above my God."

Samya: What do you mean by power?

Dr. DiNicola: Power? Control: when *you* say something, everybody else jumps. You were here when your father said, "I love my daughter before my God, before my country." That's power . . .

Samya: I didn't ask for it!

———

Khaled states that he wants to work on the issue voluntarily, not forced by law, and that if the agency doesn't withdraw, he will challenge them in court. I urge caution about that, as I believe that the real issue is not the imposition by the agency but rather Samya's confusing and inconsistent answers as to what she wants and needs.

Rakia: Why doesn't she want to live at home?

Resident: There are some questions that we can't answer in this session. Maybe that's something me and you and Samya need to talk about.

We had negotiated for the child psychiatry resident to do some mother-daughter work with Rakia and Samya. She calms Rakia and makes an appointment for the three of them for the next week.

Dr. DiNicola: Samya, is yes still yes?

Samya (exasperated): YE-ES!

Dr. DiNicola: So when are you ready to have your first home visit?

Samya: Next week!

"ARRIVAL AND DEPARTURE"

The fifth session is full of all the turbulance that made this family's therapy so difficult. Samya is not present at the outset, opening a window on how the family experiences her absence. Concerned about her absence, I choose to observe the family behind the one-way mirror while the resident conducts the session. I call the agency to determine why Samya has not arrived. Present are the grandfather, both parents, Soha and the two youngest children, and Jack. What we see appears to be a family in chaos. Salim, the toddler, shouts and cries throughout the session. Khaled threatens to leave the family to go fight for Iraq in the impending Gulf War. Rakia seems troubled and helpless in the face of Khaled's irrational behavior. I occasionally call in to the resident and the family on a telephone.

The family—and the session—is very organized around Samya's absence and their anger at the agency. On my recommendation, the resident asks for everything to be translated for the grandfather. This serves as a brake on a process that appears on the verge of collapse or a dangerous emotional escalation. As we watch the slow process of translation provided by Soha, I ask the team behind the mirror: who is the audience for translation? There are many answers to this question. The stated reason for translating the sessions is to communicate with the grandfather. This opens space for his authority and gives the rest of the family some reflective distance from their immediate reactions. But the parents constantly enlist Mr. Massoud in their opinions. His own voice doesn't come through unless we pointedly ask him direct questions and insist on his answers.

Note, in the interactions below, the family members' concern over who is in charge and their repeated demand that I "take charge" in order to remove the agency's legal mandate for Samya's care.

Khaled: Who's in charge here? Dr. D. in charge or agency in charge?

Resident (to Soha): Can you explain that to your grandfather—that your father wants to know who's in charge?

Soha translates.

Resident (to Soha): What does your grandfather think is the right answer to that?

Rakia translates, Khaled translates.

Khaled (translating for Mr. Massoud): He said that he doesn't feel Dr. D. in charge. He doesn't feel that anything is happening, it's becoming worse and worse.

Resident: I see, OK. It's important to let your father-in-law know that I understand that, how you could feel like that. However, there are some things legally that we can't control. We told you that last week. Maybe you can let your father-in-law know that.

Khaled translates.

Resident: But in these sessions, we're interested in the family, not the agency.

———

Resident: When you ask who's in control, we think *this* is the most important thing. All the action is here, this is where we're going to get ahead, please tell that to your grandfather.

Soha translates.

Resident: We'll make sure that Samya comes today, OK? Our understanding is that, although she's with the agency, we—Dr. D. and myself—will decide when she goes home.

Khaled translates.

Khaled: We feel you work hard, for what you see and what you feel. My father he said: the agency still control this girl because you don't make decision. . . .

Resident: Now, let me answer that. Based on our meeting with the agency, we were able to get them to agree after a long time. Initially, they wanted wardship. In effect, legally they have some control, but they will let us choose when Samya visits home.

———

Khaled: They said in the session that we were harassing her. Did you see us harassing her? I followed her in my car. We went to court for the man who raped my daughter. He had many records. I go to follow her to see if she's safe. [I'm] somebody who can defend her. That was for Samya, for her protection. Because what happened for my daughter is—agency wash its hands *(makes a hand-washing motion)*.

Resident: Let me stop you there, Mr. Shami, what's happening is that we're saying: we're letting them have control here. That's what we said last week: we're giving them too much control. Now this is our time. We should focus on the family. . . .

———

Khaled: I wanna left the home, stop the family session, and uh, maybe . . . take the kids to my country and then fight for our right because we feel . . . in this country, we feel this people harass us too much. We wanna take the court, we go to court, we see who . . .

I call in. After a brief conversation, the resident stops the action.

A SAMYA-SHAPED HOLE IN THEIR HEARTS

Resident: Mrs. Shami, Dr. DiNicola wants to talk to you.

Rakia: He want to talk to me? *(takes the phone)* Hello . . . I understand what you said.

Resident (to Soha): Tell your grandfather that your mother is talking to Dr. D. and he said that nothing that we say here in words is useful.

Rakia (tries to repeat what I am telling her): OK . . . he say: we don't trust English and agency—they don't trust Arabic.

Khaled: Agency not English, French!

Rakia (to me on phone): Nobody English over there, only French. *(repeating my words):* You don't trust English *or* French—and you almost give up on Italian!

EVERYBODY LAUGHS. THERE IS AN EXCHANGE IN ARABIC BETWEEN THE PARENTS.

Rakia: Yeah, I know what you say. And we're not even hearing Hindi! *(Rakia laughs at my reference to the culture of the resident.)*

Khaled: What you want from me, doctor? You want me to go to court or you want me to give up Samya? You want me to give up the family? I ready to give up everything, I give up . . .

Rakia: He say: We have to talk Japanese or don't talk at all!

Khaled: OK, I go out . . .

Rakia: Not you, he say all of us, not you!

Khaled: We go, we feel we don't have any right in this country . . .

Resident: Tell your grandfather that Dr. D. feels there's no language that we can understand here today.

SOHA TRANSLATES.

Resident: We have two choices: we either speak Japanese, or don't speak at all.

KHALED TRANSLATES, WITH A SMILE.

Khaled: We don't agree.

Resident: You don't agree? What did your father-in-law say?

Khaled: He don't agree. There's no heart left in this country!

Resident: Did he say that? What did your grandfather say?

Khaled: We are lose, everybody . . .

MR. MASSOUD SPEAKS IN ARABIC TO THE PARENTS.

Rakia: We want to go home now, because nobody understands . . . our problem eight months not finished . . .

Rakia (tries to explain my message): Speaking Japanese doesn't mean we shouldn't talk.

The family is very distraught. I enter the room. Khaled and grandfather stand to greet me, then Rakia stands. I approach Khaled in the middle of the three, who looks very upset. He holds out his hands (even though he is upset) and embraces me, in the way of the Middle East, patting me on the back. Mother cries. Then I turn to the grandfather, who embraces me as well. I shake Rakia's hand and acknowledge Soha and Jack with a nod.

Khaled (looking like a crumpled puppet, with slack strings, starts to address me): Our family break . . .

I nod and keep moving slowly around the room and bend down to acknowledge the little ones, Samuel and Salim, then I go over to Soha and shake her hand.

Khaled (haltingly, staccato): Dr. DiNicola . . . we are . . . we are not people . . .

Then I move over to the resident, who is seated, shake her hand wordlessly and stand beside her.

Khaled: We wanna talk . . .

I slowly hold up a hand, move it in a motion across my closed mouth, and place my hand over my heart. I go over and silently sit down beside Mr. Massoud and look into his eyes and make a broad gesture toward his family and clap my hands on my knees. We look at each other; he begins to talk in Arabic. I speak to him in Italian. He continues in Arabic; nobody translates. Grandfather looks puzzled, looks around for someone to translate. Soha wants to try. Khaled says no.

Rakia: He doesn't understand.

Mr. Massoud speaks to me again; Khaled tries to talk again. I hold up my hand, gently, to quieten the room. Soha leaves with Samuel and Salim. The room is finally quiet, for the first time since the start of the session. There is an air of exhaustion; it is oddly relaxing and peaceful. After exhausting what is possible with words, we seem to have stripped things down to just sitting and enduring. It is a moment of great sharing.

After a few minutes, I crouch in front of the parents and look at them. Nonverbally, I ask Rakia about her tears. She answers with a shrug that she can't explain. After another minute or two, I ask everyone else to leave. As the rest of the family goes to the waiting room, the resident joins the team behind the one-way mirror. I sit beside Khaled and look at him and Rakia. They are finally quiet, sitting on a grief.

Dr. DiNicola: We were expecting Samya at two o'clock . . . I think *nothing that we say now means anything to you because you have a hole in your heart in the shape of Samya.* And you are trying to fill that hole with all your fears, your anxiety, your anger, until Samya comes back. So wait 'til she comes.

I also think that you two have something to do together, before you can even receive her. And I think that maybe the children and your father don't need to be here for that—maybe I shouldn't be here—because I think what you're feeling is too much for other people. Only you know what you are feeling.

As I watch them, they are very attentive. Rakia is hunched over and Khaled has dropped his ''Yes, but'' way of listening.

On the other side of the mirror, all we could hear was the baby's crying. . . . But, you know what? I think he was doing for you what you feel. He was screaming, he was crying, he was agitated. All this noise—*(speaking to Rakia)* I said to you clearly *(on the phone)*—many things were being said, but not in language *(mother crying now)*, not in words. They were being said in other ways: Salim's crying, the fact that there's an empty chair for Samya *(my hand is on the chair)*, the fact that you didn't shave *(Khaled looks haggard, red-eyed, unshaven)*. You looked better last week, today you look awful. You look like you didn't sleep all night.

———

"How you make somebody a princess." We struggled to get beyond labeling individuals (Khaled, Samya), the Shami family, or institutions (the children's agency, the court, Canadian society) as static things. My notion of Samya as a "princess" grasps a relational pattern. The emphasis is on how she became a princess, how the family raised her, the importance they gave her over other children, and what meaning this now has for all of them.

Khaled: No . . . but I have to tell you one thing . . .

Dr. DiNicola: But you always have to tell me one more thing. I'm . . . *(I place my hand gently on his shoulder)* I'm offering you to sit with the worst feelings you have. You feel not understood. I think you're right: you're not understood. You are NOT understood. And it's an awful feeling not to be understood!

Rakia (between sobs): Uh-huh . . .

Dr. DiNicola: Sometimes you blame the world that you're in. And sometimes it's true. But nobody can take that away right now. You can do a lot of things to make it go away: you can cry, you could shout, but it won't go away. For sure, it is not going to go away with words.

> *(Looking at mother):* You are going through much pain. I cannot take that away. If Samya came home tomorrow, you would still have much pain. *(Mother nods in silent agreement.)* Samya has a lot of work to do. I tell you something and your lawyer agrees with me: if Samya comes home tomorrow, it will be a disaster. She's not ready . . . you're going to start all over again. . . .

> You made her a princess. I think I know why, but you did it and now you have a tyrant on your hands.

Rakia: How you make somebody a princess?

Khaled: A princess in my house, doctor. I'm king of my house, my wife, a queen of this house . . .

Dr. DiNicola: I don't know the Arabic history of princes and princesses, but in this Western world, we're talking about something that doesn't exist anymore. In this culture, "princess" means someone who feels more important than other people.

Khaled: That's it . . .

Dr. DiNicola: Samya feels very important and I believe that even in your world that you couldn't live with this person. She feels so important, I don't think you have enough money and enough time and enough energy to feed this princess. It seems tragic to me that this princess had to be in this world where she was given even more power than you ever imagined—that's a tragedy—

Rakia: Uh-huh . . .

Dr. DiNicola: But it didn't come first from Canada. I think you have to take it back into your heart, what has happened to you. In your pain, you want to be angry at people. Be angry . . . but keep it where it belongs. Make sure that the address of your anger is for the right place.

Khaled: Doctor . . .

Dr. DiNicola: I think you can't tolerate it. I think you're going crazy with all this stuff inside.

———

Rakia: When do you think she's ready to come home? When she's 14?

Dr. DiNicola: The answer is in your heart, once you're ready for it. You're working hard for it.

Rakia: We're working very hard, but she doesn't work very hard, she's not here . . .

Dr. DiNicola: We're still blaming Samya for the problem . . .

Khaled: The problem, doctor, not now a problem of family—a problem with our community. Yesterday, I need a few thousand dollars from someone. I talk to him, my friend who really understand our situation here, you know what he told me? Tell your daughter make you money, she can make for you $1,500, easy, on the street.

———

''*Where does honor come from?*'' People who live in the individually-oriented cultures of the West, who have not experienced the family-oriented cultures of the Mediterranean or the Arabic world, may find it hard to understand Khaled's burden of suffering. He was bound by a code of honor and obligation to protect his family, as Arabic historian Albert Hourani explains:

> It was part of a man's honour to defend what was his and to respond to demands upon him from members of his

family . . . *honour belonged to an individual through his mem-bership of a larger whole.* The women of his family—mothers and sisters, wives and daughters—were under his protec-tion, but what they did could affect his honour: a lack of modesty, or behaviour which would arouse in men who had no claims over them strong feelings that challenge the social order. *Mingled with a man's respect for his womenfolk there might therefore be a certain suspicion or even fear of women as a danger.* (1991, p. 105, italics added)

Dr. DiNicola: You want your daughter back?

Khaled: I don't think so: I think I need my name back, my family name . . .

Dr. DiNicola: I think you're impatient. I understand why, but I think you're impatient.

Khaled says he feels he is neither dead nor alive.

Khaled: I need peace of mind, in my heart. I am a man of honor. In this problem, I lost my honor. I don't have my daughter, I don't have any respect. If an Arab lost his honor he don't have a right to live!

Dr. DiNicola: Where does honor come from: from the outside or from the inside?

A knock on the door: Samya arrives. An ironic moment—has honor returned to this family? Someone escorts her to the waiting room. I continue.

We have to have the inside and the outside. Right now, you don't have the outside, so you have to look inside. What have you got? You've got your wife. I'm not sure you're really letting her help you, to support you and help you feel better. I'm not sure you're letting your father-in-law help you. Maybe you've lost your reputation in your community, maybe with the agency. You still have yourself, you still know what you did do and didn't do. Your wife believes you.

Khaled: For how long? My spare finish, I don't have money in my pocket.

Dr. DiNicola: I think that by the end of three months, Samya will be home.

Khaled: I give you 45 days . . . I want her home before her 14th birthday.

Dr. DiNicola: I can't promise that, it's not in my power . . . Let's say she won't come . . . you're prepared to gamble everything on this?

Rakia and Khaled (in unison): Yeah!

———

Dr. DiNicola: What's happening in 45 days?

Khaled: My family come to visit. Give me some honor . . . I've lost every respect in my community, all my honor. I live like animal—eat, sleep, I don't see nobody!

Dr. DiNicola: Let's look at it another way: what if she was home and this thing started again?

Khaled: Let me handle it . . . I know my daughter well.

Dr. DiNicola: I believe you will find the answer . . . I think you have to rebuild your house.

Khaled: I know my daughter what she wants exactly and I give her what she wants, tomorrow Samya be home . . .

They are prepared to let her do whatever she wants to get her to come home.

Dr. DiNicola: That's how you make a princess. I'm offering you a way to live together that's acceptable to you so that you're not dying inside, so that you not only have honor in your community, you also have honor inside.

You convinced one group of people that you are not harassing your daughter . . . now I think you have to convince yourselves and be gentle and kind with yourselves, use the resources in your life for support, like your wife.

Khaled: I wanna leave my wife and kids and I wanna go to my country.

Dr. DiNicola: Do you want your husband to go?

Rakia: He never listen.

Dr. DiNicola: I'm helping you—talk to him and tell him.

Rakia (crying now): If you help me here, somebody gonna help me at home?

Dr. DiNicola: Your father.

Rakia: Nobody can do nothing.

Dr. DiNicola: Do you want him to leave?

Rakia (voice shaking): He know that I don't want him to leave.

Khaled: I have no choice!

Dr. DiNicola: Every human being has a choice!

Khaled: I leave everybody, I have no honor . . .

Dr. DiNicola: What about the honor of Soha and Salwa?

Khaled: What I can do?

Dr. DiNicola: You can stay and be a man. Do what a man does. . . . What a man does is stay with his family!

Khaled: I don't care, I no more care . . . I'm a crazy man, I don't know what happened to my house! *(pause)* I'm finished, doctor!

Rakia (to husband): You think I'm gonna live here like this, that's what you think?

Khaled: I want to go back to fight in honor [for] my country, I wanna go to Iraq.

Rakia: They won't take you!

Dr. DiNicola: If you go there, you could get killed.

Khaled: Yes, of course, I wanna get killed. Why a life with no honor?

Dr. DiNicola: Your wife needs you more than Saddam Hussein needs you.

Khaled: I leave everybody, I don't have honor, no nothing . . . empty! One girl, 13 years old, play everybody, five lawyers, two judges!

Dr. DiNicola (to resident behind the mirror): Let's bring Samya in. *(To Rakia)* When he talks like this, do you believe him?

Rakia: Sometime, yes.

Dr. DiNicola: Do you believe him now?

Rakia: Now, finished.

Khaled gives an angry, standing oration on his predicament, pacing around the room. Samya returns with her grandfather and the resident.

Samya: What's going on?

Dr. DiNicola: Your father's going to leave.

Samya: Where?

Dr. DiNicola: Canada.

Samya: Why?

Dr. DiNicola: Because he's tired.

Samya: With the whole family?

Dr. DiNicola: He's tired because he has no honor. *(to mother)* Please translate for your father.

     RAKIA TRANSLATES.

Samya: Is he taking everybody?

Dr. DiNicola: No, he's going alone.

Samya: Why?

Dr. DiNicola: He has nothing left to live for.

Samya: He has a lot to live for . . .

Dr. DiNicola: This is not what I feel; this is what he told me.

Samya: . . . that's what I always say . . . I say I have nothing to live for, but it's not true *(sounding sad for the first time)*.

Dr. DiNicola: He thinks that as long the situation is the way it is now, he has no honor.

Samya: What do you mean, ''as long as it is the way it is now''?

Dr. DiNicola: With you out of the home, not happy to go home, he has no honor in Canada. He can't work, he's depressed, he looks ten years older today than he did last week. Your grandfather looks better than he does. He's getting older day by day, he feels awful, he has nothing to live for, so he's going to go and fight in the Gulf War.

     RAKIA SOBS, SIGHS LOUDLY.

Samya (defiantly): He's not going to go fight!

Dr. DiNicola: That's what he would like to do. I think they won't take him, but that's what he would like to do . . .

Khaled: So, what do you think?

Samya: I don't know.

Dr. DiNicola: Your mother feels terrible. She's going to be left with five children, alone.

Samya: No, she's not! If he's going to leave, he takes everybody with him.

Dr. DiNicola: Who's everybody?

Samya: He's not going to leave Soha and Salwa, alone.

Dr. DiNicola: All those children? What about you?

Samya: I don't want to leave Canada, but if . . . he can't leave, because then he won't have any honor if he leaves.

Dr. DiNicola: That's what I think, but he told me I don't understand Arabic culture.

Rakia: Do you understand Arabic culture, Samya?

Samya: Me?

Dr. DiNicola: Your father says, "I've already lost my honor, I've nothing more to lose."

Samya: He's got a *lot* to lose!

Dr. DiNicola: Like what?

Samya: Honor . . . if he goes back to his country, he'll lose all his respect from his brothers, if he leaves his wife and his children.

Dr. DiNicola: Well, that's what your father wants to do. What do you say?

Samya: I say no!

Dr. DiNicola: You say no what?

Samya: No, he's not going to leave!

Dr. DiNicola: And what are you going to do about it?

Samya: I can't do nothing if he wants to leave . . . *(exasperated, at a loss)* I don't want him to . . .

Dr. DiNicola: Let's put your father aside for a moment. Remember last week I asked you a question?

Samya: You asked a lot of questions!

Dr. DiNicola: I asked you one question over and over again.

Samya: If I want to go visit the place.

Dr. DiNicola: What's "the place"?

Samya: Home?

Dr. DiNicola: What was your answer?

Samya: Yeah . . .

Dr. DiNicola: You do want to visit. Can you imagine one day going back home?

Samya: No.

Rakia: If you don't want to go back home, where do you want to live?

Samya (defiantly to her mother): I'll explain you one thing: the agency will take care of me. Don't say they won't 'cause you don't know, you haven't been under their care. There's a lot of children I know who are under the agency's care.

Rakia: Like they care about you!

Dr. DiNicola: But the agency does not enjoy having children under their care: it's the second choice, the second best. The first choice is for children to be with their families.

Samya: Yeah, that's true.

Resident: I'm sitting here confused. Dr. D. asked if you ever imagined, ever, a time for you to go back home and live there, you said "no."

Samya: I thought he meant now. Not now. Maybe in the future.

Rakia: Can you ask her how old she needs to be to go back home?

Samya: When I'm old enough to understand everything I don't understand myself.

Resident: But you see Samya, I suspect that your family can help you understand that . . .

Samya: No, no one can help me understand but myself! I have to help myself understand my own self. Nobody can help me, not you, not all the doctors in the world, not nobody but myself!

Rakia: Until now you don't understand yourself? Eight months and you still don't understand yourself?

Samya: No. You can't understand yourself during eight months, no way . . .

Dr. DiNicola: Well, I think it's going to stop today.

Samya: What?

Dr. DiNicola: These sessions.

Samya: Why?

Dr. DiNicola: I think no one feels that there is any hope that you will come home, so I think they are going to give up.

This is an example of what I call "enhancing uncertainty." Others call this "provocation" (Andolfi et al., 1983, 1989), a "paradoxical prescription" (Selvini Palazzoli et al., 1978b), "prescribing the symptom," "amplification" (Andolfi, 1979), and so on. I think it's one of those statements that's so close to the felt truth, to the lived reality, that it is neither paradoxical nor an intentional provocation. But the act of saying it enhances uncertainty: it is an example of our fears spoken aloud, our private worries made public.

Samya: I just want to work on a relationship with them first.

Rakia: We waited for 13 years, Samya! You don't work on any relationship with us?

Samya: I never got along with you.

Rakia: Any girl, she's doesn't get along with her mother.

Samya: I never got along with you at all. Me and you are always fighting.

Rakia (calmly): Yeah . . . but about what?

Samya: I don't know, I don't remember what, but I know we're always fighting.

Rakia: About . . . about the work at home, that's why we're always fighting . . .

Samya: And about letting me go outside . . .

Rakia: Yeah, we don't want you to go outside the home.

Samya: See, there you go . . .

   Khaled says something in Arabic . . .

Dr. DiNicola: Say it in English . . .

Samya: Don't tell me everything's changed, because you can't change everything overnight.

Khaled: . . . but when I wanna talk, she stop me . . . today the last day. I wanna talk about this . . . to your heart, your mind. What has happened is some mistake between you and your mother, between me and you, OK. . . . Last time I talked to you I tell you: we can understand each other when we love each other. But if you don't love me, if you don't love your mother, if you don't love your sisters, your brothers . . .

   If we have love, everything we can solve, no problem. If you are against your parents, your family, this is not work. . . .

   We work for it. If you wanna repair this, if you have something you need, discuss it with us, what I want, what you want, and make bargain between us, and go work for it, and go back to united family, perfect family, is no one against the other.

   Is you not want to repair this, if you're not ready to love, to care, why you waste time, why you hurt all this people? Why do we need you home?

Dr. DiNicola: It's a very good question.

Khaled (passionately but calmly, sweetly): I need you home for love each other, to understand each other, if you fall down, he can somebody pick you up. If something happen to you at the agency, it washes hands *(makes washing motions):* ''Not my fault, her fault.'' But if you are home, I want to take responsibility for you, because we can help. If something happen to you, I can't wash my hands and say "Not my fault, it's all her fault" . . . we stand behind you!

Khaled is now calm, rational, seems to have regained his confidence, his reasons for living, for keeping the family together.

Dr. DiNicola: Your father is saying, very generously, "I'm not sure what I did wrong, but if I hurt you, I'm sorry."

Khaled: . . . if I'm too strict, I'm sorry. . . . You're on the street . . .

Samya (*indignantly*): I'm not on the street!

Dr. DiNicola (*quickly*): Can I translate here? For your family's culture "on the street" means you're not at home, not in the family.
(*In a different, calmer, authoritative tone*): We have to stop. I think your father said some warm, honest, sincere things to you. He's making you an offer. I think you're not comfortable yet to accept his apology.

Samya: I accept it. I just don't want to go home. Is that a crime?

Rakia: It's a big crime for us.

Samya: No, it isn't a crime!

Dr. DiNicola: No, it's not a crime, Samya. It's a pain. It's a hurt for your family. I think that's something you don't recognize yet Samya. . . . Something that nobody in this family understands yet: the great amount of power you have over each other to hurt, or also, to help each other. You hurt your family. I don't say you did anything wrong: you made some choices. When you say, "I don't want to go home," I don't think you recognize how powerful that makes you and how much pain you cause other people. I am sure, also, that other people have caused you pain. Your father said something true: "We have all paid for this."
You feel hurt and you feel that you're not being understood . . . but you're hitting back very hard. When you chose to go to school, instead of coming to the session, this is hitting back hard. . . . Your empty chair in the session here is a kind of hitting. . . .
If you don't work this out with the people in your family, it will follow you all your life. Let me tell you something personal: I never met my father. . . .

Samya: So, why are you telling me this?

Dr. DiNicola: Because my father's shadow is the biggest influence in my whole life. . . . I think if you leave your family now, it will leave a shadow over your whole life, it will follow you around your whole life. . . . I know about this, because I've been through it. . . .

"SYSTEM VS. SYSTEM VS. SYSTEM"

The sixth session. Present are Mr. Massoud, Rakia, Khaled, and Soha, along with the therapists. Three key things happen: (1) Samya is absent; (2) we negotiate a new plan to reinvolve Samya; and (3) we use the session to discuss the rest of the family's reactions to Samya's charges for the first time.

1. *Samya's absence.* Both the family and the treatment team are upset by Samya's failure to attend the session. The group home reported that she was sick. In fact, she had an episode of hyperventilation, at worst, a symptom of anxiety. This is an example of how a simple behavior can be read so many different ways. Even within the agency, the group home workers and Samya's social worker did not see things the same way. Her social worker had committed herself to Samya attending sessions and was unaware that the group home had kept Samya home. As a result, the different perceptions created a situation that we called "system (the agency) vs. system (the family) vs. system (the treatment team)."

2. *Three strikes and . . .* When faced with competing perceptions, I slow things down and ask for clarification. My recommendation to the parents is to suspend judgment for now. I ask the parents to have no contact with Samya for two weeks. We would invite Samya to return to family therapy. I would give her two weeks to decide. I have used the "three strikes rule" in my clinical work for twenty years. She had missed two sessions so far; I would offer her one more chance. If she chose not to attend or did not respond, we would withdraw our services from Samya. (We would continue to work with the family, as needed.) Samya's absence had the power to upset us only if the expectation for her to attend came only from us. Our invitation to her would turn that around: she would have to make a commitment.

3. *Samya's charges.* I start the session by frankly discussing my disappointment. I felt that we had worked very hard together to create a working environment for new perceptions. As I talk, I manipulate the prayer beads Khaled gave me, underscoring my concern.

Dr. DiNicola: If Samya was here, we were going to say, "Samya what do you want?"

It took us three months, not really to begin working on the problem, but to say hello. To get to know you, how you are as a family, what it means to be who you are, we didn't even get to the problems.

SOHA TRANSLATES.

It's not much, but at least I can say honestly I tried to know this family's world . . .

SOHA TRANSLATES.

. . . but while we're trying to do that, Samya lives in a different world.

SOHA TRANSLATES.

And in that world, they're not so interested. . . . Now that we're ready to talk about real problems, Samya's not here. That's why I feel very discouraged.

SOHA TRANSLATES.

Khaled: Now we can talk about real problems.
Dr. DiNicola: I feel discouraged, though . . .
Khaled: Doctor, we can talk about real problems . . .
Khaled: Of course, we make mistake with Samya, we don't let her go out, maybe I don't understand teenagers for this generation . . .

Doctor, I cry too much for my daughter, I lose part of my heart. My daughter . . . what happened to her when she out of home, nobody believe, is nobody believe it! *(He is very bitter about the agency's complaints about him.)* "Mr. Shami very strong man. Mr. Shami fight. Mr. Shami angry." *(sarcastically)* Mr. Shami, his daughter raped in foster home, under protection!

Well, how you cannot be angry with these people? How we

can be gracious with these people? This girl—virgin girl, family girl—taken from home, put on the street, look at her behavior! I don't need nothing, I need justice . . .

Dr. DiNicola: This is where we started, with these very difficult questions. You called them human questions . . .

Khaled: Many professionals, many lawyers, social workers . . . is anybody understand? Nobody understand!

Dr. DiNicola: I understand. I'm discouraged about what I can do about it. *(addressing Mr. Massoud)* I spent three months getting to know this family. Now I want to know what happened.

SOHA TRANSLATES.

————

Taking my cue from Khaled's insistence that they were ready to talk about their "real problems," I explored the charges that Samya had made and how they felt about them now. I found them all remarkably composed and direct. Soha's story became very clear. She did not believe that her father had touched her sister sexually. I wondered how she could be so sure but she responded that they used to share a room and were always together. I said, without doubting her sincerity, that it would be hard to know the truth.

Soha: There is a truth. Samya told me to say to the social worker that my dad touched me.

Dr. DiNicola: Did he?

Soha: No.

Dr. DiNicola: Your dad never touched you? Didn't touch you how?

Soha: Didn't touch me sexually.

We explored the meaning of sexual abuse, including touching, comments, looks, and feelings. Soha had a clear understanding of all these things and denied that they had occurred.

————

Khaled: I don't know why Samya said this word, this is hurt me.

Dr. DiNicola: What word?

Khaled: Touch her. Really, doctor, this hurt me. Really, I want to talk to you. She's my daughter. I hug, I love my daughter. I hugged her in front of you last time.

Dr. DiNicola: Did you hit her?

Khaled: Yes. I say the truth.

Dr. DiNicola: In this society, the agency does not find that acceptable. The physical abuse was an issue, too.

Resident: It was an issue but that's not really what the charges were. The charges were not around that issue.

Dr. DiNicola: If Samya were to come home, would you hit her again?

Khaled: No . . .

Dr. DiNicola: Would you hit the other children?

Khaled: No.

Dr. DiNicola: It's very important that you are clear about that.

A cultural reconstruction. These are some possible narrative reconstructions, based on my cultural and therapeutic translations of the Shami family's predicament. As a young child, Samya had enjoyed her special status with her father (''above God''), who treated her throughout her childhood as a princess. However, when she entered puberty, she started looking beyond the family and her father for affection. Samya had suggested (inconsistently and vaguely) that she had been sexually active before anything occurred with her father (which was similarly vague and contradictory at different tellings). In my reconstruction, Samya's sexual awareness (and possible activity) set off a power struggle with her father, who experienced her as a changeling (changed, transformed by Western culture and damaged by the perceived loss of her virginity) and as unavailable to him.

Using the language of Western family therapy, the agency workers had felt quite uncomfortable with the father's lack of boundaries with his maturing daughter (''psychological incest''), his sense of ownership of Samya (''paternalism''), and his instrusiveness into her emotional experiences (''enmeshment''). These perceptions are deeply embedded in Western cultural assumptions about children, families, and sexual behavior. In Chapter 7, I offered alternative language for some of these perceptions: ''enmeshment'' is a label for familism seen out of cultural context; ''paternalism'' is, in my cultural translation, Khaled's wish to protect his daughter, something the agency utterly failed to do (she was raped in their care); ''psychological incest'' is a very complex notion, given to many possible distortions, and one for which I see no simple alternative. It would be simpler to observe interactions and ask those involved, father and daughter in this case, to describe their own behavior.

Using the metaphors of his culture, Khaled labeled Samya as "betraying" him, and as a "*sharmuta*" and "ruined" when she (appeared to have) acted out her proscribed sexuality. Although no one could ascertain exactly what had happened, it is possible that since she was "spoiled" in his eyes, Khaled acted out his distress and culturally sanctioned disgust toward her by violating her trust and making sexual advances to her. Alternatively, to Samya her father was a kind of mirror reflecting back to her a crucial source of esteem. Is it possible that, in seeing herself "damaged" in his eyes, she offered to prove her "loyalty" and "innocence" (virginity)? In a more complex alternative, father and daughter may have experienced fears and fantasies that could not be contained within the boundaries of the incest taboo. The "spillover" may have been partly imagined fantasy and partly acted-out events on either or both their parts. The girl's charge of sexual abuse may represent any combination of fact and fantasy, guilt and fear.

Certainly, the father-daughter interactions in the family sessions were filled with many highly charged, ambivalent, and anxious exchanges. Although Samya almost certainly distorted some aspects of her relationship with her father, and asked her sister to make a false charge of sexual abuse, we refused to see this in black-and-white terms of whether it occurred or not, and at no time did we invoke the notion of a false memory or outright malingering. We saw Samya as having been deeply injured in some way; much of her behavior could be read as a confused reaction to that injury. The injury was likely more emotional than physical, at least in the home. My guess is that, like many of the stories of young people in this book, she could not reconcile the choices available to a growing girl in Canadian society with the traditional rules of her family culture. As her family had never denied her anything up to that point, she had no way to cope with their harsh responses, which she experienced as a personal injury. We can only speculate as to how she experienced sexual situations outside her home.

Rakia tended to side with her husband and appeared to be angry with Samya. Perhaps her anger was about the privileged relationship between her daughter and her husband; perhaps it was because Samya brought shame upon the family. Both female and male observers of the sessions commented on what seemed, from a Western perspective, to be the mother's lack of sympathy for her daughter's distress. For this reason, we negotiated for a therapist on the team to work with the two of them on mother-daughter issues in separate sessions.

"THE LETTER"

The seventh session is a meeting with just the two parents. I have important feedback from my meeting with the agency the day before. They are more relaxed and lead off with surprising news: their daughter Soha was invited to go to Iraq to visit the President, Saddam Hussein. She had written a letter to the newspaper about the Kuwaiti crisis and her father sent a copy to the Iraqi Embassy in Ottawa.

Dr. DiNicola: I guess it's painful to consider how Soha is doing and then to think about Samya.

The day before, I had a meeting with the agency. I tell the family that it is hard to stay open to all the possibilities with so many lawyers and others with strong opinions. For the first time, the agency acknowledged that they are stuck and don't know what to do. The agency wanted to transfer control of Samya's care to me. I refused. Then they suggested that they would tell her to attend sessions or send her home. Again, I said no. The family would have her home, but at what price? They would just be waiting for the next crisis. I repeated that my commitment is to the whole family. The agency was beginning to understand that they had no moral authority with Samya and her family, no positive influence, only power. It became clearer to me as time went on that anyone who has this power cannot help this family. This is a strange predicament for a family therapist: everyone wanted to give me control over Samya's fate, from the court and the agency to the family. It was never so clear to me just how empty such power would be.[1] I explained this to the family.

Dr. DiNicola: If Samya is forced to come home now, you'll get your honor, but nothing else. Soha decided to rejoin the family. *Samya* has to decide to rejoin this family. That's all, it's very simple, forget the lawyers, forget the judge. . . .

Samya is in between two worlds, and Soha is learning to be comfortable with two worlds. Samya grew up in a traditional Arabic family, then she sees these other girls acting very differently . . .

The agency had asked me a question: is this is a cultural conflict? Is Samya using an excuse to act more "Canadian" than "Arabic" as an excuse to get out of the family? They are beginning to wonder: maybe we are letting Samya act out in a dangerous way so that she doesn't have to accept the family's set of rules.

What I want is a way for Samya to take responsbility for her choices.

Rakia: But she doesn't want to take it . . .

Dr. DiNicola: I have a plan. You write a letter to Samya, get Soha to help you, inviting Samya to come back to family therapy.

Khaled: Doctor, I don't need this. I need her by force to come; she can't make a decision. I want to ask you a question: what reason for Samya to stay outside home? The one that take her out of home should get her back home.

Dr. DiNicola: They don't know how to do that. I can't agree that my job is to bring Samya home. What I will try to do is to create the circumstances where you can talk to each other.

Khaled: You give her power.

Dr. DiNicola: I'm not giving her power, I'm giving her responsibility. You tell her: "We need you to be part of our family. Let's start by your coming to family therapy." Don't promise her anything, just say you want to talk. Everything she wants to talk about you will listen to.

Khaled: How can they do this?

Dr. DiNicola: It's a misapplied solution. It's a solution that didn't work, they are beginning to see that.

"Garbage." At times, under the influence of their intense emotions, Samya's parents referred to her in very degrading terms, such as

sharmuta (prostitute) or "garbage." They also constantly referred to her being "on the street." The therapeutic team found it hard to hear these things and we worried about being an audience for such sentiments without comment. I made three choices: (1) I chose the moment to open this subject with them, (2) I started with "garbage," the least emotive English word they had used, and (3) I directed my comments to Rakia, who I believed was less categorical and more open to redescribing her daughter in positive terms.

Dr. DiNicola (to Rakia): I want to talk to Mrs. Shami. Do you think your daughter is "garbage"?
Rakia (leaning forward in her chair): Yeah.
Dr. DiNicola: Is there a way for her not to be garbage?

Khaled intrudes throughout. I humor him, but gently deflect his comments and keep focused on Rakia. Finally, I change chairs with him. The whole time the tone is very friendly and he accepts my redirections.

Dr. DiNicola: Is she garbage to you?
Rakia: For me, yeah.
Dr. DiNicola: Forever?
Rakia: Forever!
Dr. DiNicola: She can't change?
Rakia: She can't change *because she's not living with her family!*

I consider that a profound statement about the sources of the self and what family culture really means to the Shamis.

Dr. DiNicola: That's the best reason for her to be home again.

Khaled intrudes again, so we switch chairs.

Dr. DiNicola: Is there any way you can change your opinion about your daughter? Can she do anything that will make you feel better about her?
Rakia: If she come home and listen to what we say to her.
Dr. DiNicola: And then she can change, she's not garbage anymore?

Rakia: We need to save her from the street.

Dr. DiNicola: Let's say that Samya comes home and changes her behavior, can you imagine that she becomes a valuable person to you again?

Rakia: Valuable?

Dr. DiNicola: Someone "good" for you, worthy of your respect.

Rakia: If she changes . . .

Dr. DiNicola: What you're saying is clear: if she continues as she is, it's hard for you to respect her.

Rakia: For sure.

Dr. DiNicola: But *can* you respect her again?

Rakia: If she changes.

Notice how the dialogue has shifted from absolutes ("garbage," "*sharmuta*") to shades (value, respect) through negotiation. We have moved from how Samya is perceived to what she can become. We are talking about change and what we keep bumping up against is the family's "final vocabulary"—that irreducible set of values that generates meaning for them. I never challenge that. In fact, I value it, I support it, I encourage it. Once family members feel you are talking in their language, in their final vocabulary, you can have a real dialogue, which makes everything else negotiable! This is cultural translation—talking in the family's final vocabulary. And what cultural translation makes possible is the transformation of experience through therapeutic translation. In other words, getting people to move beyond what they usually imagine as their final vocabulary.

Dr. DiNicola: OK, now—for Khaled. Is it possible for him to respect her again if she changes her behavior?

Rakia: Yeah.

Dr. DiNicola: You see, this is what other people hear from you: "She's garbage," "She's a *sharmuta*." They don't hear the other part that I hear: the commitment to family, your values. I also would like to know if Samya thinks that you can ever respect her again?

Rakia: Samya, she doesn't believe herself, how's she gonna believe her family?

Dr. DiNicola: What do you say to her? Do you always call her *sharmuta*?

Rakia: We never call her that.

Khaled: Never.

Dr. DiNicola: Do you make her feel like that? Do you say other things that make her feel like garbage?

They both deny that.

Dr. DiNicola: So we're clear, if Samya comes home and changes her behavior, you could learn to respect her again. Write her a letter, put your heart in this letter. The message should be simple: ''We recognize that things need to be different for you to come home.''

RESPONSE TO THE LETTER

The next session, the eighth family meeting, was a brief one. We convened a meeting of the parents, Samya and her social worker, and the two co-therapists. The social worker announces that Samya said she will make a plan and respect that plan.

Samya: I said I'll come to have a better relationship with my family, but quit bugging me about going home and everything like that. I'll come every two weeks, two hours a session. All I do is translate for my grandfather, but I'll come in order to establish a better relationship with my parents.

The parents get into a verbal tug of war with Samya and the social worker—every week, not every two weeks, and so on. The team is amazed by the total unwillingness of the workers at the agency to negotiate with this family, even with our help. The agency never misses an opportunity to have a disagreement with the family. Once again, I intervene to create a bridge.

Dr. DiNicola (to Samya): What I am committed to is for this family to do what your parents have invited you to do, what you have agreed on, what we're offering, and what the agency is supporting.

This family has been flattened, now we have to rebuild the house. I am for recreating the atmosphere here where you can be honest, open, and recapture the love that I think you have for each other and a way to live together so that you don't hurt each other so much.

Khaled challenges the social worker about whether she agrees, whether she has changed her mind about the family.

Khaled: I don't want every day the family have hope—build up, then fall down. All the family hurt for this.

We are making a plan for Samya to attend family sessions. Khaled and Samya get into a fight. I try to calm each of them gently, then more firmly. Finally, I stand up and declare that if they don't stop, I will leave and the session will be over. I announce a break and the agency social worker leaves. After a break, we agree to have family meetings every two weeks, with individual sessions for Samya with the resident on alternate weeks. On occasion, we plan some home visits as well.

"THE RETURN OF THE PRODIGAL DAUGHTER"

The ninth session occurs just before Christmas and the agency has a great Christmas gift for the family. The team had conducted a home visit with Samya, her first contact with her family home in almost a year. Samya was delighted to be home and this opened up a flood of feeling for her. Soon after, she started playing with the idea of returning home, expressed with her usual ambivalence and inconsistency. The agency social worker asks to be present at the session so that she can give the family members an answer to their request for Samya to go home. She waits in my office until we have a chance to prepare the family. Samya, Soha, both parents, and the grandfather are present.

The family has surprises of their own. They bring me a Christmas card (from a Lebanese-Palestinian Catholic/Muslim family to an

Italian student of Judaism—will cultural ironies never cease?). Khaled announces that he is taking Soha and Samya to Baghdad to pursue Soha's project for peace with Iraqi President Saddam Hussein. Furthermore, Khaled says that the agency has agreed to discharge her from their care and Samya now desperately wants to return home.

Dr. DiNicola: I don't understand. This family is going through something major. A major trauma. Soha only just returned and Samya's not home yet.

Soha: I returned eight months ago.

Dr. DiNicola: Yes, but that's a short time in family life. And Samya's not home yet. I have a great sense of a lack of direction here. What do you want? You're going through a major problem. It's not finished by any means . . . and now you want to rush off to Baghdad.

Soha: It's for peace. That's why I'm going there. I've been asking the Ambassador if I can meet the Iraqi president. I'm still waiting for a reply. Why don't you like it?

Dr. DiNicola: It's not that I don't like it. I'm raising questions about what this means for your family right now.

You have major family problems and this is a diversion of energy. And not a useful one as far as I can tell. . . . Plus it's dangerous, war could break out any day.

Soha: The war will be in the Gulf, not in Baghdad.

Dr. DiNicola: I don't understand why you would undertake this mission at this time.

Khaled: Me, I say this plan good for us.

Dr. DiNicola: What do you think, Rakia?

Rakia: I lived in Beirut during the civil war . . .

————

Dr. DiNicola: So what's your plan?

Khaled: We need your help to be united again . . . I wait for you. Everybody help her go out from home, why nobody help her go home? Yesterday, the director of the agency said she can go.

Dr. DiNicola: If Samya wants to go home, I would like to support her to do that. But to reverse her mind suddenly and demand to go back home overnight does not seem healthy.

What I had discussed with the agency was what is typically done in such situations: a slow return home, starting with overnight visits, graduating to weekends at home. I am concerned about the speed with which things are changing and whether the family has had enough time to grow into the changes. But Samya short-circuits all our caution with a simple statement—

Samya: I want to go home.

Dr. DiNicola: Yes, I hear you, Samya. If you go home, do you think you will argue with your father? Is it possible that when you argue with your father, you will have those thoughts again?

Samya denies this. She is as adamant about returning home now as she was before about staying away. Having expressed my concerns aloud, I bring in the agency representative. In fact, I believe that, considering everything, there would be no benefit in prolonging Samya's stay in the group home. The session is overwhelmed by the family's joy when I make the dramatic announcement—

Dr. DiNicola (to Samya): Tell your grandfather you are going home tonight.

As Samya tells her grandfather, he beams a smile and raises his hands, holding his prayer beads.

"A DISILLUSIONED MAN"

A month later, the end of January 1991. Our tenth session. All of the Shami family is present. The children are playful, relaxed—a bubbling, "happy" family.

Dr. DiNicola: I haven't seen everybody in a while—it's been a long time.

(*To Mr. Massoud*): How's the family? How are Soha and Samya getting along?

He says well to both. They all agree.

Dr. DiNicola: Things are better now, things are back to normal?

Rakia: They fight too much.

Dr. DiNicola: Samya and her father?
Rakia: Yes.

———

Dr. DiNicola: Do you still need my help? What's our goal? I would like to know what he thinks is good for this family.
Rakia (translates for her father): He doesn't know.
Dr. DiNicola: Samya made the choice to come home. You look happy together, she looks happy.
Rakia: She doesn't like things like before. She doesn't want to stay home.
Dr. DiNicola: She wants more privileges.
Rakia: My father say, "There're no balance." He wants balance. Samya wants to go outside too much.
Dr. DiNicola: Do you want things to be just like they were before, or to move on?
Rakia: Not exactly like before.
Khaled: More balance . . .

As a group, the family is definitely happier. There's more space for Rakia. She seems more of a partner, with a clearer voice. Not just in a support role, but expressing herself. Samya seems to have returned to her role as the older sister, playing with children, especially the younger ones. This is important, because it was one of her complaints in the past—feeling she was used as a baby-sitter.

Dr. DiNicola: Let me see if I understand: a balance between the very traditional Lebanese style and the more permissive Canadian style. It can't be too permissive.

THEY ALL AGREE.

Dr. DiNicola: If you have a balance, who will be happy with the balance?
Rakia: Everybody.

I ask each of them in turn. They are pleased with the idea. Then I turn my attention to Khaled, who does not appear very happy. He is very preoccupied with the Gulf War. Khaled feels blamed for what is happening there by other Canadians and tells a story about how some Arabic children were victimized by other children at school because of the feelings emerging from the Gulf War.

Dr. DiNicola: It's a painful time for you, I see that. Most Canadians will forget about this sooner or later.

Khaled: We hurt too much, this pain stay here, then come another pain.

Dr. DiNicola: Does the pain from the outside, from the war for example, make the other pain that you had any different? Does it change your other pain?

I spend a great deal of time patiently listening to his concerns about his recent ordeal as a father with the agency and courts and now as an Arab in Canada. This is both personally genuine on my part and therapeutically important. At no time do I want to suggest that the very real trauma of his legal problems or his vicarious emotional participation in the Gulf War can be understood in other terms. Nonetheless, I am concerned about his state of mind and his apparent depression. I want to validate his distressing social experiences while expressing concern for his personal health. This goes on for over an hour.

At one point, Khaled says he is still not working, another troubling sign. He says he stays "at home like women," to which Samya responds, "Women work too, you know." Samya and Soha give their father a history lesson about women's rights in the West. Khaled listens with a mixture of curiosity and pride. Khaled explains the different sense of duty and obligation that Arabic men feel toward their families, in contrast to the lack of responsibility toward family he perceives in Canadian society.

Dr. DiNicola: The traditional sense is that families are responsible for each other. . . . In the West, it's a different world now, where people are more responsible for themselves. Many people are not comfortable with what's happening in Western society, there's such a stress on the individual. We're losing a sense of family, of community. It's not only your problem, we're all struggling with that.

Khaled: It's very materialistic.

Dr. DiNicola: The challenge is to maintain your humanity, your way of being human, wherever you are.

Khaled: How do *you* feel, are you a part or not a part?

———

Before I can answer this personal question, the observing team knocks on the door and Dr. John Theis, a psychologist and family therapist, offers me a consultation.

Dr. Theis: I've been on the other side of the mirror. We were going to send a message.

   (Speaking to Khaled): What we were saying is that you're really very disillusioned. What we saw was that Dr. DiNicola was spending a lot of time trying to get you "jacked up," that he was very concerned about you.

   We didn't know if anybody else in here is as concerned about your disillusionment as he is. So that's a question that we had. And then we wondered how far back the disillusionment goes? Do you know how far back it goes?

Khaled: Yeah, I know . . .

Dr. Theis: Years and years?

Khaled: One year ago, exactly.

Dr. Theis: It started a year ago, but it's big, huh?

Khaled: Yeah. *(Khaled tells his story.)*

Dr. Theis: I don't have any difficulty understanding in the last year you got really disillusioned, but does it go back further than that?

   (Speaking to everyone): The question at the back of my mind is, it was a big sacrifice coming to this country. He came here for his family so that it would be a peaceful place to live, and I wonder if from the beginning this country has been a disappointment?

   (To Khaled): And, if you've struggled inside yourself with this disappointment for years and years, now, you just got burned out . . .

Khaled: Yeah.

Dr. Theis: So it's longer than a year. Let me just check *(looking around at other family members)*. Do you think he was disappointed before?

Soha: No.

Dr. Theis: Do you know who in this family can help you with your disappointment?

Khaled: No.

Dr. Theis: I think when people get disappointed they need somebody. I think that was what Dr. D. was asking . . . I think you need support. Can they give it to you?

Khaled: No.

Dr. Theis: How come?

Khaled: I need to support my family.

Dr. Theis: But you looked tired. I don't think you can support anybody. At one point, you couldn't hold your head up. You know how to solve problems, but right now, you don't have the energy. I think Dr. D. was giving you support . . .

Khaled: Dr. DiNicola . . . I feel he's a friend, not a doctor, we trust each other, I think we learn from each other very much. One point, he can't help me and I can't help myself—for 14 months my social life finished.

Dr. Theis: I think the big issue is: what you're looking for in this country you need to find in your family.

Khaled: We are part of this country, we are Canadian just because we have citizenship . . .

Dr. Theis: I wouldn't worry about Canada before I'd worry about this room. I think it's more important to worry about this room. Today you've been very, very down and I'm not so sure they're doing anything for you. I don't know if they think they can.

Khaled: No.

Dr. Theis (motioning to Samya): She's falling asleep. Father is disappointed, sad, low in energy—she's falling asleep!

Khaled: Nobody has to give support for me.

Rakia: The children don't want to know what happened.

Dr. Theis: Maybe all I can do is give you a challenge. You have been a very energetic, very enthusiastic man. You have things to say, you have ideas, you've lived in different cultures. And sometimes you get very strong and I see what happens is people put a wall up, you know—"We'll just control that"—they don't listen so much . . .

Khaled: I need somebody stronger than me . . . if I die, my family finished . . .

Dr. DiNicola: Do you know the story of Job? Job was tested by God.

Khaled: God tested me!

Dr. DiNicola (nodding): God's testing you . . .

Khaled: Why not you, why not somebody else, why me? Why God choose me, to test me?

Dr. DiNicola: That's right, that's what Job asked . . .

Khaled: I supported a hundred families, I never did something bad. My home never closed for people that come: welcome, a warm welcome! Now I can't support my family.

Dr. DiNicola: Khaled, let me tell you the story of Job. It's very moving. The Devil was talking to God and God was saying, "Look at my servant Job. He's a good man." And the Devil said, "Well, sure. Sure, he's a good man. He's got a family, he's rich, he's got his health. Why shouldn't he believe You and why shouldn't he serve You well? What would happen if your servant Job didn't have his health, didn't have his family, he lost his money?" . . . All the things that happened to you, Khaled! And God said, "Well, see what happens." And so the Devil sent all these trials to Job and Job said, "Why me, what did I do? I never did anything wrong!"

Rakia (following along, nodding): Yeah . . .

Dr. DiNicola: And I don't have the answer to that question, Khaled. I don't have the answer . . .

Khaled: Nobody has . . . Doctor, I am a rich man, believe me. I am inside rich *(pointing into his chest)*, in here *(pointing to his head)*. If something happens to me and I die, my God takes me, I don't mind, everybody is going to die one day. But you see around me, everything died . . .

Dr. DiNicola: Not yet, your family's still very much alive, Khaled. You asked for my help   .   .   .   and you worked it out. You have your family, whole, again. You accomplished this: you are rich, you're rich inside and in your family. But I can't convince you of that, I tried for an hour today. You have to convince yourself.

Soha: He won't listen to us . . .

EVERYBODY IN THE FAMILY NODS, SADLY AND WITH RESIGNATION.

FALLOUT FROM THE GULF WAR

At the next meeting, the eleventh session, there is a mixture of themes. Khaled, Rakia, and her father are present. The family has a terrible sense of mistreatment in Ottawa as a result of the Gulf War with Iraq. Someone killed their cat and left it at their door with a note that this is how they will deal with Arabs.

Dr. DiNicola: Are you afraid to be victimized because you are an Arab in Canada?
Rakia: Yes.

Nonetheless, it seemed that Rakia was trying to soften Khaled's statements, with a gentle flow of comments in Arabic.

Rakia: We didn't come to talk about politics.
Dr. DiNicola: I'm not sure it's just about politics. He's scared.
Khaled: I'm scared for my kids, not for myself.
Dr. DiNicola: I know you are a brave man, Khaled. Are you worried about him, Rakia?
Rakia: Yeah.
Dr. DiNicola: Every week he's more depressed, more upset.
Rakia: Every day, every day, he becomes more and more . . .

I ask if Khaled has seen his own doctor. Khaled saw his doctor, who prescribed medication for depression. Khaled is sitting with his head in his hands, sighing, holding his prayer beads. There has been a slow shift in the past few sessions, evident today. Rakia is more open, more vocal, and supportive of Khaled, who is more receptive.

They tell me that Samya is doing better at home, and they are focusing their energy on other things. Although he can barely focus his attention, Khaled says that Samya wants to visit Lebanon when the school year ends. The family has always treated Samya as very special, as their "princess," and now the word has a new meaning for them. They see her as selfish and lacking empathy for others. They described their daughter as manipulative and seductive. I redirect them to their positive gains.

Dr. DiNicola: Samya's very sociable. In many ways, the problems have improved: she's home, she's behaving herself, she's not doing the things that made you so upset before. Now you have other problems: you worry about the political situation, about how the community treats you. You have work and business problems.

KHALED'S SOLUTION:
"THE GEOGRAPHIC CURE"

At the twelfth and final session, the parents have come alone with Samya. The family members are finding a new level of comfort with each other. Samya continues her psychotherapy sessions, which Rakia sometimes also attends to work on mother-daughter issues. Samya and Khaled are about to embark on a trip to the Middle East. Khaled's plan is to take Samya there for a year. That's his solution based on his perception of their predicament, a kind of "geographic cure." They plan to fly to Paris, then rent a car there and drive to the Middle East to visit Lebanon and a number of other countries for business. They sense my reservations about the plan.

Khaled sends Samya out for a coffee for him. The parents express concern that she is "out of control," "doing nothing" but watching TV all day.

Khaled: Please, doctor, I don't want to lose my family . . . again!

Rakia: Nobody like her at home, even Salim [the toddler], he screamed when she took his hand . . .

Khaled: Vincenzo, do you have another solution?

Dr. DiNicola: Well, the other solution is to do what we've been doing: to meet with the family, work with the family . . .

Rakia: But she doesn't respect anyone, not in the home, not outside the home. She want to do like the girls on the street. What they are doing, she wants to do . . .

Dr. DiNicola: I want to respect your family, your culture, your way of doing things. I'm not sure I would do what you are planning to do. I can't say yes, I can't say no. But I'm here for you.

Khaled: I talk to you now, not like doctor, I talk to you like friend.

SAMYA REENTERS THE ROOM.

What I want to do is present her to her cousins, her family. I want to make solutions, I'm damaged. Last week, I don't have money to buy bread. This the first time I tell anybody else: I lose everything.

Dr. DiNicola: How can you afford such an expensive trip?

Khaled: I have an American Express card!

Dr. DiNicola: You're hoping for some business contacts. Will it be safe for you to travel there?

Khaled: I work for many years in the army. I don't think about do I have safe or not have safe.

Dr. DiNicola: I hope it works out for you.

Khaled: Tell me your ideas, I'm ready to accept any ideas.

Dr. DiNicola: I'm afraid I don't know very much about that kind of thing. I'm a doctor, that's all I know how to do. I'm a doctor, I'm not a businessman. If that's what you feel you have to do, that's what you have to do. It's going to be a long trip for you and Samya.

Khaled: Sixty days. Now, I'm free, I have no money, I don't care . . .

Dr. DiNicola: Why don't you take your father-in-law along with you?

Khaled: I have two problems—business problem, family problem.

Dr. DiNicola: I'm not sure if your plan is a solution for the second problem. Write me and let me know—how do you say it? *Kotub*?

Rakia: In Arabic, a letter is *maktub*.

Dr. DiNicola: Thank you. I'll wait for your *maktub*.

We stand to say goodbye. In spite of their concerns, Samya is very different. She is more pleasant and respectful towards her parents. She is appropriately but fashionably dressed. Rakia stands beside her husband on a more equal footing. Khaled wants to know if I will see Rakia and the children in his absence. I told them what all the people of the Mediterranean say, what I always say at change points of therapy: *My door is always open.*

What can we make of this choice? This family was constantly rewriting their story. Here was a new fork in the path where no paradigm could guide me. Instead, this session has its own rationality—a *syntagm*—presenting new choices with new opportunities for making meaning. Was Khaled abducting his daughter? He had threatened to do so before. But he was now one of her legal guardians again. Was he bribing her? I had cautioned them about making her a "princess" throughout our therapy sessions. By returning to the presenting culture, I constructed a more meaningful answer.

Salman Rushdie's (1983) passionate and disturbing novel, *Shame*, was his response to the tragedy of a Pakistani father who murdered his daughter in London over honor, pride, and shame. The novel is not set in London, however, but in Pakistan, where the characters are animated by the social, cultural, and religious sources that make their lives meaningful, if tragic, and not just shocking head-lines. Rushdie's choice reflects a profound insight about cultural context and offers a key as to what forks in the path the Shami family perceived at this juncture. In the face of their distress, the family naturally turned to their own culture for healing. If Samya and her family are to have a chance to heal their injuries and to normalize their relationship, the norms will have to be generated by a culture they can all accept and integrate. Khaled and Rakia have stumbled in that attempt in Canada. The solutions offered by Canadian authorities only amplified their suffering. Now they were guiding their daughter to their home base in the Middle East for nurturance and replenishment. And what of Samya?

A *MAKTUB* FROM THE MIDDLE EAST

A month later, I received Samya's *maktub*, her letter, from the Middle East.

> Dear Dr. DiNicola:
> Hi! How are you? I'm just fine and so is my father. We're in [the Middle East] now. It's great, a little old fashioned but still great
> . . .
>
> I saw all my family and they all loved me and I'm always kept busy here . . .
>
> Everybody loves me here and they show it too. Today, I'm going to meet my father's cousin, who is Vice President . . . and tonight we're having dinner at the house of the General of the . . . Police, who is a very kind man.
>
> My Arabic is getting better every day. I really don't know what else to say, but see you soon,
>
> Yours truly,
>   Samya Shami
>
> P.S. My father thanks you for your help and he hopes you and your family are doing great. Thank you.

Chapter 10

THE WEB OF MEANING

Metaphor and the Transformation of Experience

Without the metaphor of memory and history, we cannot imagine . . . what it is to be someone else. Metaphor is the reciprocal agent, the universalizing force that makes it possible to envision the stranger's heart.

—Cynthia Ozick
(1989, p. 279)

Metaphor and its power to transform experience is the subject of this chapter. Metaphor allows us entry into the "web of meaning" of other lives, an alternative to narrower views of family therapy. A Portuguese immigrant family's story illustrates the possibilities of narrative transformation through my eighth conceptual tool, multiple codes. *These are the complex messages encoded in metaphor (figurative language) and somatics (embodied meaning), illustrated by the Figueroa family's experience of loss, pain, and overcoming. The chapter closes with an overview of the key metaphors for culture, families, and therapy constructed throughout this book.*

METAPHOR—"THE RECIPROCAL AGENT"

In Chapter 4, I suggested that the judgment that some people live in "a world beyond metaphor" is a harsh one. It is harsh regarding the capacities of our clients and, to the extent that it is accepted, it is

293

a severe limitation on how therapy is imagined. Without metaphor, therapy is nothing more than talk, with little capacity to transform our experiences. Many of the tools for conducting CFT are ways of allowing us to talk to each other meaningfully, setting the stage for an encounter—spirals of negotiation, peering through masks (cultural costume and camouflage), and playing with how we see each other (insiders and outsiders). But to do more, to foster change, requires new descriptions of family predicaments. As soon as we get into translation issues, concrete and literal descriptions fall short. The other tools of CFT—creating a lexicon of the family's language (cultural translation) and finding a common language for new experiences (therapeutic translation)—require the figurative language of metaphor. And the further we go into the change-oriented phases of therapy—when we examine cultural strategies and help the family build bridges—the more we rely on the inventiveness of metaphor to open space for the family.

What is metaphor? Since Aristotle, metaphor has been defined in terms of one thing representing another (Barker, 1996). By bringing two things together through figurative language, a metaphor is a *novel representation* (Gordon, 1978). Metaphor is a reminder that our description of the world is always incomplete and a great part of what makes our individual experiences unique is how we fill in the holes. This, in turn, makes all communication a form of translation into our known ways of thinking. In intercultural encounters, metaphor serves to bring alien experiences closer to home and gives us novel representations of what is familiar. Metaphors are translations.

Where does metaphor fit into theories of family therapy? In his study of metaphors, Paul Rosenblatt (1994) examines not only the relationship between metaphor and theory in family therapy, but the metaphors of family systems theory. His book is a constant reminder that what are commonly taken as givens, even theories, are better understood as metaphors. Rosenblatt (1994) deconstructs the metaphors in the name of our field, examining the American cultural resonances of "family" and "therapy." In my view, therapists and theorists tend to underplay Rosenblatt's key point that our ways of thinking are metaphoric. If our theories are metaphors, they are "metaphors that are meant," sometimes quite concretely and rigidly.

Therapists are divided, above all, about which domain they give primacy to in their theories of how problems are generated and in their theories of change. What has primacy—affect, behavior, or cognition? Change the behavior and the feelings and thoughts will follow, say the behaviorists. Cognitive therapists argue that cognitive schemas are the generators of our actions and feelings. Emotion-focused therapists (this covers a huge territory from psychoanalytic therapy to experiential approaches) point to the salience of affect in coloring all our thinking and our actions. All three general approaches have been applied to family therapy. I no longer believe these are resolvable quarrels. Outcome studies of therapy may show the improved efficacy of one approach over another for a specific problem, as conducted and tested in that particular study. This does not enable us to generate overall guidelines for judging the claims of these general approaches to human predicaments. Furthermore, except for graduate students committed to completing their research, hardly anyone is convinced or converted by such research data. Our choice of models of human predicaments is deeply embedded in our social histories and personal preferences, the impact of mentors and formative training experiences. Our preferred models are metaphors for our view of the world.

In this book, I espouse yet another approach: a meaning-centered view of human predicaments and of culture—what Clifford Geertz (1973b) calls the "web of meaning." Metaphor allows us entry into the web of meaning of other lives, an alternative to a more narrowly defined grounding of family therapy in behavioral, cognitive or emotional domains. In Chapter 2, I outlined why general psychology must be based on a cultural psychology whose unit of analysis is relationships rather than individuals, following the work of Richard Shweder (1991), Jerome Bruner (1990), and others. Cultural psychology provides a meaningful set of lenses to re-vision family therapy. Cultural family therapy is the product of tracking through cultural psychology and other societal and theoretical changes in anthropology, psychology, and psychiatry. In this approach, meaning has primacy in the crucible of human consciousness. Any model of affect, behavior, or cognition that does not integrate meaning is a less than comprehensive account of human being. And when you get to meaning, unless you are doing theology or metaphysics, you get to metaphor, what American Jewish writer Cynthia Ozick (1989) calls "the reciprocal agent." Metaphor makes strange worlds accessible by making them imaginable. Any other world, any other future, must first be envisioned.

The Figueroa Family:
"I Am Myself What I Have Lost"

Kingston, mid-1990s. Isabel Figueroa is a 15-year-old adolescent living with her Portuguese immigrant parents in nearby Gano-noque. A year before, she was admitted to hospital for suicidal ideation. What underlies this is a family crisis. Mother, Cristina, is chronically "depressed." Cristina and her three daughters have been in therapy for many years, with little evident benefit. Eduardo (Eddy), the father, drinks; Cristina and Eddy have chronic marital discord. But he has rarely attended any consultations or the endless therapy sessions. All of these features put Isabel at risk for a mood disorder and suicidal behavior.

Isabel has two older sisters, now both married. When Marta got engaged to be married last year, the family seemed to go collectively into crisis. Two patterns have been reported for children in families with a mood disorder (see DiNicola, 1989): children who adopt the role of "emotional caretaker" for symptomatic family members and children who "opt out" of the family. Opting out can range from self-absorption in productive academic or social activities to acting out and running away. Isabel wants to "opt out"—and she has explored almost every possible way of doing that, from absorption in school activities, to wanting to live with her sister Marta, to more potentially harmful fantasies of running away, and worst of all, suicidal thinking and behavior. Isabel has never been tempted to take on a caretaker role for her mother or her parents; it is too onerous for her. Instead, she and Marta huddled together on their own, both imagining ways to leave home. Marta's engagement sent Isabel into despair.

After completing my psychiatric assessment of Isabel, I was ready to make my first and most important intervention. I convened a family meeting and let everyone express their concerns. At a blackboard, I compiled everyone's list of problems, from personal concerns to interpersonal problems. No one thought that Isabel had a psychiatric problem (I agreed). Everyone agreed that her distress was a response to family problems—the parents' marital discord, father's drinking, and Marta's imminent move out of the family and away from Ganonoque. Isabel was discharged from hospital. The plan for follow-through care included family therapy and referrals for an alcohol assessment for father and marital therapy for the parents.

"Doing the laundry." The daughters were angry with their father over his drinking. And each successive daughter was angrier. To make discussing it more tolerable, Isabel and Marta had a metaphor for Eddy's drinking. In response to my question about how things were at home, they said Eddy was "doing the laundry a lot lately." Misunderstanding, I said it was great that he was helping out more at home. They burst into laughter. Marta clarified: "There are only two things in the basement—the laundry and the wine cellar. Guess what my father was doing down there?" "Doing the laundry" is a predicament expressed in the figurative language of metaphor. It serves to externalize the problem of father's drinking in a traditional family culture that does not easily tolerate open criticism of parental figures. It demonstrates my eighth conceptual tool for CFT—*multiple codes*, indicating the multiple meanings that can be encoded in *metaphor* or figurative language. Sometimes metaphor can serve to put pain at a safe distance or allow the indirect expression of what cannot be openly and directly stated, as in this example. At other times, metaphor can bring intolerable suffering closer, opening space within by redescribing the self in larger, more embracing terms. This is the obverse of Michael White's concept of "externalizing the problem." I call this process *somatics* or embodied meaning, illustrated in Cristina's story.

The somatics of saudade. Mother was distressed by the impending departure of her daughter. Feeling trapped in an unhappy marriage, Cristina can only see loss in her daughter's marriage, not any gain. This loss summons other losses for her: her first daughter's marriage, the death of her brother when she was a teenager (whom she still mourns), the loss of her native land and language, and the bitterness she feels toward her husband for refusing to visit Portugal, as a result of which she never saw her parents alive after they emigrated.

Cristina's mourning has a nostalgic quality. All languages have ways to express this; the Portuguese call it *saudade*, a bittersweet resignation to loss, deepened through longing and reflection. For immigrants, their *saudade* is not just about their homeland and their families, or their culture and their language. All these are important, all are critical, but emigration adds something else to these losses—there is a loss of their expectations. Their lives took a different path: in thinking about the places they left behind, they encounter other possible lives. If their lives are working for them, this creates a sense of nostalgia, a bittersweet feeling for other places. If their lives haven't worked out, they experience something much more bitter—regret, a sense of "what if," tortured walks down the roads not taken. Writing about her own migrations, Eva Hoffman (1990, p. 115) remarked that "loss is a magical preservative"—Cristina's nostalgia for the past is as fresh as a new razor blade and brings the pain back to her daily.

In one of the family sessions, Eddy was dismissive of Cristina's nostalgia for Portugal. "I don't understand this obsession with the old country," he said bluntly. "There are two flights a week to Portugal. Jump on one and go." Yet he had refused to visit Portugal in the past and had no desire to do so now. This makes for a marital stalemate. Cristina lives in the past, killing the present; Eddy lives in the present, denying the past. Two bridges, side by side, of the same river, each with its own purpose, never meeting.

Although Cristina had her own therapist, I met with her and Isabel shortly after that session with her husband to listen to her concerns. I had selected something for her to read in Portuguese. In a striking sonnet, the Portuguese poet Fernando Pessoa compares himself not to Boabdil, the last Moorish king as he fled Granada, but to his backward glance. (This is the "Moor's last sigh" of Salman Rushdie's novel of that name.) Pessoa (1942, pp. 45–46) identifies himself with the king's regret for what he is losing, moving on to an even bolder identification:

> Hoje sou a saudade imperial
> Do que já na distância de mim vi . . .
> Eu próprio sou aquilo que perdi . . .

> Now I am that imperial longing
> For what I saw of myself then in the distance . . .
> I am myself what I have lost . . .
> > —Fernando Pessoa,
> > *Passos da Cruz. VI,*
> > "Stations of the Cross. VI"
> > (my translation)[1]

She read it with tears streaming down her face. She felt that the poem grasped her feelings better than anything she could say. The last line in particular speaks to her experience and she repeated it to me in Portuguese: *Eu proprio sou aquilo que perdi*—I am myself what I have lost. It was a moment of lucidity for her. Echoing Pessoa's haunting sonnet, Cristina made a subtle but emotionally daring connection. She realized that what she had lost in all these years of sorrow and regret was much closer than she had allowed herself to imagine: a part of herself, her capacity to live in the present and hope for the future. "I am myself what I have lost" is a redescription of Cristina's self, a metaphoric transformation that creates intimacy by bringing experience closer to her known self. Such redescriptions work best when they are "concrete metaphors"—what Gregory Bateson (1972) called "metaphors that are meant," such as the Catholic belief that "the bread is the body and the wine is the blood of Jesus." The more abstract the metaphor, the more tenuous the physical connection to our bodies. The more concrete the metaphor, the more easily we can use it to redescribe our own selves. That is why I call this process of multiple coding *somatics* or embodied meaning.

In witnessing this moment, Cristina's daughter served as an audience for her story. Cristina cannot leave her pain behind; she is her pain. But Cristina is learning to move from perceiving this as an impossible predicament to a livable one. How? By making sense of the pain. Like many of the predicaments described in this book, this is not an act of courage but an act of meaning. This is a radically different story from the one Isabel grew up hearing from her mother. And the active process of witnessing her mother's new story has the potential to open doors for Isabel, too.

LISTENING AS A FOUNDATION

Readers may find the Figueroa family story unfinished (it is!) or unsatisfying (that's our problem, not necessarily the family's), especially after reading the Shami family's detailed narrative. It is like the difference between a novel and a short story. A novel draws you in entirely, creating a complete world. In a short story, you do not completely enter the minimal world sketched out in a few pages. It is an inconclusive world which we complete by joining it back into our own lives.[2] Brief narratives like this one are useful for teaching and for reflection. If everything appears resolved and clear, then there is little for the reader (or therapist) to do.

With the Figueroa family, I want to say something about the power of just listening to an evolving story and helping the family members to find words to convey their experience. Therapy, too, is a metaphor. Maybe we need new metaphors for what we do when we sit with other people. Rosenblatt (1994) suggests the metaphor of listening: "Listening is a foundation for the co-construction of reality" (p. 196). In order for our interventions to be meaningful, we have to check our impulses always to act. Physicians have a great temptation to reach for the prescribing pad; therapists want to make a treatment plan. With this family, I have done a lot of listening, punctuated by occasional interventions such as gathering the extended family to generate solutions.

Does the account lack hope? Does it lack a treatment plan? By listening to the narrative, I sit with them and help them to endure what they are going through. Together, we wait for an opening, the start of a new story. My choice to listen to (and co-edit) their narrative challenges the metaphor of "therapy" as an active, directive, change-oriented process. Let's listen in again.

ALTERNATIVE MEDICINE

After the poetry session with Cristina and Isabel, an opening took place in this family. Cristina took her husband to a Portuguese *ervanaria* in Toronto. The herbalist spoke to Eddy, admonished him against drinking alcohol, and gave him a variety of natural substances. Isabel was critical of this folk approach and tried to enlist me in her doubts, but I pointed out that her father was actually listening to the herbalist in Toronto, whereas he had been unwilling to work with the addictions agency that had assessed him in Kingston. In fact, Eddy decreased his drinking significantly and, although he was still irritable, he was no longer violent.

While I did my best to support this healthy change realistically, I also know that alcoholics make many attempts to stop their drinking before they accomplish that. It was also true that Eddy's drinking was only their most prominent concern, not their sole one. After several months, both Cristina and Isabel were disconsolate. When Eddy was drinking, this gave his family a target and a focus to their complaints. Without this distraction, they all had a chance to reflect on their lives. Isabel started to fail in school again, thinking again only of leaving home. The school issues were easy to resolve through a case conference that led to a commitment from Isabel and a close monitoring plan for her school attendance and work. The family story will not be able to change much without creating a space where the family can reflect in safety on other possibilities. Cristina started thinking seriously about seeing a lawyer for a divorce. Isabel has moved in with her oldest sister. This has already created healthier options for them than what they had experienced before—Cristina's chronic hopelessness and helplessness and Isabel's suicidal behavior. And what of Eddy? He can make choices that may allow his daughter to return home and to deal with his marital problems.

If my experience of the Figueroa family can be constructed as a family narrative without therapy, it was at least guided and co-edited by me as a therapist. Can we go further in challenging our metaphors of therapy? Can we imagine a family narrative of transformation without therapy and without a therapist?

"ENVISIONING THE STRANGER'S HEART": A COLLECTION OF METAPHORS

By collecting the metaphors of the family stories in this book, can we begin to recognize the story elements we need to understand families across cultures? Perhaps that is too ambitious. Can our readings of other stories at least teach us enough about our own humanity to be better prepared for cultural family therapy? In Chapter 1, I suggested that the stories of our families in therapy hold up a mirror to our own selves.

In writing about my "orphan cases" in Chapter 8, I was surprised by the extent to which, even in brief consultations and psychotherapy, I painted the individual on a broader canvas, depicted in family, social, historical and cultural brushstrokes. Surprised, too, by how many individuals in this book are lonely people, cut off from their moorings:

• Gregory, a Caribbean exile, a Black King Lear, facing a lonely old age, the wages of narcissism;
• Samya, both transgressed and transgressing, having betrayed

the honor of her family and her Arabic culture, struggling to (re)acquire her Arabic and her family's culture of origin;

- Hannah and her sisters, struggling with the comforting continuity of their faith as Jehovah's Witnesses against the appeals of a broader world and the price of "disfellowship";
- Musa's mother, moulting a layer of Somalian culture, turning on her own tradition, still possessing her jealously guarded secret of joy, rapidly moving into a new world, with promises of new joys;
- Isabel's mother, Cristina, spending a life in a foreign language mourning another country, finally acknowledging losses much closer to home; and
- Antonella, whose story provides a title for this book, a foundling from Milan who was adopted and raised in a border town in Northern Italy where the culture is part Italian, part Austrian, unsure of her racial heritage, always suspecting she was half Japanese, a true stranger in her own family, in her culture of origin, in Canada her adopted country, and in the end, in her own failed marriage. Antonella finds meaningful attachments only with her husky dogs.

Some of the people in these stories, however, are not cut off only because of migration and relational problems, but also because of alienating symptoms of mental illness. We can understand these symptoms as metaphors, to infuse meaning into their suffering, but for them, before these metaphoric transformations—what I call cultural and therapeutic translation—their raw experiences resisted any easy translation:

- Claudia lives in what Mara Selvini Palazzoli calls "schizoland"[3]—a world of fog where words are thick handles swirling by, which she grasps momentarily for orientation and loses in the next moment.
- Part of Nikolai is trapped in the "frozen sea" of his family, but another part is lashing out angrily, his mind full of violent urgings.

Some of my clients lived in wordless worlds:

- Pina and Rita suffered silently in families where to talk is to make a choice, an impossible situation, with betrayal on either side.

- Ismet could not articulate her predicament and her bodily distress was "a pain with no name" to her doctors until a translation could be made into another expressive channel.

Others never had the chance to own their own past:

- For Erica, her own personal and family history is "a foreign country" because her parents could not find a way to convey the stories of their past.
- River, "the White boy who thought he was Cree," was impoverished in the narrative resources of mainstream Canadian culture, finding himself with the recipes of Cree culture from Northern Canada which left him starving in Southeastern Ontario.

The metaphoric transformations that family members constructed for each other were often striking:

- For Khaled, his daughter Samya was "above my heart, above my God," but later, less charitably, also *sharmuta*, a prostitute.
- For the Mandels, Nikolai was nicknamed "Krolik" (rabbit in Russian)—an endearing "bunny" or something less than human?
- For Hannah's family and the elders of her congregation, she was raised "from the cradle" to be a Jehovah's Witness.
- Isabel's family rendered the father's drinking more tolerable by calling it "doing the laundry."
- Erica was described by her boyfriend's father as a "used bicycle," a demeaning term that distances her as a real person, making her into a "safe" object.

Therapeutic metaphors for their family experiences include:

- Thami: Is his drawing like "an African harlequin" or like poet Derek Walcott's "divided child"?
- Claudia's family lives on both sides of "the Berlin Wall."
- The Brissa family lived through "a Japanese earthquake."
- Alicia was "a Caribbean Cordelia"; her father, a Black King Lear.

And, overall, the metaphor of *storytelling*, and the metaphors used in the telling of stories:

- metaphors for intercultural encounters: "meeting strangers," "spirals";
- metaphors for acculturation: "culture shock," "mourning," "anxiety";
- metaphors for living together: "créole blending," "syncretism" (see next chapter);
- metaphors for translation: "bridge," "map,";
- metaphors for therapy: "translation," "cultural bridge," "threshold therapy";
- a metaphor for the unfolding, unfinished nature of therapy: "a garden of forking paths."

In the next chapter, "Strangers No More," I explore another metaphor for families by telling my own story. It is a family narrative with neither a therapist nor therapeutic goals. And yet, telling the story has had a deeply transformative impact on my life, creating new metaphors and new possibilities. These possibilities encourage me to adapt narrative techniques in family therapy and, at the same time, to challenge the meanings we give to the metaphor of therapy. When family stories are fragmented and memories are "outtakes" from a life, cultural family therapy consists of "suturing"—stitching the pieces together into a coherent whole.

Chapter 11

STRANGERS NO MORE

A Family Therapist Meets His Father

To care for the soul, then, we might make every effort to keep stories alive and to provide opportunities for the family to get together to renew its culture. We might pass on to our spouse, our children, and our friends the stories of our own experience with family and its early history. This narrative not only promotes intimacy with those close to us, it also keeps us in touch with that large piece of our own soul that is located in the family.

—Thomas Moore,
Soul Mates
(1994, p. 86)

This closing chapter tells one more family story—my own. It comprises several narratives: a memoir of the journey to meet my father in Brazil, how I stitched the fragments and "outtakes" of my knowledge of my father into a portrait of my parents' marriage to create a coherent narrative of my family, concluding with reflections for therapists about how we heal ourselves. My memoir is interwoven with the story of Totò from the Italian film, Cinema Paradiso, *an illustration of intertextuality. If family predicaments are "stories gone awry," then suturing—the ninth and final conceptual tool I offer, is cultural family therapy as story repair. Is this family therapy? Family of origin work? Neither. Both. Suturing is the (re)construction work we do on our family narratives. It is like sifting through a family photo album, lingering in the past and juxtaposing it with the present, imagining many possible futures.*

Em memória do meu irmão
(In memory of my brother)
Julio César DiNicola
(1959–1996)

A DOUBLE PORTRAIT

A man is born three times in his life. He is born of his
mother, he is born of his father, and finally he is born of his
own deep self.

—Guy Corneau (1991, p. 181)

"How will I recognize him?" I asked my wife on the way to the
airport in Toronto. After the anguish of deciding to meet him and
all the practical preparations—rushing to get Brazilian visas, immu-
nizations for typhoid, vaccinations for yellow fever, prophylaxis
against malaria—it dawned on me that I was about to meet my
father for the first time in my life. I had kept myself too busy to
wonder, "What does he look like, this stranger?" My wife Vicky
did not hesitate for a moment, "You'll know each other. He'll be
looking for a man and a ten-year-old boy, and you'll be looking for
the man in the portrait. Only older."

Much older—more than forty years! Among the few tangible re-
membrances of my father were some faded photographs of him as
a young man in the late 1940s and early 1950s. The portrait my wife
referred to was hanging in our living room. It is a photographic
double portrait of my father and my mother, when they were both
in their early twenties. Until now, that portrait represented all I
knew and felt about my parents as a couple: presumably seated,
they are incomplete, only busts. My mother, on the left, is smiling
naturally, looking to the right, past the camera lens; my father, on
the right, is expressionless, his unfocused gaze directed to the left,
into the distance somewhere. They are placed side by side, but
their bodies are oriented away from each other.

So many clues cluster within this frame: although they are placed
together, the portrait is actually a composite of two separate black-
and-white photographs, so retouched that they look like charcoal
sketches. The composite lacks a context: its background just a flat

grey wash, without any perspective. But there is much more to the history of this portrait, which tells the story of my parents' marriage by proxy and my mother's deep ambivalence about it. More recently, recollections of my childhood led to the restoration of this portrait and reevaluations of my own family relationships. Memory and longing, restoration and reconciliation—all have become etched into this portrait.

As we settle on the plane bound for Brazil, my son Carlo wonders aloud, "It must be strange not knowing your father." My father's absence is odd to Carlo, who has always been with me, but it was all I knew. Whenever I had thought about it, I had imagined this as my personal odyssey—Telemachus retracing the steps of his father Odysseus, lost on a voyage of discovery and danger. Just three weeks earlier, on Carlo's tenth birthday, I had made my first contact with my father. The only thread I had to follow was an old letter from one of my half-brothers in Brazil received more than a decade ago. With this information, we worked with the international operators until we found my father's telephone number. My wife dialed the number, spoke my father's name and handed me the phone. Almost in a trance, I searched her eyes, placed the phone next to my left ear, and heard my father's voice for the first time.

In that first telephone conversation, my father had asked if I wished to meet him. In a dreamlike state, I told him, yes, I would. "Bring your family," he said. "We have a large house, there is room for everyone." Gently, I demurred. It was my journey, I told him. But after I hung up, trying to imagine going alone to Brazil, I realized I had to connect the past to the present; I knew that my son could help me do that. Carlo was thrilled. With the support of Vicky and our daughter, Nina Mara, Carlo and I were soon on our way. From the airplane, we call my mother, who gave me her blessing for the journey, confiding that she wished she could join us!

During the trip, I talk to Carlo about the strange yet familiar gaps in my family. My family portrait was only half full. Unable to put a face to the image of my father, I was never able to say the simple word *father* in any of the tongues I learned. My childhood was full of my father's absence, and my mother's family artfully worked around that absence. Sensing my mother's pain, I learned how to avoid bringing attention to the missing man in the portrait. My imagination, however, was free to roam, taking me to exotic, strange, sometimes wonderful, sometimes alien places in my search for my father.

As a child, I made these vicarious journeys through the literature, films, and music of other places. The long flight to São Paulo allows time for me to recall the imaginary journeys of my childhood. Half-asleep, both excited and tired, I dream of Totò, the little boy in the Italian film, *Cinema Paradiso*, who has grown up to be a filmmaker, returning home for the funeral of *Alfredo*, the film projectionist who became a father to him (Tornatore, 1994).[1]

In my waking life, back in Canada, I am a child psychiatrist and family therapist. Unlike Totò, I am not an artist who can make films or paint or sculpt to convey my experience. Instead, I spend my working day listening and talking, struggling with a few, fragmentary pieces of the lives of children and families to help them make a coherent, meaningful story of their lives. After my journey to meet my Italian father in Brazil where he has lived for many years, my father wrote to me, eager to know how I felt:

> *Figlio, dimmi sé possibile qualcosa di te, di Vittoria e dei bambini. Principalmente vorrei sapere qualcosa al tuo rispetto—dopo la venuta qui in Brasile e di conoscere a noi, come ti senti? E stato per te un risultato positivo di conoscermi? Sei riuscito con serenità a superare tutto quello che ti affligeva il cuore? Io spero di sí, anche perchè il contrario sarebbe più male . . .*

> Tell me, son, if you can, something about yourself, Vittoria, and the children. Above all, I'd like to know something about you—after coming to Brazil and getting to know us, how do you feel? Was it a positive experience getting to know me? Did you succeed peacefully in overcoming all that was afflicting your heart? I hope so, especially because the opposite would be worse . . .

Like my composite portrait of them, I am reconstructing, from the few, fragmentary images I have gleaned, what meeting him and what my parents' brief marriage mean to me.

THE LAST STRANGE PLACE

We are born, so to speak, provisionally, it doesn't matter where. It is only gradually that we compose within ourselves our true place of origin so that we may be born there retrospectively and each day more definitely.

—Rainer Maria Rilke[2]

Thousands of people await the passengers disembarking at Guarulho, São Paulo's international airport. As I leave the controlled area of the airport, with Carlo by my side, the first thing that comes into focus in a sea of people is one man's face. In the few seconds it takes to push our baggage cart in his direction, a guess becomes a certainty. The kindly man with gray hair is hugging me tightly, welcoming me in a gentle, Italian voice. I feel the great warmth of his first word to me—"*Figlio!*" Son! I surrender to his embrace. Minutes seem to go by, each moment carrying a different tone of feeling, but I am sure it is only seconds later that he says, "*Perdonami!*" Forgive me! What a burden he must have carried for forty years.

As we relax our embrace, I become aware of my father's family. Mira, my father's wife, is a *brasileira* with a broad, beaming smile. She welcomes me in Italian softened by a Brazilian lilt. Shortly, I will coin my own name for her, *Mira-Mãe*, Mother Mira. My father's Italian name is Giuseppe, remembered by my mother as Peppino, but his wife calls him Nicola, shortening the family name. Now that I have recognized my father, I have to find a name for him. I am still wondering what I will call him when I meet my youngest brother, Julio, who calls him *pai* (father, in Portuguese). Julio, who could have stepped out of my parents' portrait, is tall and gaunt. He speaks English and immediately takes Carlo under his wing, buffering the shock of my son's first encounter with a different culture.

A tall, striking woman who resembles Mira introduces herself in Portuguese as *sua irmã*, your sister, Silvana. I search her face for familiar features but decide she is her mother's daughter, a *brasileira*. She is the oldest of my father's Brazilian children. As I get to know her, I find similarities of temperament with my father and myself. I do not think of Julio and Silvana, the children of my father and his Brazilian wife, Mira, as half-siblings. I embrace them fully as my siblings. Next we meet Silvana's daughter Vanessa.

Later, I will meet another brother, José Carlos, and his family. Missing here in Brazil is Luis Eduardo, who emigrated to Milan. Luis was the thread that led me to find my father. Over a decade earlier, I received a letter in English from him that had been the beginning of this quest. In it, Luis introduced himself as my half-brother in Brazil, expressing a wish to get to know me. Luis's letter reached me in Montreal at another crossroads in my life. I had just started my training in psychiatry and Vicky and I were about to be married. Luis's letter was an invitation to enter an unknown past. I did not respond to the letter. At the time, I was not ready, although for many years I have felt a sense of regret for not responding to Luis's hand reaching over the length of the Americas; regret for not taking my own first step in my father's direction.

As I take that first step, my encounter with my father proves surprisingly easy, flowing comfortably, liberating my thoughts and energy. I had come hoping to close a chapter of my early life. Instead, any questions that were afflicting me, as my father puts it, took on new meanings face to face. Instead of closing a chapter, Brazil opened a whole new book: a new language, a new culture, and a more complete and larger sense of family than I had known.

In my cross-cultural work, I have played with the theme of "the strange and the familiar." My father's absence in a distant continent, my mother's family's move to Canada (when I was five years old), growing up in a community of immigrants, all provided a backdrop of strangeness. As soon as the opportunities were available, I chose to travel for my education and my work. I nurtured a special interest in transcultural psychiatry, in immigrants and refugees—those people, like me, whom George Steiner (1976) calls "extraterritorial," whose personal identities move beyond the borders of their birthplace.

Perhaps this is the most important legacy of my father: that his absence led me to be a searcher (just as he went searching), engendering an ability to set aside my own starting points to enter other people's lives as a family therapist (he designed and built houses), to learn new languages (he learned Spanish and Portuguese as a young man), and to explore new cultures (he lived in Venezuela, Argentina, Brazil).

After all this searching, Brazil was, for me, the last strange place. Now that I have met my father and been welcomed by him, my emotional vocabulary is shifting from a preoccupation with alienation and estrangement to belonging and meaning. I feel less strange, more at home now. For me, home means a connection to all my family. With all these people in so many places—Canada, Italy, Brazil—my home is spread out, somewhere in the spaces between me and each part of my family.

"OUTTAKES"

The recollections of my childhood work like a primitive motion picture projector. A few static images flashed quickly in sequence create the illusion of movement. This is what memory is like: a few still photographs, juxtapositions, artificial lighting.

In the Italian film, Cinema Paradiso, *Totò, a fatherless boy growing up in postwar Sicily, is befriended by the gruff Alfredo, a childless man who is the projectionist at the parish movie theatre. The local priest screens all the movies, making Alfredo cut out all the embraces, kisses, and signs of affection between men and women before the audience can view the film. Alfredo is supposed to splice these "outtakes" back into the films. Somehow, they just remain in his booth, long strands of celluloid hanging like black vines, creeping into Totò's imagination. Totò sneaks the "outtakes" home, viewing the still frames against a lantern, recalling the dialogue and the action.*

When I was growing up, my knowledge of my father was based on "outtakes" from other people's lives: scraps of memory—what my mother, Nena, remembered or chose to tell me about him, stories told in unguarded moments during family gatherings; and recovered objects—a few photos saved by my mother, grabbed at the last moment and thrown into a suitcase on our way out of our home in Italy before setting out for Canada.

One of the objects was her portrait with my father. I can remember when I was five years old, my mother taking off her shoe and smashing the frame with her high heel, sending shards of glass flying. My recollection of this is vivid: I had a fever that heightened my awareness and burned the event into my memory. As I watched, I felt detached from my mother's intense turmoil. Oblivious to the glass fragments, she extended an elegantly gloved hand and pulled out the portrait, damaged with a heel mark across my father's chest. For my mother, it was a final, forced leave-taking. In her intense ambivalence about him, she saved the photo, unable to leave it behind.

> When Totò grows up, Alfredo vehemently tells him to put this place behind him and never come back. Totò unquestioningly obeys, leaving behind Alfredo, his mother, and memories of his first love. Years go by. Totò has become a filmmaker in Rome. Whenever his mother calls, there is a new female voice on the telephone: Totò is living the "outtakes" of his childhood. This time, his mother informs him Alfredo is dead. Totò leaves immediately for Sicily.

Until I went to Brazil, these "outtakes" were all I had to splice this man into my life. Brazil—for me this single word stands for a culture, the country where my father lives, a state of mind, a symbol of what is unreachable and what is reached; Brazil suddenly created an opening. Because I did not want to be hurt, I prepared myself to expect nothing. And as I wanted to accept whatever I found, I wanted to be ready for anything. In Brazil, this dizzying openness, a kind of "hunger of memory" in Richard Rodriguez's (1983) evocative phrase, was tempered by the impossibility of somehow reliving my childhood with my father, of telescoping forty years into four weeks. Brazilians have a word for this sentiment, *saudade*: an indefinable longing, homesickness, nostalgia.

> After the funeral, Totò receives Alfredo's final gift, a can of celluloid "outtakes" from his childhood, spliced together. In the kitchen with his mother, he admits, "I've always been afraid to come back. And now . . . I thought I was stronger, that I'd forgotten a lot of things. But in fact, I find I'm right back where I

was . . . as if I'd never been away." Back in Rome, Totò watches the soundless visual legacy that Alfredo has left him. Overwhelmed, Totò cries. Saudade. *From beyond the grave, Totò has finally allowed Alfredo to touch him. We sense that he is ready to integrate Alfredo (a man without a child), his mother (a woman without a man), and the "outtakes" of his childhood into his work as a filmmaker and into his life.*

EMOTIONAL ALCHEMY

To this meager cache of memories and objects, my father has added some significant items: a framed picture of himself in Brazil at the age of 25; the ring of his voice in my ear from our telephone conversations; a 30-year-old fountain pen with his name engraved on it; my own memories of his house, which he designed and built; the experience of the two of us alone; walking around his city, meeting his friends; and our final, intimate conversation in his car on a beautiful, sunny day, our last day together in Brazil. With these threads, I do a kind of emotional alchemy, spinning them into the gold of my life. I take what has been handed down to me haphazardly and arrange it meaningfully.

Conducting therapy, learning a language, entering another culture are activities that require childlike qualities—the ability to see things freshly, to suspend one's disbelief. Meeting my father required that I put aside some of the things I had been taught: basic instincts, habits of the heart, family myths. I had to be ready to reconstruct my personal myth. Doing so proved to be much easier than I could have imagined. Not undertaking it earlier was a failure of imagination, an inability to think that my future could take a different shape than the one into which my mother had kneaded our shared past.

At the time of my journey, I was strolling in an obscure woods of my life, driven by something I could not give words to. Looking back on the path that took me to Brazil, I perceive a fork in the woods, cleaving my life. The reason it flowed so easily, and why I linger through these woods, is that I was ready to make a choice and follow a new path. My turn was outward, not inward. In Brazil, I learned the meaning of my longing: not nostalgia for the past, but a wish to be more fully in the present. I went there not to retrieve my childhood, nor to magically to relive it with my father. I wanted to end my childhood. But to do this, I needed my father's blessing.

A NIGHT IN SÃO PAULO

My sister Silvana is a real *Paulistana*, born and bred. Being half-Italian, she fits the ethnic joke about São Paulo: half the *Paulistanos* are Italian, the other half are their children. To welcome me, she arranges a night out in São Paulo. After going to a concert, we head for the Bixiga district. With cafés, bookstores, and arty boutiques open all night, the Bixiga is just the kind of place for Silvana and me to get to know each other.

We start a nightlong conversation over coffee and dessert. It is slow at first, since we lack one really fluent language in common. We watch each other closely, shape the air with our hands for emphasis, mixing a cocktail of Spanish, Italian, and Portuguese. We laugh a lot. In spite of language, we are really communicating. We move on to a bookstore, where we point out our favorite authors. We get to know each other even better by comparing musical tastes and by our reactions to photographs and paintings at an art gallery.

With these new perceptions, we begin a more intimate conversation. Silvana says she has known about me for a long time. She tells me I have done a good thing for *pai*. She had always felt there was something missing in him. As we are talking, she gives me a picture, covering the back with a long dedication in a flowing ornate hand, "*Para o meu amado irmão . . . por quem esperei 39 anos para abraçar e conhecer. . . .*" For my beloved brother . . . for whom I waited 39 years to embrace and to know. . . .

Everywhere here, something is incomplete. In Brazil, too, there has been a family legacy of gaps. My sister tells me that *pai* has been waiting for me. She has also been waiting for something. Like my mother's, Silvana's marriage ended early, leaving her with a daughter. Like me, Silvana is filling in her family portrait. My arrival spurs her own search for meaning. In my search for my father, I had not imagined that I might be a missing character in this Brazilian family drama.

''[E]very exit [is] an entrance somewhere else,'' says a character in
Tom Stoppard's *Rosencrantz and Guildenstern Are Dead* (1967, p. 28).
When my father left my mother's life, he entered another. In the
other life he has built here in Brazil, I became an offstage character.
If not quite present at the table, I nonetheless had a place set for me.
Coming to this table, in my father's house, I find myself an actor in
their family drama. Moved, shaken, I lose my cue, fall silent.

When my father had asked for my forgiveness, I do not know
how to respond to him meaningfully in words. Now, I sense something similar in my sister—a searching soulfulness. Long into the
night, exhilarated, exhausted, words—my old friends—fail me. Another fork in the path; my chance to become an adult. Another
cafezinho—Brazilian espresso. We talk about . . . what else? The
missing pieces of our lives. What *pai's* absence meant to my mother
and me, beckoning me to faraway places. What his presence meant
to Silvana and her mother, with parts of his heart and mind in
other places.

As we talk about our marriages and our children, we wordlessly
recognize a family pattern of meaningful absence (like the missing
men in the family) and senseless presence (when husbands and
fathers do not speak of their pain, and wives and children must
find another language for their longing). I begin to understand my
father's plaintive invitation to bring my family, and Silvana's wish
to meet Vicky. Vicky and I are to them the image of a complete
family, keeping alive their own hopes. Silvana extends her hand.
When I absentmindedly admire a silver bracelet, she places it on
my wrist. I'll accept it, I say, for Vicky.

In the morning, I will call home to invite Vicky and Nina Mara to
come to meet my father and his family. It is my gift to them. Their
hopes and needs draw me deeply into this family. After a month-
long stay, I am not sure that I have entirely returned to the known
world of my family in Canada or left the new world of my family in
Brazil. I'm extraterritorial.

SYNCRETISM

To the Northerner, Brazil is a country of extraordinary contradictions living side by side. Most meaningful for me is the Brazilian

intermingling of peoples of *vária côr*, multicolor, to forge a "Luso-tropical culture" and the syncretic blend of diverse religions, layered with the symbols of Portuguese Catholicism, French spiritism, and Afro-Brazilian *Candomblé*. Syncretism is an evocative metaphor for splicing together what seem to be incongruities.

Vicky's arrival in São Paulo with Nina Mara is cause for another celebration with the whole family. At the table, there is an intermingling of Brazilian and Italian foods, languages, and families. *Pai* and *Mira-Mãe* are delighted by Vicky and Nina Mara. Later, Vicky and my father go for a walk, during which he tells her of his struggle over how to talk about the past, how to find forgiveness. Vicky encourages me to lighten his burden.

In Salvador da Bahia in *O Nordeste*, the Northeast, Vicky and I enjoy an immersion into Afro-Brazilian culture. We attend a coming-out ritual called a *saida*, a young man's confirmation of faith in *Candomblé* (see Wafer, 1991). When he is in a deep trance, covered in the blood of an animal sacrifice, the *orixá* or spirit assigned to him enters his body as he leaps into the air. In the cramped quarters of the *terreiro*, packed with celebrants and visitors, a Belgian student anxiously fends off the experience as improbable. "These celebrants," I whisper to her in French, "accept your Catholic belief that Jesus enters your body during communion." Religion here is syncretic, layered with the symbols of diverse faiths. The *orixás* of *Candomblé* have their counterparts in Christian saints. This is deeply resonant for me, offering powerful confirmation of my hope that we can learn to live with competing claims on our allegiances and our hearts.

Syncretism has a profound resonance in my meeting with my father. I had grown up with my mother's story of her marriage to my father. Now I felt a terrible conflict of loyalties. Even wanting to meet my father felt like a betrayal of my mother. And yet, I needed to hear his story. In Brazil, I had the chance to hear my father's story. They are stories told and retold, worn smooth like pebbles from constant handling.

At home, we had displayed my parents' portrait. That portrait is frozen in time. Here in Brazil, I have recognized my father and find comfort in calling him *pai*. The opportunity for healing the damaged family portrait has passed on to another generation: to Silvana, to me, perhaps to the others. A few years ago, before I went to Brazil, my mother gave me the portrait of my parents. It had lain in the suitcase my mother brought from Italy. I doubt that she had ever looked at it in Canada. In passing it on to me, she had completed her act of preservation. For me, it was just starting.

The portrait sat in a trunk in my basement for a few years. After telling my family story during my family therapy training in Rome with Maurizio Andolfi, I resolved to have it restored and framed. Upon my return to Canada, I asked my mother to join me in taking the portrait to a photographic restorer. Examining the portrait, he told us that the superficial scratches could be fixed, but the emulsion had been badly damaged in one spot. When he wondered how it had occurred, I told him the story. Intrigued, he thought that the heel mark had become ''part of the story of the picture.'' He advised us not to repair it. We agreed. After it was restored, I had it beautifully framed. My wife and I agreed to hang it in a prominent living space in our home until I could meet my father. It was a ritual of confirmation; it was a rite of separation. It confirmed my mother's way of responding to my father, simultaneously separating my own possible response. It honors my mother's experience, freeing me to have my own.

''BYE, BYE, BRAZIL''[3]

My last day in Brazil was momentous. The night before, at a party for Vanessa's sixteenth birthday, all the family and many friends arrived. Vanessa and her friends taught us to dance the *samba*, that uniquely Brazilian musical beat, a kind of tropical blues animated by the feeling of *saudade*. It was a unique opportunity to take pictures and videos of the family together.

The next day, my father and I took time to be alone together and talk. We sat in his car overlooking the city from a hill near his home. He was prepared to answer my questions, but he had a wariness about opening the past with me. He did not want to hurt the memory of people I loved. Perhaps he was right. After meeting each other, what did we need to say about other people and the failed connections of the past? They would be the same worn pebbles I had been handed down from my mother's family, all the sharp edges smoothed down from repeated handling over the years.

Memory serves different needs for my father and me. The waves of recollection have lapped on the shore of his memory, softening and shaping the landscape into a safe harbor. As a character says in Brian Friel's (1981) play, *Translations*, "*To remember everything is a form of madness*" (p. 67). From this conversation, I began to understand my father and his sense of where he came from, his struggle in his own family. His self-revelations about his pain and anger as a young man have the ring of truth. He had promised himself that he would leave his family and his town as soon as he could. It was a long time before he returned.

What made me sad that day was not what my mother had led me to expect, not some tragic flaw in my father's character or some awful secret. My father told me, "Your mother was the love of my life." Theirs is the story of two young innocents, both dreaming about a different world than the one they knew. My father went to follow his dream in South America, hastily becoming engaged to the sister of his friend, before he left. After establishing himself in Venezuela, my father resolved to have his fiancée join him. Due to his resentment toward his own family, he did not want to return to Italy, so my parents were married by proxy.

Separated by many miles and months, they entrusted their happiness and well-being to the meddling and invidiousness of family and friends. Each was told malicious stories about the other. Half-true, distorted, or fabricated, the impact of these stories was amplified by their separation. As my father tells it, he decided to confront the truth directly by returning home. My parents were united for a brief time. Still unsure, bewildered, my father left again, not yet knowing I was conceived. Neither of them, it seems, could completely decide to take charge of their lives. Instead, they let themselves be guided by the fears, fantasies and plans of other people. Although they speak warmly of each other even now, they complain about others, about circumstances.

Now, I understand that there is a broader truth for me than what my parents can say. It is more profound than the truths that are spoken about families: it is what stays when words have had their say. It is the truth about the spaces between people, like the silences that shape the sounds of music. My truth is the story I can live with, one that is both believable and meaningful to me. This is neither wholly my mother's story nor my father's. My truth allows me to love my mother for all her pain, her sacrifice, and, in the end, her rescue of that parental portrait as my legacy. It allows me to accept my father for who he is and to learn to love him, realizing that what he needs from me is forgiveness. Finally, it allows me to tell my story as a complete person—someone with a mother and a father. The "outtakes" have been spliced back into the whole life. Now I can see my mother as a woman. I know my father, a living mirror of my own face. Now I can do what everyone else seems to have had a chance to do: to let the story of my parents seep deeply into me and to emerge in my own relationships.

Still, with each of them remarried and happy, I did not wish events from so long ago to continue to cast their shadow on our lives. In that moment, I forgave him. I came to understand that to forgive is to live in the present instead of the past.

———

This journey ended in a peculiar way. We were traveling in two cars to the airport in Guarulhos. Fortunately, my father was following my sister's car closely when it broke down on the highway. We had to shift all the luggage to my father's car and to say our goodbyes hurriedly. I hugged *Mira-Mãe* with affection and kissed my soulful sister Silvana and my niece Vanessa goodbye. I looked at my brother Julio, whose gauntness and lethargy I now know were part of a fatal illness, fearing it would be our last embrace.

At the airport, shortly before boarding, while we were immersed in our farewells, our camera bag with all our films and videos was stolen! With my father busy making a report to the airport police, we were again forced to go through hurried goodbyes to register for boarding. My father, filled with longing and regret for many things, including now the loss of our cameras and films, hugged me one last time, expressing his love for me, his gratitude for coming to him, and asked me yet again to forgive him.

During the flight home, I reflected on the cameras and films. After all these years, to be leaving without a single photograph of my meeting with my father was heartbreaking. I had to console myself by making some meaning of their loss. The meaning could not come from the outside or from someone else; it had to be my own. If my trip was to have any meaning, I could not allow even this loss to wrench away what I had finally found.

In spite of the importance to me of our photographs and videos of my Brazilian family, the meaning I gave to their loss is that one cannot replace forty years with one month. No alchemy of transformation can give me the childhood with my father that I never had. And even the lush tropical rhythms of Brazil's *sambas* could not assuage the *saudade*—longing—I felt on leaving.

For me, making sense of this misfortune was an act of meaning. Physical images are vulnerable, like my parents' damaged portrait, like the emotional "outtakes" from Totò's films and the stolen record of our trip to Brazil. But once spliced into the context of our lives, given a meaningful ordering of events, they are burned into our memories in a way that no one and nothing can remove them.

―――――

Memory is not a running movie but a series of discrete images, "outtakes" from a life. A few images, carefully chosen or perhaps all that is available, tell our most important stories. Like my childhood, only a few images remain of my meeting with my father. One that endures is from my first days in Brazil. Silvana and I are in the kitchen of my father's home, conversing in a *minestrone* of languages. We are getting to know each other, describing little things that reveal so much—favorite foods, daily habits, quirks of temperament.

At breakfast, my father had been a little harsh with Silvana about her divorce. He told her she is "difficult" and that she must move on with her life. Although I only partly understood the exchange, I felt that Silvana had been hurt. Later, I try to reassure her that, when it comes to relationships, we are all "difficult," we all need to move on. We start talking about our marriages. We talked for some time before we notice that *pai* has entered the kitchen.

Pai stirs the language soup, sampling the conversation, translating a phrase here and there, adding spice. I am no longer immersed in my childhood fantasies now; I'm among familiar strangers. Our stories, only freshly told to each other, are already becoming interwoven. When he hears me talking about myself and my difficulties, my father laughs and shrugs knowingly. "*Claro,*" he says in Portuguese, laughing. "Of course—you're a DiNicola!"

"BRINGING IT ALL BACK HOME"

In the end, stories are what's left of us, we are no more than
the few tales that persist.

                                    —Salman Rushdie (1995, p. 110)

Writing these stories—a memoir about meeting my father and a
commentary on how it affected me as a family therapist—trans-
ported me back to the woods of my Brazilian experience. "Woods"
is Umberto Eco's (1994) metaphor for narratives based on a story by
Jorge Luis Borges, "The Garden of Forking Paths" (1964). With
each story I faced a different fork in the path. Each story offers a
different point of view. If the key metaphor of family life in my
memoir is "outtakes" for the fragmentary nature of our lives, then
the key metaphor for family therapy is "suturing," splicing or sewing together the fragments into a whole.

Brazil was a gift to me, enriching my narrative resources. It is a
new metaphor in my life. "Brazil" is a book I open to read all the
stories of my life. It is where I go to revisit the journey to meet my
father, where I remember my past without him, and now, revision
a different future, one that he and my Brazilian family are part of.
I can even choose among alternative selves and stories lived by
these other selves. In "Brazil," I can collect these alternative selves
and repatriate them into me as parts of my distributed self. Like a
film festival where a filmmaker's body of work is given a fresh
perspective through a new audience, sometimes showing different
versions—the "director's cut," with the "outtakes" restored—
"Brazil" is playing my life.

My first wish was to tell the story of my trip from the point of
view of the person who made the trip. That person is not a family
therapist but a man who went to Brazil to meet his father. After my
trip, I returned to work. Now I was a family therapist who had
journeyed to meet my father. I made the resolution to keep myself
continually open to the experience, allowing it to resonate in my
personal relationships and to enrich my professional life. My experience is multilayered, syncretic. And the best way to convey that
the man who went to Brazil and the family therapist have overlapping and congruent—but different—experiences is to structure the
text this way: memoir and postscript.

The stories have different potential readers. For family and friends, the memoir is a walk in the woods with someone they know. Some see themselves in the woods I describe, others are reminded of their own walks in the woods. Each reader took different turns in the Brazilian woods of my memoir. And each conversation became a mutual story-telling, a shared walk in the woods. We gave one another permission to disclose something about ourselves. As I discovered in my family therapy training and in my therapeutic work, these intimate walks always bring us back home.

SUTURING AS STORY REPAIR: THOUGHTS FOR FAMILY THERAPISTS

Professional readers will want to know about the impact of the Brazilian experience on my work. What does it mean to me as a family therapist?

1. *Things take time.* It took seven years to fulfill a promise I made during my family therapy training in Rome to meet my father. Why so long? Personal and interpersonal changes take time. It takes time, it seems, to live fully in the present: to integrate the past so well that it does not kill the present. Each language has words of longing that keep us anchored in the past: English and Italian call it *nostalgia*; in Brazil I learned to call it *saudade*. The director of *Cinema Paradiso* maintains that, "the best way to cut the bridges with our past is to go back over them" (cited in Vermilye, 1994, p. 250). We need to imagine such processes fluidly, over time: a journey, a path, an evolution, an unfinished narrative. In the light of this, what meaning can "outcome" have in the limited time of most courses of therapy? Perhaps "outcome" in therapy is like the "outtakes" of my memoir—representative selections at best, disembodied snapshots of a life at worst.

2. *We see fragments.* Some of my friends and colleagues have a sense of incompletion in the memoir, expressing curiosity about the people I have introduced, wanting to know more. But this is not a capsule autobiography, nor even a complete account of my trip to Brazil. How the memoir fits into the whole is continually emerging,

enriching me with fresh vistas. This, too, is like therapy: we view fragments of our clients' lives, we walk along with them for part of the road, and then we let them get on with their journey on their own. It can be difficult to let go.

As I wrote in Chapter 1, in *Six Characters in Search of an Author*, a family insistently shows up to demand of Luigi Pirandello (1952), the playwright who imagined them, that he finish their story so they can know the meaning of their existence. The families I have seen in therapy sometimes pay me imaginary visits to ask such questions. The difference between fiction and reality is that fiction has to make sense. The demands of "sense-making" within both fiction and therapy can be usefully provocative. To keep yourself humble, try making sense of some part of your own journey by writing it out. It will help you to be open to the unfolding story of your clients and decrease the Procrustean temptation to impose premature closure on their stories.

3. *The distributed self.* At times in the memoir, the narrator going through the experience and his childhood self are strangers to each other. Most of us are familiar with that kind of strangeness: the remembrance of things past. Truly dislocating for me was my discovery of a different, alternative self in Brazil. A version of me was constructed by my father and his family in my absence. Silvana most clearly articulated this version of me, the brother she "waited 39 years to embrace and to know." In Brazil, I met another part of my "distributed self" (Bruner, 1990), one who speaks and dreams in Portuguese, who dances *samba*, and who has always known his father and his Brazilian siblings and their mother.

Because it can encompass more than one perspective, more than one context, family therapy can lead us to fresh constructions of the very idea of the self. By attending to the "situated nature" of family life in place and across time, cultural family therapy opens space for a more social view of the sources of the self. In therapy, do not dismiss the blind alleys, unfinished journeys, and other roads not taken: parts of the family are living there. Salman Rushdie (1991) captured this exquisitely in *Midnight's Children*: "Most of what matters in our lives takes place in our absence" (pp. 14–15).

4. *Desafinado/out of tune.* How does my personal growth fit in with my professional preparedness? While I was preparing to meet my

father, was I somehow incomplete as a family therapist? Can we do our work without knowing ourselves? These are false notes—*desafinado* in Tom Jobim's song, out of tune. *Desafinado* was Jobim's response to Brazilian musical traditionalists with "perfect pitch" and "privileged ears."[4] We do not come to our work with perfect pitch or totally integrated. For at least part of our lives, we are all out of tune. What we need is not perfection or even healing to do our work. We need to nurture the personal capacity to accept our own imperfections to do our work. This grants us the patience to view the fragments of a family's life and to take time to understand their experience. Have you ever heard yourself on tape? It is an awful experience; we hear ourselves "out of tune." Have you reviewed your session notes? Are they incomplete, impressionistic, overly detailed, or missing the point? Mine too.

5. *When words fall short*. The description of the night in São Paulo with my sister reveals a moment of loss. Andolfi and his associates (1989) call this "embarrassment," a sense of "awkwardness, bewilderment and perplexity which grasps a sense of personal fragility and insecurity" (p. 73). Alone with my sister whom I had just met, after the usual social rituals had been exchanged, there came a moment when words felt inadequate. I had never heard this story or one quite like it. And a new kind of story calls for a new emotional vocabulary. My sense of loss exposed a narrative impoverishment. What do you do when words fall short? You enter your predicament more deeply; you start using words differently. Instead of describing a story I already knew, I had to start telling a new one in a strange new language.

Now I listen more attentively in therapy, attuned to moments of loss and how they get filled with clichés and stereotypes, what novelist Milan Kundera (1988) calls the "nonthought of received ideas." How do you breach such a wall of words in therapy? You find an opening and enter it, little by little; there is no other way through. Words are part of the narrative resources that we learn from our families as "storying cultures." Listen for lost words, the orphan words and phrases that slip through the net of sentences that maintain family myths. The meaning of a session, of any encounter, cannot be discovered or taught, only constructed. As Richard Rorty (1989, p. 94) has said, "Solidarity has to be constructed out of little pieces, rather than found already waiting."

6. *"Science is nothing but the finding of an analogy,"* wrote William James.[5] In the Japanese film, *Rashomon*, by Akiro Kurasawa, different stories emerge from a shared experience.[6] A lot is made of the "Rashomon" effect (see Elizur & Minuchin, 1989) or "double description" in family therapy (White, 1986). This notion of multiple perspectives is a cornerstone of postmodern thought. But how do you live a coherent life with a "multiphrenic" identity? (Gergen, 1991). It is one thing for me to see different stories in my parents' portrait, but what I need is a story about my parents that I can live with, a story that generates sense-making in my life. After I presented my memoir with video selections from *Cinema Paradiso*, a woman warmly approached me to say, "Goodnight, Totò!" When one story is embedded in another, like the story of Totò within my own, literary theorists call this *intertextuality*. When it happens between people, like the night in São Paulo when my sister and I were (re)writing our overlapping family drama, we call this *intersubjectivity*, the co-construction of social reality. What is missing in many accounts of postmodernism and in much of family therapy is an understanding of our common need for *making meaning*. In addition to *Rashomon*, I offer family therapists *Cinema Paradiso*, Giuseppe Tornatore's (1989) homage to the history of film, a film about parts and wholes (Gergen's "saturated self"), about our scattered selves (Bruner's "distributed self"), about what we leave behind ("outtakes") and what meanings we can reconstruct by splicing them back into our lives (re-editing personal and family myths) and by putting our lives in "order" (narrative).

7. *"To remember everything is a form of madness,"* warns a character in Brian Friel's play, *Translations* (1981, p. 67). The classical notion of memory was of a comprehensive repository of the past. Instead, I offer recollection as an active meaning-making process, a "projector" where you load up still images by hand. You place them in the order that the story demands. On their own, sometimes, these images make no sense. By rearranging them or rearranging our

lives around them, the sense emerges. We must be active in this process of sense-making, like the meaning I "wrenched" from the loss of my photos. If we take them as they are handed down, "like pebbles worn smooth by handling," they become myths. When you try to get detailed family histories, do you get confusing and contradictory information? Good: the family members have brought you the "damaged portraits" of their lives. All you have to do is "frame" them and display them as I did. Are you getting a lot of "pebbles" handed to you—well-rehearsed stories whose function is to preserve the family and its myths? When this happens in therapy, I hope that you will be as curious about how those sharp-edged stones became pebbles as you are about your own family story.

8. *A shared walk in the woods.* I discovered the releasing power of my memoir as a way to deepen my personal relationships. Self-disclosure is mirrored interpersonally. How can this be used in our therapeutic work? Brief, thoughtfully selected stories can have a powerful impact in therapy. Practice retelling stories from folktales, literature, cinema—whatever offers a mirror to the family. When you are comfortable, tell stories about yourself and people you know. Learn to be aware of your own feelings about them and how other people hear them. Try them out in supervision or with your colleagues. Do not tell stories if you do not want other people to imagine different endings for them.

9. *Story repair.* Many meaningful metaphors can be made from our personal experiences. My own teach me to understand family predicaments in terms of "outtakes" or fragments and family therapy as a way to suture or splice them into the whole of our lives. Using the narrative metaphor, George Howard (1991) suggests that psychopathology and family predicaments are "life stories gone awry" and that therapy is an exercise in "story repair." *Suturing* as story repair is the ninth and final tool for cultural family therapy. The danger, of course, lies in repairing the story or suturing the tapestry according to a known paradigm. An alternative to familiar paradigms is the semiotic notion of *syntagm*, which implies that meaning comes out of the contiguity and juxtaposition of elements. What does this mean? Sometimes we just have to let the fragments sit

there and see what comes from viewing them side by side, like two different stories of the same relationship.

Whatever metaphors we choose, the work of therapy demands that family life be imagined over time and in the context of place. Any given slice or "outtake" may make families seem fragmented and out of tune. Finding the right analogy or metaphor, learning new words, can help us wrench meaning from even bizarre and accidental events. And mutual story-telling is one way to make therapy a collaborative encounter that confirms and deepens our humanity, rather than an exchange of technical solutions or an exercise in knowledge and power.

10. *A closing thought.* Just as we do not listen to music to hear the finale, we cannot listen to family stories with an eye on the horizon, as if we know who or what will come into view. In family life, we must always be ready for the next chapter to change everything. There is an ageless tension between those who say, "You can't go home again" (novelist Thomas Wolfe, 1940) and those who say, "You can and should go home" (family therapist James Framo, 1976). I say: *You never leave home, and like a snail bound to its shell, you carry it with you wherever you go.*[7]

NOTES

Introduction

1. The Italian film, *The Passenger*, was directed by Michelangelo Antonioni in 1975.

Chapter 1

1. See my overview of family therapy and transcultural psychiatry (DiNicola, 1985b, pp. 94–95).

2. For a review of the cultural aspects of Maurizio Andolfi's work in this period, see DiNicola (1985a).

3. This clinically useful distinction was introduced by psychoanalyst Donald Spence (1982).

Chapter 2

1. For a review of how these issues play to family therapy's mainstream audience, see the theme issue on "multiculturalism" of *The Family Therapy Networker* (July–August 1994). The lead article is a broad overview by Laura Markowitz (1994), which includes a discussion with Monica McGoldrick about *EFT*. McGoldrick offers her frank assessment that, "A lot of the book seems a little naive today. Maybe that's what made it palatable to a large audience" (p. 23). For her personal review of multiculturalism, see McGoldrick's (1994) essay in the same issue.

   EFT (McGoldrick et al., 1996) came out in a second edition just as this book was going to press. This edition makes no mention of Maranhão's (1984) significant critique, nor any others. It has dropped the more thoughtful chapters of the "Special Issues" section in the first edition and streamlined the "Conceptual Overview" section to one chapter. The first edition's "Paradigms" section of ethnic families has been greatly expanded to become a sort of ethnic encyclopedia for family therapists, written (as far as I can tell) exclusively by family therapists. To give just one example that I am intimately familiar with, the chapter on Italian families restates just the kind of ethnic stereotypes that made cultural scholars cringe, characterizing Italian American families *generally* as "enmeshed." I dispute both the usefulness of the term and its generic application to a whole group. As I point out in Chapter 7, this is a cultural misperception of the familism imported by Italian immigrants from an earlier era. It is as instructive as studying Frank Capra's films for a definitive sociology of mid-century America.

While the second edition of *EFT* is filled with many interesting perspectives, it still exhibits limited constructions of culture and how they shape family experiences. Cultural anthropology and transcultural psychiatry are just as absent in this edition as they were in the first, bolstering Maranhão's (1984) ironic conclusion that "EFT failed to convince us that family therapy needs anthropology" (p. 275).

2. My overview (DiNicola, 1985b, 1985c) appeared in *Transcultural Psychiatric Research Review* (*TPRR*), the first and longest running journal in its field, established by the founders of transcultural psychiatry at McGill University in 1956. *TPRR* also published four detailed and thoughtful responses: two by family therapists, Mara Selvini Palazzoli from Milan (1986a) and Celia Falicov from California (1986), one by an American cultural psychiatrist, Armando Favazza (1986), and one by a Canadian anthropologist, Barry Martin (1986). My synthesis, four published responses, and another unpublished response by an Israeli Canadian family therapist, Esther Gelcer (1986), were accepted as my thesis for the Diploma in Psychiatry at McGill University in 1986.

3. From Raymond Prince's lectures in transcultural psychiatry at McGill University (1983–1985).

4. Other journals specializing in cultural aspects of mental illness have included (some are no longer being published): *Antropologia Medica* (in Italian), *Culture, Medicine and Psychiatry, Curare, Ethnopsychiatrica, Ethos, Journal of Cross-cultural Psychology, Medical Anthropology, Journal of Operational Psychiatry, Journal of Psychological Anthropology,* and *Psychopathologie Africaine* (in French). Transcultural psychiatry societies were established in Britain, the United States, France, Italy, and Cuba.

5. "Gloria" is a composite of several cases in order to highlight typical features of eating disoders and the need for a multidisciplinary approach.

Chapter 3

1. Carlos Sluzki (1982) offers an illuminating example of the problems of cross-cultural perception. His fascinating study of "the Latin Lover" examines one particular aspect of the intercultural encounter between the Anglo cultures of North America and the Latin cultures of this hemisphere.

2. The notion of "global flows" was developed by the Rand Corporation to identify large-scale movements of people, ideas, and cultures throughout the world (Brown, 1983).

3. My subtitle was inspired by a painting by Giorgio de Chirico, "The enigma of arrival" (1912) and V.S. Naipaul's (1987) evocative novel of the same name about cultures undergoing change and decay.

Chapter 4

1. See Fritz Simon and associates (1985) for mini-essays on these terms.

2. The Italian film, *Il Postino (The Postman)*, was directed by Michael Radford in 1994.

3. This section is based on my review of the transcultural research on expressed emotion (DiNicola, 1988a).

4. Mary Douglas has applied sociolinguist Basil Bernstein's ideas brilliantly in her anthropology (1978) and has written a fine short introduction (1975a) to his work.

Chapter 5

1. American novelist Alice Walker (1992) has written a moving fictional exploration of female genital mutilation, *Possessing the Secret of Joy*. Walker collaborated with Indian-British filmmaker Pratibha Parmar to make a documentary on this subject throughout West Africa, *Warrior Marks*, which is captured in the written account of their journey (Walker & Parmar, 1993). For a discussion of female genital mutilation in the context of culture and psychiatry, see Armando Favazza (1996).

2. For cultural and historical background on Indians as migrants in the Western Hemisphere, including Guyana, see Thomas Sowell (1996, pp. 332–344).

3. "River Running," the name I have chosen for this child, echoes the parent's own sentiments, as they had named him after a river in Cree country. It has the added resonances of sounding like a Native name (as does his real name) and echoing Heraclitus and James Joyce, in the

wrap-around opening and closing sentence of *Finnegans Wake*—"river-run, past Eve and Adam's . . . " (Joyce, 1939, p. 3).

Chapter 6

1. I have elaborated these three hypotheses in detail and outlined the requirements for a comprehensive model of anorexia nervosa in other works (DiNicola, 1990a, 1990b).

2. There are a number of child psychiatric disorders for which available research data suggest covariance with culture (see my overview, Di-Nicola, 1992, for more details and references):
    1. Anorexia nervosa
    2. Elective mutism
    3. Infantile autism
    4. Suicidal behavior
    5. Self-mutilation
    6. School refusal
    7. Disruptive behavior disorders—the controversy over diagnosis and prevalence of attention-deficit hyperactivity disorder vs. conduct disorder.

Culture-reactive constructs and other child and family phenomena whose patterns and qualities require further intracultural and intercultural studies include:
    1. Attachment and bonding
    2. Selective child attachment
    3. Extracultural adoption
    4. Parenting styles
    5. Child abuse
    6. Sex differentials in the treatment of children
    7. Gender roles and behavior
    8. Child temperament studies
    9. Vulnerablity-invulnerability
    10. Games and toys as culture; the use of toys and soft inanimate objects or "transitional objects"
    11. Bilingualism and education
    12. Adolescent turmoil
    13. Children as/of migrants, immigrants, and refugees
    14. Children as/of victims of war, torture, and other severe traumas
    15. Comparative epidemiology of child disorders

Chapter 7

1. Mara Selvini Palazzoli, personal communication, 1984.

2. The American film, *Terms of Endearment*, was directed by James L. Brooks in 1983.

3. Inpatient family treatment is unusual. Three groups have reported this in the U.S.—Murray Bowen's experimental inpatient family work at NIMH in the 1950s, a family treatment unit in Colorado from 1964–1969 (Pittman et al., 1971), and short-term hospitalization of whole families in Philadelphia (Combrinck-Graham et al., 1982). Norway is another country where this has been practiced. In Norway, this was necessitated by the long distances of the sparse population from regionalized hospital services (Johnsen, 1968).

4. My interpretation of Takeo Doi's work is based on his presentation at McGill University in 1986 and my reading of his work. The case illustration is based on conversations with Tazuko Shibusawa, L.C.S.W., now a doctoral student at UCLA.

5. Laurence Kirmayer, personal communication, 1985.

6. My editor points out that this is similar to Bowen's concept of differentiation, defined as "the ability to be in emotional contact with others yet still autonomous in one's emotional functioning" (Kerr & Bowen, 1988, p. 145).

Chapter 8

1. Source of the William James quote: Plaque in the entrance of William James Hall at Harvard University.

2. This heading is inspired by Margaret Atwood's novel, *Life Before Man* (1979).

3. See George Steiner's (1982) provocative essay on Germany after the Nazis, "The Hollow Miracle."

4. Alexithymia and *pensée opératoire* are dealt with in Chapter 3.

5. See Barbara Grizzuti Harrison, *Visions of Glory* (1978). In critical discussions of Jehovah's Witnesses, there is much reference to the work of social psychologist Leon Festinger and his associates, *When Prophecy Fails* (1964), criticizing the teachings of the Witnesses for inaccurate predictions.

6. Pierre Leichner, "Effects of childhood abuse." Grand Rounds Presentation, Dept. of Psychiatry, Queen's University, February 16, 1996.

Chapter 9

1. This had a profound impact on the voluntary philosophy of the Adolescent Eating Disorders Program I later established at Queen's University.

Chapter 10

1. I have provided a more literal translation of part of this beautiful sonnet in order to highlight the links in Pessoa's metaphors. A more poetic

translation of the last line is: "I am myself the loss I suffered," which somewhat blurs the fact that a part of the self is lost (Pessoa, 1971, p. 67).

2. This well-known analogy was articulated particularly well in a review of a book of short stories by William Trevor (Lesser, 1996).

3. Selvini Palazzoli's description of the predicament of schizophrenia as "schizoland" can be found in my review of her work on psychosis in the 1980s (DiNicola, 1984b).

Chapter 11

1. The Italian film, *Cinema Paradiso*, was written and directed by Giuseppe Tornatore in 1989. The filmscript is available in English (Tornatore, 1994).

2. This quote from the poet Rainer Maria Rilke was found on the Internet.

3. My subtitle was inspired by the Brazilian film, *Bye, Bye, Brazil*, directed by Carlos Diegues in 1980.

4. "Desafinado" (Off Key) appears on the compilation, *Antonio Carlos Jobim*, Verve Jazz Masters 13, PolyGram Records, 1993. John Krich (1993) places Jobim's music in cultural context in his delightful musical tour of Brazil.

5. Cited in "Mindworks" (1991) exhibit. Toronto: Ontario Science Centre.

6. *Rashomon* is a Japanese film directed Akiro Kurosawa in 1951.

7. This formulation of our relationship to home is from German philosopher Martin Heidegger via Czech novelist Milan Kundera (1988):

> Heidegger characterizes existence by an extremely well-known formulation: *in-der-Welt-sein*, being-in-the-world. Man does not relate to the world as subject to object, as eye to painting; not even as actor to stage set. Man and the world are bound together like the snail to its shell: the world is part of man, it is his dimension, and as the world changes, existence (*in-der-Welt-sein*) changes as well (p. 35).

REFERENCES

Allodi, F. (1989). The children of victims of political persecution and torture: A psychological study of a Latin American refugee community. *International Journal of Mental Health, 18*(2), 3–15.

American Psychiatric Association. (1994). *Diagnostic and statistical manual of mental disorders,* Fourth edition. Washington, DC: American Psychiatric Association.

Andersen, T. (1991). *The reflecting team: Dialogues and dialogues about the dialogues.* New York: W. W. Norton.

Andolfi, M. (1979). *Family therapy: An interactional approach* (H. R. Cassin, Trans.). New York: Plenum Press.

Andolfi, M. (1994). The child as consultant. In M. Andolfi & R. Haber (Eds.), *Please help me with this family: Using consultants as resources in family therapy* (pp. 73–89). New York: Brunner/Mazel.

Andolfi, M., & Angelo, C. (1981). The therapist as director of the family drama. *Journal of Marital and Family Therapy, 7*(3), 255–264.

Andolfi, M., Angelo, C., & de Nichilo, M. (1989). *The myth of Atlas: Families and the therapeutic story* (V. F. DiNicola, Ed. and Trans.). New York: Brunner/Mazel.

Andolfi, M., Angelo, C., Menghi, P. et al. (1983). *Behind the family mask: Therapeutic change in rigid family systems* (H. Cassin, Trans.). New York: Brunner/Mazel.

Andolfi, M., & Haber, R. (1994). *Please help me with this family: Consultation resources in family therapy.* New York: Brunner/Mazel.

Archard, D. (1993). *Children: Rights and childhood.* London: Routledge.

Arendt, H. (1968). On humanity in dark times. In *Men in dark times* (pp. 3–31). New York: Harcourt, Brace & World.

Ariès, P. (1977). The family and the city. *Daedalus, 106,* 227–235.

Atwood, M. (1979). *Life before man.* Toronto: McClelland & Stewart.

Atwood, M. (1995). *Strange things: The malevolent North in Canadian fiction.* New York: Clarendon Press/Oxford University Press.

Baldwin, J. (1955). *Notes of a native son*. Boston: Beacon Press.

Banfield, E. C. (1958). *The moral basis of a backward society*. Glencoe, IL: Free Press and University of Chicago.

Barankin, T., Konstantareas, M. M., & de Bosset, F. (1989). Adaptation of recent Soviet Jewish immigrants and their children to Toronto. *Canadian Journal of Psychiatry, 34*(6), 512–518.

Barker, P. (1996). *Psychotherapeutic metaphors: A guide to theory and practice*. New York: Brunner/Mazel.

Bateson, G. (1972). A theory of play and fantasy. In *Steps to an ecology of mind* (pp. 177–193). New York: Ballantine Books.

Bateson, G. (April 21, 1978). The double-bind theory—Misunderstood? *Psychiatric News*, 40–41.

Bateson, G., Jackson, D. D., Haley, J., & Weakland, J. (1956). Toward a theory of schizophrenia. *Behavioral Science, 1*, 251–264.

Baumeister, R. F. (1986). *Identity: Cultural change and the struggle for self*. Oxford: Oxford University Press.

Beiser, M. (1989). Migration and mental health. *Annals of the Royal College of Physicians and Surgeons of Canada, 22*(1), 21–25.

Bellow, S. (1982). *The dean's December*. New York: Harper & Row.

Benjamin, W. (1968). *Illuminations*. New York: Schocken.

Berger, B., & Berger, P. (1984). *The war over the family: Capturing the middle ground*. Garden City, NY: Anchor/Doubleday.

Berry, J. W. (1992). Acculturation and adaptation in a new society. *International Migration, 30*, 69–85.

Berry, J. W., Kim, U., Minde, T., & Mok, D. (1987). Comparative studies of acculturative stress. *International Migration Review, 21*(3), 491–511.

Bhatti, R. S., Janakiramaiah, N., & Channabasavanna, S. M. (1980). Family psychiatric ward treatment in India. *Family Process, 19*, 193–200.

Borges, J. L. (1964). The garden of forking paths. In D. A. Yates & J. E. Irby, (Eds.), *Labyrinths: Selected stories & other writings* (pp. 19–29). New York: New Directions.

Boscolo, L., Cecchin, G., Hoffman, L., & Penn, P. (1987). *Milan systemic family therapy: Conversations in theory and practice*. New York: Basic Books.

Boswell, J. (1990). *The kindness of strangers: The abandonment of children in Western Europe from Late Antiquity to the Renaissance*. New York: Vintage Books.

Boszormenyi-Nagy, I., & Spark, G. (1973). *Invisible loyalties: Reciprocity in intergenerational family therapy*. New York: Harper & Row.

Bowlby, J. (1979). On knowing what you are not supposed to know and feeling what you are not supposed to feel. *Canadian Journal of Psychiatry, 25*, 403–408.

Bradley, S., & Sloman, L. (1975). Elective mutism in immigrant families. *Journal of the American Academy of Child Psychiatry, 14*, 510–514.

Braverman, S. (1995). The integration of individual and family therapy. *Contemporary Family Therapy, 17*(3), 291–305.

Brodsky, J. (1986). The child of civilization. In *Less than one: Selected essays* (pp. 123–144). New York: Farrar Straus Giroux.

Brown, B. S. (1983). A new perspective on the political and psychological nature of borders and sovereignty. *Canadian Journal of Psychiatry, 28,* 597–601.

Brown, G. W. (1959). Experiences of discharged chronic schizophrenic mental hospital patients in various types of living group. *Millbank Memorial Fund Quarterly, 37,* 105–131.

Brown, G., & Harris, T. (1978). *Social origins of depression: A study of psychiatric disorder in women.* New York: Free Press.

Brumberg, J. J. (1985). "Fasting girls": Reflections on writing the history of anorexia nervosa. *Monographs of the Society for Research in Child Development, 50 (4–5, Serial No. 211),* 93–104.

Bruner, J. (1990). *Acts of meaning.* Cambridge, MA: Harvard University Press.

Bullrich, S. (1989). The process of immigration. In L. Combrinck-Graham (Ed.), *Children in family contexts: Perspectives on treatment* (pp. 482–501). New York: Guilford.

Calvino, I. (1977). The castle of crossed destinies (W. Weaver, Trans.). New York: Harcourt Brace Jovanovich.

Calvino, I. (1978). Invisible cities (W. Weaver, Trans.). New York: Harcourt Brace Jovanovich.

Canetti, E. (1962). *Crowds and power* (C. Stewart, Trans.). London: Victor Gollancz.

Canino, I. A. (1988). The transcultural child. In C. J. Kestenbaum & D. T. Williams (Eds.), *Handbook of clinical assessment of children and adolescents* (Vol. II, pp. 1024–1042). New York: New York University Press.

Canino, I. A., & Spurlock, J. (1994). *Culturally diverse children and adolescents: Assessment, diagnosis, and treatment.* New York: Guilford.

Cardinal, M. (1983). *The words to say it: An autobiographical novel* (P. Goodheart, Trans.). Cambridge, MA: VanVactor and Goodheart.

Carter, E. A., & McGoldrick, M. (Eds.) (1980). *The family life cycle: A framework for family therapy.* New York: Gardner Press.

Cavell, S. (1976). The avoidance of love: A reading of *King Lear.* In S. Cavell, *Must we mean what we say?* (pp. 267–353). Cambridge: Cambridge University Press.

Cayley, D. (1995). *Modes of thought.* Transcript of a four-part series in the CBC Radio "Ideas" program broadcast April 10, 11, 17, 18, 1995. Toronto: CBC RadioWorks.

Cederblad, M. (1981). Getting an identity: Transracial, inter-country adoption. In L. Eitinger & D. Schwarz (Eds.), *Strangers in the world* (pp. 317–330). Bern: Hans Huber Publishers.

Cohen, L. (1963). *The favorite game.* New York: Viking.

Combrinck-Graham, L., Gursky, E. J., & Brendler, J. (1982). Hospitalization of single-parent families of disturbed children. *Family Process, 21,* 141–152.

Corneau, G. (1991). *Absent fathers, lost sons: The search for masculine identity* (L. Shouldice, Trans.). Boston: Shambhala.

Crystal, D. (1987). *The Cambridge encyclopedia of language*. Cambridge: Cambridge University Press.

D'Andrade, R. G. (1989). Cultural cognition. In M. I. Posner (Ed.), *Foundations of cognitive science* (pp. 795–830). Cambridge, MA: MIT Press.

Dawkins, R. (1976). *The selfish gene*. Oxford: Oxford University Press.

de Chesnay, M. (1986). Jamaican family structure: The paradox of normalcy. *Family Process, 25*(2), 293–300.

de Zulueta, F. I. S. (1984). The implications of bilingualism in the study and treatment of psychiatric disorders: A review. *Psychological Medicine, 14*, 541–557.

Devereux, G. (1980). *Basic problems of ethnopsychiatry*. Chicago: University of Chicago Press.

DiNicola, V. F. (1984a). Review of *Ethnicity and Family Therapy*, M. McGoldrick, J. K. Pearce, & J. Giordano (Eds.). *Transcultural Psychiatric Research Review, 21*(2), 115–118.

DiNicola, V. F. (1984b). Road map to Schizo-land: Mara Selvini Palazzoli and the Milan model of systemic family therapy. *Journal of Strategic & Systemic Therapies, 3*(2), 50–62.

DiNicola, V. F. (1985a). The acoustic mask: A review of "Behind the Family Mask," family therapy workshop with Maurizio Andolfi, M.D., Montreal, Quebec, April 12–13, 1984. *Journal of Strategic & Systemic Therapies, 4*(1), 74–80.

DiNicola, V. F. (1985b). Family therapy and transcultural psychiatry: An emerging synthesis. Part I. The conceptual basis. *Transcultural Psychiatric Research Review, 22*(2), 81–113.

DiNicola, V. F. (1985c). Family therapy and transcultural psychiatry: An emerging synthesis. Part II. Portability and culture change. *Transcultural Psychiatric Research Review, 22*(3), 151–180.

DiNicola, V. F. (1985d). Le Tiers-monde à notre porte: Les immigrants et la thérapie familiale [The Third World in our own backyard: Immigrants and family therapy]. *Systèmes Humains, 1*(3), 39–54.

DiNicola, V. F. (1986). Beyond Babel: Family therapy as cultural translation. *International Journal of Family Psychiatry, 7*(2), 179–191.

DiNicola, V. F. (1988a). Expressed emotion and schizophrenia in North India: An essay-review. *Transcultural Psychiatric Research Review, 25*(3), 205–217.

DiNicola, V. F. (February 26, 1988b). *Lost across cultures, found in translation: Family therapy in cultural context*. Lecture at The Anthropological Perspective in Psychiatry Residency Training, McGill University, Montreal, Quebec.

DiNicola, V. F. (1989). The child's predicament in families with a mood disorder: Research findings and family interventions. *Psychiatric Clinics of North America, 12*(4), 933–949.

DiNicola, V. F. (1990a). Anorexia multiforme: Self-starvation in historical and cultural context. Part I: Self-starvation as a historical chameleon. *Transcultural Psychiatric Research Review, 27*(3), 165–196.

DiNicola, V. F. (1990b). Anorexia multiforme: Self-starvation in historical and cultural context. Part II: Anorexia nervosa as a culture-reactive syndrome. *Transcultural Psychiatric Research Review, 27*(4), 245–186.

DiNicola, V. F. (1990c). Contrasting visions from Milan: Family typology vs. systemic epistemology. *Journal of Strategic and Systemic Therapies, 9*(2), 19–30.

DiNicola, V. F. (1990d). Family therapy: A context for child psychiatry. In J. G. Simeon & H. B. Ferguson (Eds.), *Treatment strategies in child and adolescent psychiatry* (pp. 199–219). New York: Plenum Press.

DiNicola, V. F. (1990e). A stranger in the family: Culture, families and therapy (Presentation at the Annual Meeting, Surrey, England, October 6, 1989). *Society for the Study of Psychiatry and Culture (SSPC) Newsletter, 8*(1), 5–6.

DiNicola, V. F. (1992). De l'enfant sauvage à l'enfant fou: A prospectus for transcultural child psychiatry. In N. Grizenko, L. Sayegh, & P. Migneault (Eds.), *Transcultural al issues in child psychiatry* (pp. 7–53). Montreal: Éditions Douglas.

DiNicola, V. F. (1993). The postmodern language of therapy: At the nexus of culture and family. *Journal of Systemic Therapies, 12*(1), 27–41.

DiNicola, V. F. (1994). The strange and the familiar: Cross-cultural encounters among families, therapists, and consultants. In M. Andolfi & R. Haber (Eds.), *Please help me with this family: Using consultants as resources in family therapy* (pp. 33–52). New York: Brunner/Mazel.

DiNicola, V. F. (1995a). Estranei non più: Un terapeuta familiare incontra suo padre. *Terapia Familiare, 49,* 75–89.

DiNicola, V. F. (1995b). On the rights and philosophy of children. *Transcultural Psychiatric Research Review, 32*(2), 157–165.

DiNicola, V. F. (1995c). Strangers no more: A family therapist meets his father. *The Calgary Participator, 5*(2), 53–63.

DiNicola, V. F. (1996). Ethnocultural aspects of PTSD and related disorders among children and adolescents. In A. J. Marsella, M. J. Friedman, E. T. Gerrity, & R. M. Scurfield (Eds.), *Ethnocultural aspects of posttraumatic stress disorder: Issues, research, and clinical applications* (pp. 389–414). Washington, DC: American Psychological Association.

DiNicola, V .F. (in press). Changelings: Children and families in cultural transition. In S. O. Opkapu (Ed.), *Clinical methods in transcultural psychiatry.* Washington, DC: American Psychiatric Press.

Doi, T. (1973). *The anatomy of dependence.* New York: Kodansha International.

Donne, J. (1962). *Donne.* New York: Dell.

Douglas, M. (1975a). Humans speak. In *Implicit meanings: Essays in anthropology* (pp. 173–180). London: Routledge & Kegan Paul.

Douglas, M. (1975b). Self-evidence. In *Implicit meanings: Essays in anthropology* (pp. 276–318). London: Routledge & Kegan Paul.

Douglas, M. (1978a). To inner experience. In M. Douglas, *Natural symbols: Explorations in cosmology* (pp. 40–58). New York: Penguin Education.

Douglas, M. (1978b). *Natural symbols: Explorations in cosmology.* New York: Penguin Education.

D'Souza, D. (1992). *Illiberal education: The politics of race and sex on campus.* New York: Vintage Books/Random House.

Earls, F., & Eisenberg, L. (1991). International perspectives in child psychiatry. In M. Lewis (Ed.), *Child and adolescent psykchiatry: A comprehensive textbook* (pp. 1189–1196). Baltimore: Williams & Wilkins.

Eco, U. (1994). *Six walks in the fictional woods.* Cambridge, MA: Harvard University Press.

Edwards, J. (1994). *Multilingualism.* London: Routledge.

Eitinger, L. (1980). Jewish concentration camp survivors in the post-war world. *Danish Medical Bulletin, 27*(5), 232–235.

El-Islam, M. F. (1983). Cultural change and intergenerational relationships in Arabian families. *International Journal of Family Therapy, 4*, 321–329.

El-Islam, M. F., Abu-Dagga, S. I., Malasi, T. H., & Moussa, M. A. (1986). Intergenerational conflict and psychiatratric symptoms. *British Journal of Psychiatry, 149*, 300–306.

Elizur, J., & Minuchin, S. (1989). *Institutionalizing madness: Families, therapy, and society.* New York: Basic Books.

Ellison, R. (1952). *Invisible man.* New York: Vintage Books/Random House.

Engel, M. (1976). *Bear.* Toronto: McClelland & Stewart.

Engels, F. (1972). *The origins of the family, private property and the state.* New York: International Publishers.

Epstein, N. B., Rakoff, V., & Sigal, J. J. (1964). *Family categories schema.* Unpublished manuscript.

Erickson, G. D. (1988). Against the grain: Decentering family therapy. *Journal of Marital and Family Therapy, 14*, 225–236.

Erikson, E. H. (1960). Identity and uprootedness in our time. In *World Federation for Mental Health, Uprooting and resettlement.* Geneva: World Federation for Mental Health.

Falicov, C. J. (Ed.) (1983). *Cultural perspectives in family therapy.* Rockville, MD: Aspen Systems.

Falicov, C. J. (1986). Comments on DiNicola's "Family therapy and transcultural psychiatry: Parts 1 and 2." *Transcultural Psychiatric Research Review, 23*(2), 165–169.

Falicov, C. J. (1988). Learning to think culturally. In H. A. Liddle, D. C. Breunlin, & R. C. Schwartz (Eds.), *Handbook of family therapy training and supervision* (pp. 335–357). New York: Guilford.

Falicov, C. J. (1995). Training to think culturally: A multidimensional comparative framework. *Family Process, 34*, 373–388.

Favazza, A. R. (1986). Commentary on DiNicola's "Family therapy and transcultural psychiatry." *Transcultural Psychiatric Research Review, 23*(1), 86–87.

Favazza, A. R. (1996). *Bodies under seige: Self-mutilation and body modification in culture and psychiatry, Second ed.* Baltimore: Johns Hopkins University Press.

Feldman, L. B. (1992). *Integrating individual and family therapy.* New York: Brunner/Mazel.

Fernando, S. (1988). *Race and culture in psychiatry.* London: Croom Helm.

Ferreira, A. J. (1963). Family myth and homeostasis. *Archives of General Psychiatry, 9,* 457–473.

Ferreira, A. J. (1964). Family myths: The covert rules of the relationship. *Confinia Psychiatrica, 8,* 15–20.

Ferreira, A. J. (1967). Psychosis and family myth. *American Journal of Psychotherapy, 21,* 186–197.

Festinger, L., Riecken, H. W., & Schachter, S. (1964). *When prophecy fails: A social and psychological study of a modern group that predicted the destruction of the world.* New York: Harper Torchbooks.

Foucault, M. (1980). *Power/knowledge: Selected interviews and other writings 1972–1977* (C. Gordon, Ed.). New York: Pantheon.

Framo, J. L. (1976). Family of origin as a therapeutic resource for adults in marital and family therapy: You can and should go home again. *Family Process, 15*(2), 193–210.

Fresco, N. (1984). Remembering the unknown. *International Review of Psycho-Analysis, 11,* 417–427.

Freud, A. (1946). *The ego and the mechanisms of defense.* New York: International Universities Press.

Freud, A. (1958). Adolescence. *Psychoanalytic Study of the Child, 13,* 255–278.

Freud, S. (1924). The dissolution of the Oedipus complex. In J. Strachey (Ed. and Trans.), *The complete psychological works of Sigmund Freud* (Vol. XXI, pp. 173–179). New York: W. W. Norton.

Freud, S. (1927). *The future of an illusion.* In J. Strachey (Ed. and Trans.), *The complete psychological works of Sigmund Freud* (Vol. XXI, pp. 5–56). New York: W. W. Norton.

Friedlander, S. (1980). *When memory comes.* New York: Avon Books.

Friedman, E. H. (1982). The myth of the shiksa. In M. McGoldrick, J. K. Pearce, & J. Giordano (Eds.), *Ethnicity and family therapy* (pp. 499–526). New York: Guilford.

Friel, B. (1981). *Translations.* London: Faber and Faber.

Fromm-Reichmann, F. (1959a). Loneliness. *Psychiatry, 22,* 1–15.

Fromm-Reichmann, F. (1959b). *Psychoanalysis and psychotherapy: Selected papers of Frieda Fromm-Reichmann.* Chicago: University of Chicago Press.

Fuentes, C. (1989). Words apart. In L. Appignanesi & S. Maitland (Eds.), *The Rushdie file* (pp. 245–249). London: Fourth Estate.

Fussell, P. (Ed.) (1991). *The Norton book of modern war.* New York: W. W. Norton.

Garfinkel, B. D., Carlson, G. A., & Weller, E. B. (Eds.) (1990). *Psychiatric disorders in children and adolescents*. Philadelphia: W. B. Saunders.

Geertz, C. (1973a). The impact of the concept of culture on the concept of man. In C. Geertz, *The interpretation of cultures: Selected essays by Clifford Geertz* (pp. 33–54). New York: Basic Books.

Geertz, C. (1973b). *The interpretation of cultures: Essays in interpretive anthropology*. New York: Basic Books.

Geertz, C. (1983a). Blurred genres: The refiguration of social thought. In C. Geertz, *Local knowledge: Further essays in interpretive anthropology* (pp. 19–35). New York: Basic Books.

Geertz, C. (1983b). ''From the native's point of view'': On the nature of anthropological understanding. In C. Geertz, *Local knowledge: Further essays in interpretive anthropology* (pp. 55–70). New York: Basic Books.

Geertz, C. (1983c). *Local knowledge: Further essays in interpretive anthropology*. New York: Basic Books.

Geertz, C. (1988). *Works and lives: The anthropologist as author*. Stanford, CA: Stanford University Press.

Geertz, C. (1995). Culture war. *The New York Review of Books, 42*(19), 4–6.

Gelcer, E. (1986). Family therapy and transcultural psychiatry: Will the synthesis reveal invariances? Reactions to DiNicola's papers. In V. F. DiNicola, *Family therapy and transcultural psychiatry: An emerging synthesis* (pp. 159–172). Diploma in Psychiatry thesis. Montreal: McGill University.

Gergen, K. J. (1991). *The saturated self: Dilemmas of identity in contemporary life*. New York: Basic Books.

Gilligan, C. (1982). *In a different voice: Psychological theory and women's development*. Cambridge, MA: Harvard University Press.

Ginzburg, N. (1989/1963). *Family sayings* (Revised from the origianl translation by D. M. Low). New York: Arcade/Little, Brown.

Giordano, J., & McGoldrick, M. (1996). Italian families. In M. McGoldrick, J. Giordano, & J. K. Pearce (Eds.), *Ethnicity and family therapy, Second ed.* (pp. 567–582). New York: Guilford.

Glazer, N., & Moynihan, D. (1963). *Beyond the melting pot*. Cambridge, MA: MIT Press.

Goldner, V. (1982). Continuing education and training: Trialogue—Philadelphia Child Guidance Clinic. *American Journal of Family Therapy, 10*(2), 65–68.

Goll, K. (1980). Role structure and subculture in families of elective mutists. In J. G. Howells (Ed.), *Advances in family psychiatry* (Vol. II, pp. 141–161). New York: International Universities Press.

Gonzalez-Wippler, M. (1992). *The Santeria experience: A journey into the miraculous, Rev. ed.* St. Paul, Minnesota: Llewellyn Publications.

Gordon, D. (1978). *Therapeutic metaphaphors: Helping others through the looking glass*. Cupertino, CA: META Publications.

Gotowiec, A., & Beiser, M. (1993–94). Aboriginal children's mental health: Unique challenges. *Canada's Mental Health, 41*(4), 7–11.

Green, H. J. (1983). Risks and attitudes associated with extra-cultural placement of American Indian children: A critical review. *Journal of the American Academy of Child Psychiatry, 22*(1), 63–67.

Greenbaum, L., & Holmes, I. H. (1983). The use of folktales in social work practice. *Social Casework, 64*(7), 414–418.

Grinberg, L., & Grinberg, R. (1989). *Psychoanalytic perspectives on migration and exile.* New Haven: Yale University Press.

Grizenko, N., Sayegh, L., & Migneault, P. (Eds.) (1992). *Transcultural issues in child psychiatry.* Montreal: Éditions Douglas.

Grizzuti Harrison, B. (1978). *Visions of glory: A history and a memory of Jehovah's Witnesses.* New York: Simon & Schuster.

Grubrich-Simitis, I. (1984). From concretism to metaphor: Thoughts on technical aspects of the psychoanalytic work with children of Holocaust survivors. *The Psychoanalytic Study of the Child, 39,* 301–319.

Haley, J. (1963). *Strategies of psychotherapy.* New York: Grune & Stratton.

Haley, J. (1976a). Development of a theory: A history of a research project. In C. Sluzki & D. Ransom (Eds.), *The double bind.* New York: Grune & Stratton.

Haley, J. (1976b). *Problem-solving therapy.* New York: Harper & Row.

Harré, R. (1979). *Social being: A theory for social psychology.* Oxford: Basil Blackwell.

Harré, R. (1984). *Personal being: A theory for individual psychology.* Cambridge, MA: Harvard University Press.

Hartley, L. P. (1953). *The go-between.* London: Hamish Hamilton.

Harvey, D. (1989). *The condition of postmodernity.* Oxford: Basil Blackwell.

Hatfield, A. B. (1987). Taking issue: The expressed emotion theory. Why families object. *Hospital and Community Psychiatry, 38,* 341.

Helman, C. G. (1994). *Culture, health and illness, Third ed.* Oxford: Butterworth-Heineman.

Herz, F. M., & Rosen, E. J. (1982). Jewish families. In M. McGoldrick, J. K. Pearce, & J. Giordano (Eds.), *Ethnicity and family therapy* (pp. 364–392). New York: Guilford.

Hines, P. M., & Boyd-Franklin, N. (1982). Black Families. In M. McGoldrick, J. K. Pearce, & J. Giordano (Eds.), *Ethnicity and family therapy* (pp. 84–107). New York: Guilford.

Hoffman, E. (1990). *Lost in translation: A life in a new language.* New York: Penguin Books.

Hoffman, L. (1990). Constructing realities: An art of lenses. *Family Process, 29,* 1–12.

Hourani, A. (1991). *A history of the Arab peoples.* Cambridge, MA: Belknap Press/Harvard University Press.

Howard, G. S. (1991). Culture tales: A narrative approach to thinking, cross-cultural psychology, and psychotherapy. *American Psychologist, 46,* 187–197.

Hsu, F. L. K. (1971). Psychosocial homeostasis and Jen: Conceptual tools for advancing psychological anthropology. *American Anthropology,* *73,* 23–44.

Ignatieff, M. (1986). *The needs of strangers: An essay on privacy, solidarity, and the politics of being human.* New York: Elisabeth Sifton Books/Penguin Books.

Illich, I. (1973). *Tools for conviviality.* New York: Harper & Row.

James, W. (1890). *Principles of psychology.* New York: Holt.

Johnsen, G. (1968). Family treatment in psychiatric hospitals. *Psychotherapy & Psychosomatics, 16*(6), 41–46.

Jonas, H. (1987). The concept of God after Auschwitz: A Jewish voice. *The Journal of Religion, 67*(1), 1–13.

Josselson, R. (1995). Narrative and psychological understanding. *Psychiatry, 58,* 330–343.

Joyce, J. (1939). *Finnegans wake.* New York: Viking Press.

Kanner, L. (1948). Early infantile autism. *American Journal of Orthopsychiatry, 19,* 416–426.

Kaplan, M. (1990). What is traditional Judaism? In J. Pelikan (Ed.), *The world treasury of modern religious thought* (pp. 343–351). Boston: Little, Brown.

Kareem, J., & Littlewood, R. (Eds.) (1992). *Intercultural therapy: Themes, interpretations and practice.* Oxford: Blackwell Scientific Publications.

Kaslow, F. W. (1982). The history of family therapy in the United States: A kaleidoscopic overview. In F. W. Kaslow (Ed.), *The international book of family therapy* (pp. 5–37). New York: Brunner/Mazel.

Kaslow, N., Celano, M., & Dreelin, E. D. (1995). A cultural perspective on family theory and therapy. *Psychiatric Clinics of North America, 18*(3), 621–633.

Keesing, R. M. (1981). *Cultural anthropology: A contemporary perspective.* New York: Holt, Rinehart & Winston.

Kerr, M. E., & Bowen, M. (1988). *Family evaluation: The role of the family as an emotional unit that governs individual behavior and development.* New York: W. W. Norton.

Kirmayer, L. J. (1984). Culture, affect and somatization. Part I. *Transcultural Psychiatric Research Review, 21*(3), 159–188.

Kirmayer, L. J. (1989a). Cultural variations in the response to psychiatric disorders and emotional distress. *Social Science and Medicine, 29*(3D), 327–339.

Kirmayer, L. J. (1989b). Psychotherapy and the cultural concept of the person. *Sante Culture Health, 6*(3), 241–270.

Kirmayer, L. J. (1995). Versions of intercultural therapy. *Transcultural Psychiatric Research Review, 32*(2), 166–177.

Kleinman, A. M. (1977). Depression, somatization and the new cross-cultural psychiatry. *Social Science and Medicine, 11,* 3–10.

Kleinman, A. (1980). *Patients and healers in the context of culture.* Berkeley: University of California Press.

Kleinman, A. (1988). *Rethinking psychiatry: From cultural category to personal experience.* New York: Free Press.

Kolvin, I., & Fundudis, T. (1981). Elective mute children: Psychological development and background factors. *Journal of Child Psychology and Psychiatry, 22,* 219–232.

Konker, C. (1992). Rethinking child sexual abuse: An anthropological perspective. *American Journal of Orthopsychiatry, 62*(1), 147–153.

Korzybski, A. (1933). *Science and sanity.* Chicago: International Non-Aristotelian Library.

Kotre, J. (1995). *White gloves: How we create ourselves through memory.* New York: Free Press.

Kracke, W. (1987). Encounter with other cultures: Psychological and epistemological aspects. *Ethos, 15*(1), 58–81.

Krich, J. (1993). *Why is this country dancing? A one-man samba to the beat of Brazil.* New York: Basic Books.

Krystal, H. (1982). Alexithymia and the effectiveness of psychoanalytic treatment. *International Journal of Psychoanalytic Psychotherapy, 9,* 353–378.

Kuipers, L. (1979). Expressed emotion: A review. *British Journal of Social and Clinical Psychology, 18,* 237–243.

Kundera, M. (1988). *The art of the novel* (L. Asher, Trans.). New York: Harper & Row.

Kundera, M. (1991). *Immortality* (P. Kussi, Trans.). New York: Grove Weidenfeld.

Kushner, T. (1994). With a little help from my friends. In J. Heffron (Ed.), *The best writing on writing* (pp. 20–25). Cincinnati, Ohio: Story Press.

Lappin, J. (1983). On becoming a culturally conscious family therapist. In C. J. Falicov (Ed.), *Cultural perspectives in family therapy* (pp. 122–136). Rockville, MD: Aspen.

Larson, R., & Csikszentmihalyi, M. (1983). The experience sampling method. In H. T. Rees (Ed.), *Naturalistic approaches to studying social interaction. New directions for methodology of social and behavioral science* (15, pp. 41–56). San Francisco: Jossey-Bass.

Laurence, M. (1963). *The prophet's camel bell.* Toronto: McClelland & Stewart.

Leff, J. (1977). The cross-cultural study of emotions. *Culture, Medicine and Psychiatry, 1,* 317–350.

Leff, J. (1981). *Psychiatry around the globe: A transcultural view.* New York: Marcel Dekker.

Leff, J. (1986). The epidemiology of mental illness across cultures. In J. L. Cox (Ed.), *Transcultural psychiatry* (pp. 23–36). London: Croom Helm.

Leff, J., Wig, N. N., Ghosh, A., Bedi, H., Menon, D. K., Kuipers, L., Korten, A., Ernberg, G., Day, R., Sartoris, N., & Jablensky, A. (1987). Expressed emotion and schizophrenia in North India. III: Influence of relatives' expressed emotion on the course of schizophrenia in Chandigarh. *British Journal of Psychiatry, 151,* 166–173.

Leichner, P. (February 16, 1996). *Effects of childhood abuse.* Grand Rounds presentation, Dept. of Psychiatry, Queen's University, Kingston, Ontario.

Lesser, W. (October 20, 1996). The casualties of deception. Review of *After Rain* by William Trevor. *New York Times Book Review,* p. 15.

Lewis-Fernandez, R., & Kleinman, A. (1995). Cultural psychiatry: Theoretical, clinical, and research issues. *Psychiatric Clinics of North America,* 18(3), 433–448.

Littlewood, R. (1990). From categories to contexts: A decade of the "New cross-cultural psychiatry." *British Journal of Psychiatry, 156,* 308–327.

Littlewood, R., & Lipsedge, M. (1986). The "culture-bound syndromes" of the dominant culture: Culture, psychopathology and biomedicine. In J. Cox (Ed.), *Transcultural psychiatry* (pp. 253–273). London: Croom Helm.

Littlewood, R., & Lipsedge, M. (1987). The butterfly and the serpent: Culture, psychopathology and biomedicine. *Culture, Medicine and Psychiatry, 11,* 289–335.

Littlewood, R., & Lipsedge, M. (1989). *Aliens and alienists, Second ed.* London: Unwin Hyman.

Lock, M., & Gordon, D. (Eds.) (1988). *Biomedicine examined.* Dordrecht: Kluwer.

MacEwen, G. (1987). *Afterworlds.* Toronto: McClelland and Stewart.

Madanes, C. (1980). The prevention of rehospitalization of adolescents and young adults. *Family Process, 19,* 179–191.

Mahler, M. S. (1963). Thoughts about development and individuation. *Psychoanalytic Study of the Child, 18,* 307–324.

Malcolm, J. (May 15, 1978). A reporter at large: The one-way mirror. *The New Yorker,* 39–114.

Maranhão, T. (1984). Family therapy and anthropology. *Culture, Medicine and Psychiatry, 8,* 255–279.

Markowitz, L. (July/August, 1994). The cross-currents of multiculturalism. *The Family Therapy Networker,* 18–27, 69.

Marsella, A. J., Friedman, M. J., Gerrity, E. T., & Scurfield, R. M. (Eds.) (1996). *Ethnocultural aspects of posttraumatic stress disorder: Issues, research, and clinical applications.* Washington, DC: American Psychological Association Press.

Martin, B. J. (1986). Some steps to further systemic holism in family theory and therapy: A rejoinder to V. F. DiNicola. *Transcultural Psychiatric Research Review, 28*(4), 328–338.

Marzorati, G. (January 29, 1989). Salman Rushdie: Fiction's embattled infidel. *The New York Times Magazine,* 24–27, 44, 47–49, 100.

Masterson, J. F. (1968). The psychiatric significance of adolescent turmoil. *American Journal of Psychiatry, 124,* 1549–1554.

Matthews, G. B. (1994). *The philosophy of childhood.* Cambridge, MA: Harvard University Press.

McDermott, J. F., Jr. (1991). The effects of ethnicity on child and adolescent development. In M. Lewis (Ed.), *Child and adolescent psychiatry: A comprehensive textbook* (pp. 408–412). Baltimore: Williams & Wilkins.

McDermott, J. F., Robillard, A. B., Char. W. F. et al. (1983). Reexamining the concept of adolescence: Differences between adolescent boys and girls in the context of their families. *American Journal of Psychiatry, 140,* 1318–1322.

McGoldrick, M. (July/August, 1994). The ache for home. *The Family Therapy Networker,* 38–45.

McGoldrick, M., Pearce, J. K., & Giordano, J. (Eds.) (1982). *Ethnicity and family therapy.* New York: Guilford.

McGoldrick, M., Giordano, J., & Pearce, J. K. (Eds.) (1996). *Ethnicity and family therapy, Second ed.* New York: Guilford.

McLean, A. (1986). Family therapy workshops in the United States: Potential abuses in the production of therapy in an advanced capitalist society. *Social Science and Medicine, 23,* 179–189.

Mead, M. (1947). The concept of culture and the psychosomatic approach. *Psychiatry, 10,* 57–76.

Mechanic, D. (Ed.) (1982). *Symptoms, illness behavior and help seeking.* New Brunswick, NJ: Rutgers University Press.

Merton, R. K. (1973). The perspectives of insiders and outsiders. In N. W. Storer (Ed.), *The sociology of science: Theoretical and empirical investigations* (pp. 99–136). Chicago: University of Chicago Press.

Meyers, S. V. (1984). Elective mutism in children: A family systems approach. *American Journal of Family Therapy, 12*(4), 39–45.

Minuchin, S. (1974). *Families and family therapy.* London: Tavistock Publications.

Minuchin, S., & Fishman, H. C. (1981). *Family therapy techniques.* Cambridge, MA: Harvard University Press.

Minuchin, S., Baker, L., Rosman, B. L. et al. (1975). A conceptual model of psychosomatic illness in children: Family organization and family therapy. *Archives of General Psychiatry, 32,* 1031–1038.

Minuchin, S., Montalvo, B., Guerney, B. G., Rosman, B. L., & Schumer, F. (1967). *Families of the slums: An exploration of their structure and treatment.* New York: Basic Books.

Moore, T. (1994). *Soul mates: Honoring the mysteries of love and relationship.* New York: HarperCollins.

Morin, E. (1982). *Science avec conscience.* Paris: Fayard.

Murphy, H. B. M. (1973). The low rate of mental hospitalization shown by immigrants to Canada. In C. Zwingmann & M. Pfister-Ammende (Eds.), *Uprooting and after . . .* (pp. 221–231, 340–341). New York: Springer-Verlag.

Murphy, H. B. M. (1977). Editorial: Transcultural psychiatry should begin at home. *Psychological Medicine, 7,* 369–371.

Murphy, H. B. M. (1982). *Comparative psychiatry: The international and intercultural distribution of mental illness.* New York: Springer-Verlag.

Murphy, H. B. M. (1986). The historical development of transcultural psychiatry. In J. L. Cox (Ed.), *Transcultural psychiatry* (pp. 7–22). London: Croom Helm.

Naipaul, V. S. (1987). *The enigma of arrival: A novel.* New York: Alfred A. Knopf.

Nann, R. C. (1982). *Uprooting and surviving: Adaptation and resettlement of migrant families and children.* Dordrecht: D. Reidel.

Neki, J. S. (1973). Guru-chela relationship: The possibility of a therapeutic paradigm. *American Journal of Orthopsychiatry, 43,* 755–766.

Neki, J. S. (1974). A reappraisal of the Guru-chela relationship as a therapeutic paradigm. *International Mental Health Research Newsletter, 6*(22), 2–7.

Neki, J. S. (1976a). An examination of the cultural relativism of dependence as a dynamic of social and therapeutic relationships: I. Socio-developmental. *British Journal of Medical Psychology, 49,* 1–12.

Neki, J. S. (1976b). An examination of the cultural relativism of dependence as a dynamic of social and therapeutic relationships: II. Therapeutic. *British Journal of Medical Psychology, 49,* 11–22.

Nichols, M. P. (1987). *The self in the system: Expanding the limits of family therapy.* New York: Brunner/Mazel.

Nichter, M. (1982). Idioms of distress: Alternatives in the expression of psychosocial distress. A case study from South India. *Culture, Medicine and Psychiatry, 5,* 379–408.

Nida, E. (1959). Principles of translation as exemplified by Bible translating. In R. A. Brower (Ed.), *On translation* (pp. 12–31). Cambridge, MA: Harvard University Press.

Novak, M. (1971). *The rise of the unmeltable ethnics: Politics and culture in the Seventies.* New York: Macmillan.

Offer, D. (1969). *The psychological world of the teenager.* New York: Basic Books.

Ojemann, G. A., & Whitaker, H. A. (1978). The bilingual brain. *Archives of Neurology, 35,* 409–412.

Okpaku, S. (Ed.) (in press). *Clinical methods in transcultural psychiatry.* Washington, DC: American Psychiatric Press.

Orbach, S. (1986). *Hunger strike: The anorectic's struggle as a metaphor for our age.* New York: W. W. Norton.

Ozick, C. (1989). *Metaphor & memory: Essays.* New York: Alfred A. Knopf.

Pande, S. K. (1968). The mystique of "Western" psychotherapy: An Eastern interpretation. *Journal of Nervous & Mental Disease, 146,* 425–432.

Paré, D. A. (1995). Of families and other cultures: The shifting paradigm of family therapy. *Family Process, 34*(1), 1–19.

Parry, A., & Doan, R. E. (1994). *Story re-visions: Narrative therapy in the postmodern world.* New York: Guilford.

Pawel, E. (1984). *The nightmare of reason: A life of Franz Kafka.* New York: Farrar, Straus & Giroux.

Perelberg, R. J. (1992). Familiar and unfamiliar types of family structure: Towards a conceptual framework. In J. Kareem & R. Littlewood (Eds.), *Intercultural therapy: Themes, interpretations and practice* (pp. 112–13). Oxford: Blackwell Scientific Publications.

Pessoa, F. (1942). *Obras completas de Fernando Pessoa. Vol. I: Poesias* (J. G. Simões & L. de Montalvor, Eds.). Lisbon: Edicões Atica.

Pessoa, F. (1971). *Selected poems. Edinburgh bilingual library (4)* (Peter Rickard, Ed. and Trans.). Edinburgh: Edinburgh University Press.

Pfister-Ammende, M. (1973). The problem of uprooting. In C. Zwingmann & M. Pfister-Ammende (Eds.), *Uprooting and after . . .* (pp. 7–18, 323–330). New York: Springer-Verlag.

Pinker, S. (1994). *The language instinct.* New York: Morrow.

Pirandello, L. (1952). *Naked masks: Five plays* (E. Bentley, Ed.). New York: E. P. Dutton.

Pirandello, L. (1952). Six characters in search of an author. In *Naked masks: Five plays by Luigi Pirandello* (E. Bentley, Ed., & E. Storer, Trans.) (pp. 211–276). New York: E. P. Dutton.

Pittman, F. (March–April, 1984). Terms of enmeshment. *Family Therapy Networker*, 59–61.

Pittman, F. S., Langsley, D. G., Flomenhaft, K. et al. (1971). Therapy techniques of the family treatment unit. In J. Haley (Ed.), *Changing families: A family therapy reader* (pp. 259–276). New York: Grune & Stratton.

Popper, K. R. (1945). *The open society and its enemies.* London: Routledge & Kegan Paul.

Postman, N. (1993). *Technopoly: The surrender of culture to technology.* New York: Vintage Books/Random House.

Prince, R. (1969). Psychotherapy and the chronically poor. In J. Finney (Ed.), *Culture, change, mental health and poverty* (pp. 20–41). Lexington, KY: University of Kentucky Press.

Prince, R. (1972). Mental health workers should be trained at home: Some implications of transcultural psychiatric research. *African Journal of Psychiatry, 2,* 277–282.

Prince, R. (1985). The concept of culture-bound syndromes: Anorexia nervosa and brain-fag. *Social Science and Medicine, 21*(2), 197–203.

Rakoff, V. (1981). Children of immigrants. In L. Eitinger & D. Schwarz (Eds.), *Strangers in the world* (pp. 133–146). Bern: Hans Huber.

Rakoff, V. (1984). The necessity for multiple models in family therapy. *Journal of Family Therapy, 6,* 199–210.

Raphael-Leff, J. (1983). Facilitators and regulators: Two approaches to mothering. *British Journal of Medical Psychology, 56,* 379–390.

Raval, H. (1996). A systemic perspective on working with interpreters. *Clinical Child Psychology and Psychiatry, 1*(1), 29–43.

Reiss, D. (1971). Varieties of consensual experience: 1. A theory of relating family interaction to individual thinking. *Family Process, 10,* 1–35.

Remnick, D. (February 6, 1995). Reading Japan. *The New Yorker, LXX,* No. 48, 38–44.

Resdin, A. R. (1979). *Reflections of the rav: Lessons in Jewish thought adapted from lectures of Rabbi Joseph B. Soloveitchik.* Jerusalem: Alpha Press.

Richler, M. (1992). *Oh Canada! Oh Quebec: Requiem for a divided country.* Penguin: Toronto.

Rilke, R. M. (1969). *Letters of Rainer Maria Rilke, 1892–1910*. New York: W. W. Norton.

Robinson, D. (1991). *The translator's turn*. Baltimore: The Johns Hopkins University Press.

Rodriguez, R. (1983). *Hunger of memory: The education of Richard Rodriguez*. New York: Bantam Books.

Roland, A. (1983). Psychoanalysis without interpretation: Psychoanalytic therapy in Japan. *Contemporary Psychoanalysis, 19*, 499–505.

Rorty, R. (1989). *Contingency, irony, and solidarity*. Cambridge: Cambridge University Press.

Rosenblatt, P. C. (1994). *Metaphors of family systems theory: Toward new constructions*. New York: Guilford.

Rushdie, S. (1983). *Shame*. New York: Alfred A. Knopf.

Rushdie, S. (1991a). *Imaginary homelands: Essays and criticisms 1981–1991*. New York: Penguin Books.

Rushdie, S. (1991b). *Midnight's children*. New York: Penguin Books.

Rushdie, S. (1995). *The Moor's last sigh*. Toronto: Alfred A. Knopf.

Rutter, M., Graham, P., Chadwick, O., & Yule, W. (1976). Adolescent turmoil: Fact or fiction? *Journal of Child Psychology and Psychiatry, 17*, 35–56.

Said, E. W. (1979). *Orientalism*. New York: Vintage/Random Books.

Said, E. W. (1994). *Culture and imperialism*. New York: Vintage Books/Random House.

Schafer, R. (1992). *Retelling a life: Narration and dialogue in psychoanalysis*. New York: Basic Books.

Scheff, T. J. (Ed.) (1975). *Labeling madness*. Englewood Cliffs, NJ: Prentice-Hall.

Scheper-Hughes, N., & Stein, H. F. (1987). Child abuse and neglect and the unconscious in American popular culture. In N. Scheper-Hughes (Ed.), *Child survival: Anthropological perspectives on the treatment and maltreatment of children* (pp. 339–358). Boston: D. Reidel.

Schlegel, A., & Barry, H., III. (1991). *Adolescence: An anthropological inquiry*. New York: Free Press.

Schwartz, D. M., Thompson, M. G., & Johnson, C. L. (1985). Anorexia nervosa and bulimia: The sociocultural context. In S. W. Emmett (Ed.), *Theory and treatment of anorexia nervosa: Biomedical, sociocultural and psychological perspectives* (pp. 95–112). New York: Brunner/Mazel.

Seltzer, W. J. (1988). Myths of destruction: A cultural approach to families in therapy. *Journal of Psychotherapy and the Family, 4*(3/4), 17–34.

Seltzer, W. J., & Seltzer, M. R. (1983). Material, myth and magic: a cultural approach to family therapy. *Family Process, 22*(1), 3–14.

Selvini Palazzoli, M. (1972). Racialism in the family. *Human Context, 4*, 624–629.

Selvini Palazzoli, M. (1963/1974). *Self-starvation—from the intrapsychic to the transpersonal approach to anorexia nervosa* (A. Pomerans, Trans.). London: Chaucer.

Selvini Palazzoli, M. (1986a). Comments on DiNicola's "Family therapy and transcultural psychiatry: Parts 1 and 2." *Transcultural Psychiatric Research Review, 23*(1), 83–85.

Selvini Palazzoli, M. (1986b). Towards a general model of psychotic family games. *Journal of Marriage & Family Therapy, 12*(4), 339–349.

Selvini Palazzoli, M., Boscolo, L., Cecchin, G., & Prata, G. (1974). The treatment of children through the brief therapy of their parents. *Family Process, 13,* 429–442.

Selvini Palazzoli, M., Boscolo, L., Cecchin, G., & Prata, G. (1978a). *Paradox and counterparadox: A new model of the family in schizophrenic interaction* (E. V. Burt, Trans.). New York: Jason Aronson.

Selvini Palazzoli, M., Boscolo, L., Cecchin, G., & Prata, G. (1978b). A ritualized prescription in family therapy: Odd days and even days. *Journal of Marriage & Family Counselling, 3*(4), 3–9.

Selvini Palazzoli, M., Boscolo, L., Cecchin, G., & Prata, G. (1980). Hypothesizing—circularity—neutrality: Three guidelines for the conductor of the session. *Family Process, 19*(1), 3–12.

Selvini Palazzoli, M., Cirillo, S., Selvini, M., & Sorrentino, A. M. (1989). *Family games: General models of psychotic processes in the family* (V. Kleiber, Trans.). New York: W. W. Norton.

Selvini Palazzoli, M., & Prata, G. (1982a). A new method for therapy and research in the treatment of schizophrenic families. In H. Stierlin, L. C. Wynne, & M. Wirsching (Eds.), *Psychosocial intervention in schizophrenia: An international view* (pp. 237–243). Berlin: Springer.

Selvini Palazzoli, M., & Prata, G. (1982b). Snares in family therapy. *Journal of Marriage & Family Therapy, 8,* 443–450.

Shaw, G. B. (1911/1946). *The doctor's dilemma.* Harmondsworth, Middlesex: Penguin Books.

Shaw, G. B. (1916/1940). *Pygmalion.* New York: Dodd, Mead & Company.

Shibusawa, T. (1992). Post-partum psychosis in a father: Japanese cultural dynamics. In N. Grizenko, L. Sayegh, & P. Migneault (Eds.), *Transcultural issues in child psychiatry* (pp. 119–130). Montreal: Éditions Douglas.

Shorter, E. (1992). *From paralysis to fatigue: A history of psychosomatic illness in the modern era.* New York: Free Press.

Shweder, R. A. (1991). *Thinking through cultures: Expeditions in cultural psychology.* Cambridge, MA: Harvard University Press.

Sifneos, P. E. (1972). *Short-term psychotherapy and emotional crisis.* Cambridge, MA: Harvard University Press.

Sigal, J. J. (1986). The nature of evidence for intergenerational effects of the Holocaust. *Simon Wiesenthal Center Annual, 3,* 363–376.

Sigal, J. J., DiNicola, V. F., & Buonvino, M. (1988). Grandchildren of survivors: Can negative effects of prolonged exposure to excessive stress be observed two generations later? *Canadian Journal of Psychiatry, 33*(3), 207–212.

Sigal, J. J., & Weinfeld, M. (1989). *Trauma and rebirth: Intergenerational effects of the Holocaust*. New York: Praeger

Silone, I. (1949). Prefazione. In *Fontamara* (pp. 19-31). Milano: Arnoldo Mondadori Editore.

Simon, F. B., Stierlin, H., & Wynne, L. C. (1985). *The language of family therapy: A systemic vocabulary and sourcebook*. New York: Family Process Press.

Simons, R. C., & Hughes, C. C. (Eds.) (1985). *The culture-bound syndromes: Folk illnesses of psychiatric and anthropological interest*. Boston: D. Reidel.

Simpson, M. (1978). The language least emotional to me. *World Medicine, 28*.

Slaff, B. (1981). The history of adolescent psychiatry. In S. C. Feinstein, J. G. Looney, A. Z. Schwartzberg, A. Z., & A. D. Sorosky (Eds.), *Adolescent psychiatry: Annals of the American Society for Adolescent Psychiatry. Developmental and clinical Studies. IX*. Chicago: University of Chicago Press.

Sluzki, C. E. (1979). Migration and family conflict. *Family Process, 18*(4), 379-390.

Sluzki, C. E. (1982). The Latin lover revisited. In M. McGoldrick, J. K. Pearce, & J. Giordano (Eds.), *Ethnicity and family therapy* (pp. 492-498). New York: Guilford.

Sluzki, C. E. (1983). The sounds of silence: Two cases of elective mutism in bilingual families. In C. J. Falicov (Ed.), *Cultural perspectives in family therapy* (pp. 68-77). Rockville, MD: Aspen.

Sluzki, C. (1984). The patient-provider-translator triad: A note for providers. *Family Systems Medicine, 2*, 397-400.

Sorel, E. (Ed.) (1990). *Family, culture and psychobiology*. New York: Legas.

Sowell, T. (1996). *Migrations and cultures: A world view*. New York: Basic Books.

Spence, D. P. (1982). *Narrative truth and historical truth: Meaning and interpretation in psychoanalysis*. New York: W. W. Norton.

Steiner, G. (1975). *After Babel: Aspects of language and translation*. New York: Oxford University Press.

Steiner, G. (1976). *Extraterritorial: Papers on literature and the language revolution*. New York: Atheneum.

Steiner, G. (1982). The hollow miracle. In *Language and silence: Essays on language, literature and the inhuman* (pp. 95-109). New York: Atheneum.

Stewart, R. H., Peters, J. C., Marsh, S. et al. (1975). An object-relations approach to psychotherapy with marital couples, families and children. *Family Process, 14*, 161-178.

Stierlin, H., Weber, G., Schmidt, G. et al. (1986). Some features of families with affective disorders. *Family Process, 25*, 325-336.

Stoppard, T. (1967). *Rosencrantz and Guildenstern are dead*. New York: Grove Press.

Sugarman, S. (1983). An interview with David Reiss. *American Family Therapy Association Newsletter, 12,* 4–8.

Super, C. M. (1980). Cognitive development: Looking across at growing up. In C. M. Super & S. Harkness (Eds.), *Anthropological perspectives on child development* (pp. 59–69). San Francisco: Jossey-Bass.

Szilard, L. (1963). Die Stimme der Delphine. In *Utopische Erzählungen.* Hamburg: Rowohlt Taschenbuch Verlag.

Tamura, T., & Lau, A. (1992). Connectedness versus separateness: Applicability of family therapy to Japanese families. *Family Process, 31*(4), 319–340.

Taylor, C. (1989). *Sources of the self: The making of the modern identity.* Cambridge, MA: Harvard University Press.

Taylor, D. C. (1985). The sick child's predicament. *Australian and New Zealand Journal of Psychiatry, 19*(2), 130–137.

Taylor, G. J. (1984). Alexithymia: Concept, measurement, and implications for treatment. *American Journal of Psychiatry, 141,* 725–732.

Thomas, C. (1957). *Leftover life to kill.* London: Putnam.

Tornatore, G. (1994). *Cinema paradiso.* London: Faber and Faber.

Treacher, A. (1986). Invisible patients, invisible families—A critical exploration of some technocratic trends in family therapy. *Journal of Family Therapy, 8,* 267–306.

Tremblay, M. (1990). *Nelligan: Livret d'opéra.* Ottawa: Leméac Éditeur.

Tseng, W.-S., & Hsu, J. (1991). *Culture and family: Problems and therapy.* New York: Haworth Press.

Turner, J. E. (1991). Migrants and their therapists: A transcontextual approach. *Family Process, 30*(4), 407–419.

Turner, V. (1969). *The ritual process: Structure and anti-structure.* Ithaca, NY: Cornell University Press.

Valsiner, J. (Ed.) (1989). *Child development in cultural context.* Toronto: Hogrefe and Huber.

Vargas, L. A., & Koss-Chioino, J. D. (Eds.) (1992). *Working with culture: Psychotherapeutic interventions with ethnic minority children and adolescents.* San Francisco: Jossey-Bass.

Vermilye, J. (1994). *Great Italian films.* New York: Citadel Press.

Wafer, J. (1991). *The taste of blood: Spirit possession in Brazilian Candomblé.* Philadelphia: University of Pennsylvania Press.

Walcott, D. (1986). *Collected poems, 1948–1984.* New York: The Noonday Press/Farrar, Straus & Giroux.

Walker, A. (1992). *Possessing the secret of joy: A novel.* New York: Harcourt Brace Jovanovich.

Walker, A., & Parmar, P. (1993). *Warrior marks: Female genital mutilation and the sexual blinding of women.* New York: Harcourt Brace and Company.

Wallace, M. (1986). *The silent twins.* London: Chatto & Windus.

Waring, E. M. (1988). *Enhancing marital intimacy through facilitating cognitive self-disclosure.* New York: Brunner/Mazel.

Waterman, A. S. (1981). Individualism and interdependence. *American Psychologist, 36,* 762–773.

Watzlawick, P., Beavin, J. H., & Jackson, D. D. (1967). *Pragmatics of human communication.* New York: W. W. Norton.

Webster's third new international dictionary. (1966). Chicago: Encyclopaedia Britannica/William Benton.

Werkman, S. (1978). A heritage of transience: Psychological effects of growing up overseas. In E. J. Anthony & C. Chiland (Eds.), *The child in his family* (pp. 117–133). New York: Wiley-Interscience.

Westermeyer, J. (1987). Clinical considerations in cross-cultural diagnosis. *Hospital and Community Psychiatry, 38,* 160–165.

Westermeyer, J. (1991). Psychiatric services for refugee children: An overview. In F. L. Ahearn & J. L. Athey (Eds.), *Refugee children: Theory, research, and services* (pp. 127–162). Baltimore: Johns Hopkins Press.

White, M. (1986). Negative explanation, restraint, and double description: A template for family therapy. *Family Process, 25*(2), 169–184.

White, M. (1995). *Re-authoring lives: Interviews & essays.* Adelaide: Dulwich Centre Publications.

Wig, N. N., Menon, D. K., Bedi, H., Ghosh, A., Kuipers, L., Leff, J., Korten, A., Day, R., Sartorius, N., Ernberg, G., & Jablensky, A. (1987a). Expressed emotion and schizophrenia in North India. I: Cross-cultural transfer of ratings of relatives' expressed emotion. *British Journal of Psychiatry, 151,* 156–160.

Wig, N. N., Menon, D. K., Bedi, H., Leff, J., Kuipers, L., Ghosh, A., Day, R., Korten, A., Ernberg, G., Sartorius, N., & Jablensky, A. (1987b). Expressed emotion and schizophrenia in North India. II: Distribution of expressed emotion co components among relatives of schizophrenic patients in Aarhus and Chandigarh. *British Journal of Psychiatry, 151,* 160–165.

Wilden, A. (1972). *Systems and structures: Essays in communication and exchange.* London: Tavistock Publications.

Wilkes, T. C. R., Belsher, G., Rush, A. J., & Frank, E. (Eds.) (1994). *Cognitive therapy for depressed adolescents.* New York: Guilford.

Wilkins, R. (1985). A comparison of elective mutism and emotional disorders in children. *British Journal of Psychiatry, 146,* 198–203.

Wilson, E. O. (1978). *On human nature.* Cambridge, MA: Harvard University Press.

Wittgenstein, L. (1953/1958). *Philosophical investigations* (G. H. von Wright & G. E. M. Anscombe, Eds., G. E. M. Anscombe, Trans.). Oxford: Basil Blackwell.

Wolfe, T. (1940). *You can't go home again.* New York: Harper.

Wynne, L. C. (1969). The family as a strategic focus in cross-cultural psychiatric studies. In W. Caudill & T.-Y. Lin (Eds.), *Mental health research in Asia and the Pacific* (pp. 463–477). Honolulu, Hawaii: East-West Center Press.

Yap, P. M. (1974). Nosological aspects of the culture-bound syndromes. In M. P. Lau & A. B. Stokes (Eds.), *Comparative psychiatry: A theoretical framework* (pp. 84–104). Toronto: University of Toronto Press.

Young, A. (1980). The discourse on stress and the reproduction of conventional knowledge. *Social Science and Medicine, 14B,* 133–146.

Zeldin, T. (1995). *An intimate history of humanity*. London: Minerva.

Glossary

Note: Terms that appear in *italics* in the definitions are defined elsewhere in the glossary.

Acculturation: cultural adaptation, a process of refocusing or changing cultural lenses, which spans the spectrum from *assimilation* or total immersion into the host culture (like the American image of the "melting pot") to *estrangement* or total separation (like the former South African policy of "apartheid"). Compare *enculturation*.

Assimilation: a form of *acculturation* that is a total immersion into the host culture (like the American image of the "melting pot"). Compare *estrangement*.

Changeling: a metaphor for children undergoing cultural dislocation, based on the fairy-tale notion of a strange child left in place of a family's own valued child.

Code-switching: sociolinguists call switches from one language to another "code-switching" (see DiNicola, 1985a; Crystal, 1987). Following code-switching in therapy with bilingual or polyglot families can reveal fundamental details about their affective and cognitive states.

Concrete metaphors: redescriptions of the self work best when they are "concrete metaphors"—what Gregory Bateson (1972) called "metaphors that are meant," such as the Catholic belief that "the bread is the body and the wine is the blood of Jesus." The more abstract the metaphor, the more distant is the physical connection to our bodies. The more concrete the metaphor, the more easily we can use it to redescribe our own selves. For this reason, I call this process of multiple coding *somatics* or *embodied meaning*.

Consultant: into the family's complex story of strangeness, the consultant is brought in as one more stranger, creating yet another level of strangeness. What the consultant can do is open the system up for the introduction of novelty. If the family is open to new experiences, this will be incorporated into their history and their repertoire of skills in a helpful and positive way. If not, this new stranger will be dealt with in their usual way: perhaps to keep rigid boundaries, to confirm survivorhood, and to legitimize and validate their pain and their reasons to prize it and retain it.

Conviviality: "individual freedom realized in personal interdependence" (Illich, 1973, p. 24).

Cultural costume and camouflage: cultural costume is the particular set of recipes the individuals or families of a community employ to give meaning and shape to their experiences through shared ceremonies, rituals, and symbols. It serves two functions—adaptive and defensive. Used adaptively, cultural costume is protective. When culture is invoked defensively as a smokescreen to obscure individual states of mind or patterns of family interactions, cultural costume becomes camouflage. See *masks.*

Cultural family therapy (CFT): an interweaving of family stories (predicaments expressed in the narratives of family life) and conceptual tools (lenses, metaphors, and clinical methods for working with and making sense of these stories in cultural context).

Cultural translation (CT): the elucidation of an individual's or a family's *idioms of distress, explanatory models of illness,* and *perceived predicaments* using family members, culture brokers and other informants when useful and language translators when necessary in a collaborative effort.

Culture: there are many definitions of this embracing and complex construct. We need varying definitions for different tasks. In Chapter 2, culture is explored in relation to families and family therapy. The definitions of anthropologists Geertz, Helman, Keesing, and Kracke are examined and other features of a comprehensive definition for family therapy are set out.

Culture-bound syndromes (CBS): a collection of signs and symptoms of disease (not including notions of cause) restricted to a limited number of cultures due to their psychosocial features. Compare *culture-change syndromes* and *culture-reactive syndromes.*

Culture-change syndromes (CCS): specific problems arising during times of cultural stress and change which express a cultural conflict. Compare *culture-bound syndromes* and *culture-reactive syndromes.*

Culture-reactive syndromes (CRS): mental illneses with a marked geographic distribution, an affinity for certain sociocultural circumstances, or an association with specific ethnocultural communities. Compare *culture-bound syndromes* and *culture-change syndromes.*

Embarrassment: in personal relationships is a kind of "awkwardness, bewilderment and perplexity which grasps a sense of personal fragility and insecurity" (Andolfi et al., 1989, p. 73).

Emotional alchemy: this metaphor is drawn from the the mystical art of transformation, of turning base elements into gold. It suggests that the "accidents" and "givens" of our lives can be experienced meaningfully.

Enculturation: a process of slowly acquiring the cultural lens of our own society; growing up in a culture; this implies that culture is transmitted from generation to generation. Compare *acculturation*.

Estrangement: a form of *acculturation* that is a total separation (like the former South African policy of "apartheid"). Compare *assimilation*.

Explanatory models of illness (EMs): generate the client's answers to basic questions about their illness such as: "Why me?" "Why now?" "What is wrong?" "How long will it last and how serious is it?" "What problems does it create for me?" "How do I get rid of the problem?" (Kleinman, 1988, p. 156).

Familism: the common ground in definitions of familism is that the family is a natural group that presents a united front to others. Ferreira demonstrated the survival value of familism, refining it further into the concept of the *family myth*.

Family-as-culture: this is a polysemous phrase, open to many meanings including the analogy of seeing families as unique cultures and using this analogy as a new "story" for family therapy.

Family myth: "a series of well-integrated beliefs, myth-like, which members of the family entertain about each other and their relationship . . . [that] is not only shared but actually promoted by all family members" (Ferreira, 1963, p. 55).

Family therapy: family therapy is the space that we open to explore the possibilities of the family. My definition of the task of family therapy is to give structure and meaning to a family's *predicament*. Family therapy offers (re)descriptions of human predicaments and tools for inventing new metaphors for family experiences.

Idioms: see *idioms of distress (IDs)* and *therapeutic idioms (TIs)*.

Idioms of distress (IDs): a concept used by medical anthropologists (Nichter, 1982) to identify the ways people express their dilemmas and their pain in their local language and folkways. "For the anthropologist, the idiom is the symptom," says cross-cultural psychiatrist Arthur Kleinman (1988, p. 70).

Insider position: as an insider, the therapist takes a position of shared common experience with the family. See *roles*; compare *outsider position*.

Intercultural communication and translation: see *cultural translation (CT)*.

Intercultural encounters: we need models of intercultural encounters to understand the experience of confronting an alien culture. Anthropologist Kracke emphasizes the intercultural encounter as a psychological process. The outcome of the encounter is shaped, to some extent, by basic conceptions of the notion of culture, which may be positive or negative.

Intersubjectivity: when one person's story is nested in another's, like the night in São Paulo when my sister and I were (re)writing our overlapping family drama; the co-construction of social reality.

Intertextuality: when one textual story (e.g., novel, film, play) is embedded in another, like the story of Totò within my own, literary theorists call this intertextuality.

Interventions in family therapy: family therapy interventions are ways of feeding back, transmitting, or transforming the information obtained from the family and the therapeutic systems. With all their interventions, family therapists do three simple things: (1) enhance uncertainty, (2) introduce novelty, and (3) encourage diversity (DiNicola, 1990b).

Language translation: the process of rendering a communication or message from one language (the source language) into the ''closest natural equivalent'' words and idioms of another language (the receptor or target language).

Levels: different conceptual levels of functioning for understanding and explaining ''mind,'' progressing from individuals, through families, to social structures and culture. Based on this, I propose a new model of levels of adaptive functioning: the adaptive mechanisms of the individual, family myths and rules, and cultural costume and camouflage.

Liminality/liminal people: being at the threshold of new experiences with many possibilities as potential insiders; people who are undergoing culture change; synonym: ''threshold people.'' Compare *marginality*. See *transitional states.*

Marginality/marginal people: being at the periphery of society; outsiders with no perceived entrance into mainstream. Compare *liminality.*

Masks: learning to read *cultural costume and camouflage* is a key clinical tool of *CFT.*

Memory: family narratives teach us that memory is how we create ourselves. It serves different needs for each person. Human memory is not an objective repository but a process of selection.

Metaphor (figurative language): metaphor is defined in terms of one thing representing another. By bringing two things together through figurative language, a metaphor is a ''novel representation.'' One of the functions of metaphor is to put pain at a safe distance or allow the indirect expression of what cannot be openly and directly stated. Metaphors are *translations.*

Metaphoric transformation: in the story of the Figueroa family, ''I am myself what I have lost'' is a redescription of Cristina's self, a metaphoric transformation which creates intimacy by bringing experience closer to her known self.

Multiple codes: a conceptual tool of *CFT*, indicating the multiple meanings that can be encoded in *metaphor* or figurative language.

Multiple descriptions: this is the postmodern alternative to categorical thinking. We need diverse vocabularies that enable multiple descriptions, *explanatory models*, and *therapeutic idioms*—what I call the postmodern language of therapy. Family therapy can make meaningful use of many concepts and distinctions from its allied disciplines.

Myth of independence: a connecting theme in mainstream Western psychological theories and therapies. Chapter 7 explores aspects of this myth to show its pervasive implications.

Myths, personal and family: in Chapter 11 I write: ''I had to be ready to reconstruct my personal myth." Personal and family myths are like pebbles worn smooth from repeated handling. Writing family stories allows us to deconstruct and reconstruct personal and family myths.

Narrative resources: the stories provided by families and other cultures that offer recipes and rules for living and give meaning to experience. The absence or relative impoverishment of narrative resources leaves people with inadequate resources for living.

Outsider position: as an outsider, the therapist can be explicit about his differences with or inequalities in relation to the family. One can either take the posture of an expert or a one-down position by acting as cultural outsider. See *roles*, compare *insider position*.

Outtakes: this is a metaphor for what is missing from the narrative of our lives. In my family narrative, this metaphor is drawn from the film, *Cinema Paradiso*, where romantic scenes ("outtakes") are censored from films.

Paradigm: the notion that there are guidelines for conducting therapy based on universal, or at least stable, truths that can be brought reliably to the session with predictable impacts and outcomes.

Predicaments: "painful social situations or circumstances," of clients and their families, that are "complex, unstable, morally charged and varying in their import in time and place" (Taylor, 1985, p. 130). We find the client's predicament through history-taking, where what we are seeking is context. The notion of predicament overlaps significantly with what family therapy means by such terms as family process and context.

Presenting culture: the stories of family life, shaped by the history and geography of their lives, are transformed by memory and myth into their "presenting culture."

Rashomon effect: in the Japanese film, *Rashomon*, by Akiro Kurasawa, different stories emerge from a shared experience. This postmodern idea of multiple perspectives has become a key metaphor in family therapy.

Roles: examining the perspectives of insiders and outsiders, one of the key tools for *CFT*, offers a useful way to map the relationship between the therapist and the family culture. As a therapist, one can take both *insider and outsider positions* or roles with families.

Saturated self: the narrator of my memoir "speaks in different voices" and is an example of the "saturated self" described by Kenneth Gergen (1991). As discussed in an essay on postmodernism in therapy, "the saturated postmodern self . . . can give way to the relational self richly informed by a pluralistic world of diversity" (DiNicola, 1993, p. 58).

Saudade: each language has words for longing and loss. In Portuguese, this word is *saudade*, defined as: "the evocation of an indefinable longing . . . homesickness, nostalgia for happier days, suffering over love lost and dreams squandered, and ultimately, a confrontation with every man's inherent state of solitude" (Krich, 1993, p. 74).

Somatics (embodied meaning): metaphor can bring intolerable suffering closer, opening space within by redescribing the self in larger, more embracing terms. This is the obverse of Michael White's concept of "externalizing the problem." I call this process somatics or embodied meaning. *Concrete metaphors* are examples of somatics.

Spirals: a way of conducting the interview in which you gently skirt around the issues and let the family lead you to what they are looking for: how they define themselves, how they define the problem, and what sorts of solutions are acceptable to them.

Stories (narrative): a conceptual tool of *CFT*, stories metaphorically express the evolving narrative of family life as "alternities of being" and therapy as "a garden of forking paths."

Stranger in the family: when strangeness comes in the form of an encounter with a family therapist, several levels of strangeness may be discerned. One or more family members is behaving strangely; they may have become estranged from themselves or from other family members; the family turns to outsiders or strangers with an experience of strangeness within the familiar. The family turns with this puzzle to a real stranger outside the family—a family therapist. There may come, in turn, other strange aspects of their encounter with a therapist: negotiating new and difficult tasks through a newly acquired language in a cultural context that can be alien and sometimes hostile to them.

Suture: the therapist may or may not be successful in alleviating families' suffering or in giving meaning to their story, but families inevitably suture the story of therapy and of the therapist into the narrative of their lives. Even the most reluctant families have stories to tell about previous encounters with therapists: the personality, the quirks, the beliefs, the perceived successes or failures of their encounter with the therapist all become part of the history and mythology of the family.

Syncretism: this metaphor is drawn from the layered religious experiences of Brazil where African *orixás* or deities have counterparts in Christian saints. Syncretism is a model for cross-cultural pollination and interpenetration and for peaceful co-existence.

Syntagm: the postmodern alternative to *paradigm* is to capture a fresh, different discourse with every family, in every session.

Therapeutic communication and translation: see *therapeutic translation*.

Therapeutic idioms (TIs): formal, systematized schemas of mental and relational disorders used by professionals to facilitate exchange. This captures not only diagnostic schemas such as *DSM-IV* but all the core concepts of each therapeutic approach. In family therapy, TIs include classical concepts such as "scapegoating," "homeostasis," and the "family myth."

Therapeutic temperament: I have identified two therapeutic temperaments among family therapists: the technocratic temperament, which stresses the techniques of therapy, and the phenomenological temperament, whose main concern is family process.

Therapeutic translation (TT): the process of rendering an individual's or a family's *idioms of distress, explanatory models of illness,* and perceived *predica-*

ments into *therapeutic idioms.* In therapeutic translation, we move from idioms of distress to therapeutic idioms.

Threshold therapy: a synonym for *cultural family therapy* when applied to working with migrants, studying culture change, liminal people, and transitional states.

Tools for CFT: the actions and thoughts of the therapist—what philosopher Michel Foucault (1980) calls a "tool-kit."

Transitional states: the predicaments experienced by *liminal people* undergoing culture change. See *threshold therapy.*

Translation: see *language translation, cultural translation (CT),* and *therapeutic translation (TT).*

Woods: a metaphor for narratives developed by Eco (1994) from a story by Borges (1964). It suggests that family predicaments are a wood with many forking paths. Family therapy is a garden of forking paths where possible futures present themselves for consideration. Therapy helps the family define, comprehend, and prepare to live in these woods.

INDEX OF FAMILY STORIES

Client: Gloria, 17-year-old female
Conducted in English by Dr. DiNicola

Chapter 3

1. "Meeting Strangers"/"A Familiar Stranger"
   Della Seta family in Montreal, mid-1980s
   Italian/Jewish immigrant family
   Client: Alessandra (Sandra), 20-year-old female
   Conducted in English and Italian by Dr. DiNicola

2. "Racism in the Family"
   Szabo family in Ottawa, late 1980s
   Hungarian immigrant husband and French-Canadian wife
   Client: Julie, 15-year-old female
   Conducted in English by Dr. DiNicola

3. "A Latin Temperament"
   Lake family in Salterton, mid-1990s
   English-Canadian mother with half-Mexican children
   Client: Paul/Pablo, 10-year-old boy
   Conducted in English by Dr. DiNicola

4. "Elephant Boy"
   Nariman family in Montreal, mid-1980s
   Indian Parsee/Zoroastrian immigrant family
   Client: Navroz, 21-year-old male
   Conducted in English by Dr. DiNicola

Chapter 4

1. "Unlovable"
   Client: Jessica, 15-year-old female with depression
   Example of cognitive formulation of a depressed adolescent
   From Wilkes and associates (1994, p. 116)

2. "Drifting Apart"
   Clients: Couple with marital maladjustment
   Example of cognitive marital therapy
   From Waring (1988, pp. 89–92)

3. "The Japanese Earthquake"
   Brissa family in Rome, 1987
   Italian family

Consultation by Tazuko Shibusawa, L.C.S.W., with Dr. Andolfi in English

Italian-English translation by Dr. DiNicola

4. "Mother's Space"
Karasimos family in Montreal, mid-80s
Greek immigrant family
Client: Chrissoula, 19-year-old woman
Conducted in English by Dr. DiNicola

5. "A Private Language"
Pasquini family in Montreal, mid-80s
Italian immigrant family
Client: Luisa, 15-year-old female
Conducted in Italian, Abruzzese dialect, and English by Dr. DiNicola

Chapter 5

1. "The Story of an African Harlequin"
Kumalo family in Ottawa, early 1990s
Xhosa/Zulu South African immigrant family from Swaziland
Client: Thami, 11-year-old boy
Child psychiatric consultation, family therapy
Conducted in English by Dr. DiNicola

2. "A Caribbean Cordelia"
Edmunds family in Ottawa, late 1980s;
Jamaican immigrant family
Client: Alicia Edmunds, 15-year-old female
Conducted in English by Dr. DiNicola

3. "A Train of Traumas"
Noor family in Ottawa, early 1990s
Somali immigrant family
Client: Musa, 10-year-old boy
Child psychiatric consultation, social work consultation, family therapy
Conducted in English and French by Dr. DiNicola with Donna Morris, M.S.W.

4. "Culture Is Not a Dirty Window"
Prasad family in Ottawa, 1980s
Guyanese family of East Indian descent
Client: Jasmine, 14-year-old female
Child psychiatric consultation
Conducted in English by Dr. DiNicola

5. "A White Boy Who Thought He Was Cree"
Running family in Ottawa, late 1980s
English-Canadian family who migrated to Cree country in Northern Ontario
Client: River, 11-year-old boy
Child psychiatric consultation, family therapy
Conducted in English by Dr. DiNicola

Chapter 6

1. "An Acoustic Mask"
Lomano family in Montreal, 1984
Italian immigrant family
Client: Rita, 12-year-old girl
Consultation in English and Italian by Dr. Maurizio Andolfi
Translation into Italian by workshop participant

2. "Mum's the Word"
D'Angelo family in Montreal, 1985
Italian immigrant family
Client: Pina, 6-year-old girl
Conducted in English and Italian by Dr. DiNicola
Supervision by Dr. Gerald Wiviott

Chapter 7

1. "Conspiracy of Silence"
Milan, Italy, 1970s
Client: Marella, 2-year-and-2-month-old girl
Conducted by Dr. Mara Selvini Palazzoli and the Milan team
(Selvini Palazzoli et al., 1974)

Chapter 8

1. "A Stranger in the Family"
Ottawa, early 1990s
Italian immigrant
Client: Antonella Trevisan, a 24-year-old recent Italian immigrant
Psychiatric consultation, marital therapy, family therapy, and individual psychotherapy
Conducted in English and Italian by Dr. DiNicola

2. "The Past Is a Foreign Country"
Montreal, early 1980s
Polish Jewish woman

Client: Erica Gershon, 33-year-old daughter of Holocaust survivors
Individual psychotherapy conducted in English by Dr. DiNicola

3. ''From the Cradle''
   Davies family in Kingston, early 1990s
   British immigrants, Jehovah's Witnesses
   Client: Hannah, 16-year-old female
   Inpatient treatment in eating disorders program
   Family sessions conducted in English by Dr. DiNicola

4. ''A Pain With No Name''
   Montreal, early 1980s
   Pakistani adolescent
   Client: Ismet Farida Aziz, 17-year-old female
   Psychiatric consultation and brief therapy conducted in English by Dr.
   DiNicola

Chapter 9

1. ''Above My Heart, Above My God''
   Shami family in Ottawa, early 1990s
   Lebanese/Palestinian immigrant family
   Client: Samya, 13-year-old female
   Conducted in English by Dr. DiNicola
   Consultations by maternal grandfather and Dr. John Theis
   Co-therapy with a child psychiatry resident
   Arabic translation by family members

Chapter 10

1. ''I Am Myself What I Have Lost''
   Figueroa family in Gananoque, in mid-1990s
   Portuguese immigrant family
   Client: Isabel, 15-year-old female
   Conducted in English and Portuguese by Dr. DiNicola
   Co-therapy with a child psychiatry resident
   Portuguese translation by family members

Chapter 11

1. ''Strangers No More''
   DiNicola family in Brazil and Canada, mid-1990s
   Family narrative intercut with vignettes of *Cinema Paradiso* (film) and
   literary quotes
   Narrative written in English, Italian, and Portuguese

2. *Cinema Paradiso*
   Italian film, written and directed by Giuseppe Tornatore in 1989, about Totò, a little boy who becomes a filmmaker, Salvatore Di Vita, who returns home to Sicily for the funeral of Alfredo, his mentor in film and living
   English filmscript by Tornatore (1994)

INDEX